THE THEORY OF IRV:
AN AMERICAN HEALTH POLICY DETECTIVE STORY

BY
GREG VIGDOR

To Our Readers: As a special thank you to our readers, we are providing a free consumer health tool for you to use to take greater control of your health care experience and make the health care system better. The Tool is a usable record of your Personal Health History. Once completed, you have this for yourself, and can choose which providers, caregivers or others to share this with- or not- based on your desires. To receive a PDF copy of Personal Health History: Control Your Future by Organizing Your Past, go to: HHPersHis.pdf (squarespace.com) The full set of WHF's consumer Health Home Tools can be found on the Current Resources Page at the Washington Health Foundation website at washhealthfoundation.org.

Copyright © 2021 Greg Vigdor

All rights reserved.

United States Copyright: TXu002222969/2020-10-05

Book Cover Design by ebooklaunch.com

Contents

1. The Year of 2020: A Bodily Beginning 1
2. Early Irv Tinsley 7
3. Irv's Investigation Begins 11
4. Go West, Young Irv 16
5. Irv Meets with the Director 20
6. Early Nancy Jones 26
7. Irv Forms an Investigation Plan 33
8. Early Irv Moves to Seattle 36
9. 1932: Patrick Jones and the CCMC 42
10. Irv Goes to Moses Lake 50
11. The Committee on the Cost of Medical Care 54
12. Early Johnny 61
13. Irv Tours Moses Lake with Ken 67
14. Early Johnny Part 2 70
15. A Discovery in Moses Lake 75
16. 1933: The CCMC Report Gets Buried 78
17. Young Irv and Johnny Look to the Future 83
18. Irv Stakes Out the Airport 90
19. Post-WWII: The Age of More in Health Care 92
20. The Formal Investigation Is Closed 100
21. 2020: A Patient Dump 106
22. Young Johnny Builds His Political Résumé 111
23. Irv Investigates Anyway 115
24. Early Mary Beth Collins 118
25. Evidence in a Sock 124
26. 2020: HealthMost Board Meeting 127
27. 1960: The Jones and Medicare 133
28. Irv Contemplates Evidence in a Sock 140
29. Young Johnny Goes to Congress 143
30. Irv Explores Insurance Numbers 147
31. Early Richard Thrust 154
32. 1966: The Age of Health Care Rationalization Begins 160
33. Young Mary Beth Meets Nancy Jones 164
34. Irv Finds Some Useful Clues 169

35.	Young Irv Ponders His Life	172
36.	Young Johnny Ponders His First Year in Congress	175
37.	Irv Takes the Investigation to Phoenix	180
38.	Trapped in Canyonlands	183
39.	Hiking Out of Canyonlands	190
40.	The Theory of Irv	193
41.	Rescue	198
42.	Westside Medical Center in Phoenix	200
43.	1980: Chris Jones Looks for Bigger Policy Answers	206
44.	2020: Patient Dumping Hearing in the Senate	216
45.	Secretary of HHS Ben Olsen	224
46.	Mary Beth and Johnny Discuss a Local Hearing	228
47.	Post Utah Irv	232
48.	Irv's Investigation Goes to DC	237
49.	Post Utah Johnny	242
50.	Irv's Investigation Goes to Hartford	245
51.	Early Sam Bridgewater	249
52.	Thrust Plots a Cover-Up	254
53.	Nelson Duncan III	259
54.	Young Irv Gets a Master's Degree	266
55.	Nelson Duncan III Stews	268
56.	Irv's Early Health Care Career	270
57.	Senator Gibson Meets with Nelson Duncan III	274
58.	Young Mary Beth Builds a Career	278
59.	1990: Beginning of the Age of Health Reform	282
60.	Young Johnny Reacts to Political Change	288
61.	Irv and Lance Review the ALI Data	292
62.	Irv Finds a Leadership Job in Public Health	299
63.	Johnny's Friends Give Him Health Care Policy Guidance	305
64.	Irv Plans to Go Undercover	312
65.	A Fissure Grows Between Irv and Mary Beth	315
66.	2010: Federal Health Reform Happens	322
67.	Mary Beth Moves to Shelton	328
68.	Irv Goes Undercover	330
69.	Mary Beth and the Mason Health Foundation	336
70.	Irv Wakes Up in Limbo	341

71.	A Public Hospital District Is Approved	346
72.	Irv In Limbo 2	350
73.	Mason Health Foundation Grows	357
74.	Irv and Jose on a Plane	363
75.	Johnny Finds His Way in Congress	372
76.	HealthMost Managers Meeting	378
77.	Irv Makes His Escape in Rapid City	384
78.	Congressman Gibson Wonders about the Senate	387
79.	Irv Meets His Friends in Denver	393
80.	Johnny Runs for the Senate	397
81.	Irv's New Investigation Plan Forms	399
82.	Mason Health Foundation Faces Money Troubles	403
83.	Irv's Public Health Job Goes Awry	409
84.	The Dump Site in Mason County	415
85.	The Evil Plan	419
86.	What Next in the Investigation?	428
87.	Thrust's Conspiracy Deepens	431
88.	Johnny's Senate Career Threatened	435
89.	HealthMost's Cover-Up Expands	445
90.	Johnny and Nancy Meet	451
91.	Irv Crashes	456
92.	Mason Health Foundation Threatened	458
93.	Nancy Confirms Johnny's Political Problem	469
94.	A Campaign Against Mary Beth	474
95.	Irv Resigns, Under Pressure	479
96.	No Confidence Vote	483
97.	Mary Beth and Irv Hook Up Again	490
98.	Planning Meeting at the Alderbrook Lodge	494
99.	Prep for the Public Hearing in Belfair	497
100.	Temporary Restraining Order	502
101.	Thrust Gets Ready for His Win	506
102.	The Hearing in Belfair	510
103.	Post Hearing Meeting with Thrust	514
104.	Lance Meets with the Secretary of HHS	525
105.	The Rest of the Friends' Discussion in Denver	532
106.	Mary Beth's Vindication	538
107.	Johnny Gets His Bill	546

108.	The Process Used to Draft the Bill	552
109.	Thrust Goes to Prison	561
110.	Bridgewater's Fate	565
111.	Irv Gets His Whole Life Together	570
112.	Johnny and the Olympic Institute	575
113.	The Theory of Irv Bill	579
114.	Afterword	585

Chapter One

The Year of 2020: A Bodily Beginning

They were an ugly and uncomfortable people, Irv concluded about the two men who walked about the inside of the small, unfurnished cabin and pointed at the body lying in the middle of its one-room hardwood floor. He could see that the body was worse for its recent wear even from his distant observation point. The men stepped around and over it, showing little respect, laughing as they mocked its grotesque features. It seemed a cheap thrill for them to be here, not a somber duty to the dead.

Gazing through the dirty window from the porch, Irv Tinsley second-guessed his harsh assessment of the volunteers at the scene. But he had seen behavior like this too many times before. Most first responders typically did their job with honor, especially while in the eye of neighbors and passersby. But some, when hidden from sight, let their true nature rise to the surface. Irv had come to realize over the years that not everyone's nature was good.

Irv knew this was a bit of an overreaction—he didn't know these men. He was in a bad mood and ready to think the worst of them. Wanting to do better, he dug within to find a more positive space before walking into the cabin and confronting them.

He had good reason for his lousy attitude, starting with the 4 a.m. phone call that woke him from a deep sleep, telling him a public health investigator was required to be at the scene of an "incident." He rarely slept through the night at the best of times, and the call broke up an opportunity to get a complete night of needed rest.

Investigator on call came with its privileges—well, one that is, the extra pay—but this was its burden. He had grown accustomed to controlling his schedule when he served as key aide to the last director of health, and getting up early as part of his recent demotion for regular office hours was not something he took to well. Being on call just added to his new time management burden. But he needed this job for now and would have to deal with it.

The cross-country car trip wasn't difficult; he beat the wicked pulse of morning rush-hour traffic in the greater Seattle region by a couple of hours. A strong cup of coffee helped clear his head for what was to come. He was still finding it hard to completely focus on the task at hand as his mind drifted instead to the events of the past several days. These weren't pleasant remembrances, so he tried to reframe his context by turning up the volume on the radio of his government car. The Band's "The Night They Drove Old Dixie Down" didn't pull him out of his sour and distracted mood, but at least it got his foot tapping.

After a twenty-five-minute drive, he took the turn off the county road he was tracking on his GPS. The house in question was just a half mile off this road in the rural sticks of Kent, Washington, down a few hundred yards along a wide gravel path. A Rural Metro ambulance and a volunteer fire department car were parked in front of the house along the edge of the rough roadway, lights swirling, sirens on mute. A county sheriff's car was ten yards farther down. Next to it was a sheriff, leaning over an open window and talking into the extended microphone of his radio.

Irv could overhear him through his open windows as he drove by and parked just beyond the sheriff's car. "Yeah, he just got here. Think they could move their ass a little faster, but that's how it works around here. If it isn't in the big city, who gives a shit. All right, gotta go. Catch up with you for coffee as soon as I can wrap up my work here." With that, the balding sheriff turned to Irv, who had opened the door to his car.

Irv pulled his six-foot frame from the vehicle. He was fifty-nine years old but looked much younger. Most thought him to be more around fifty when they first met. Irv had stayed in good physical shape, and his muscular shoulders and thick Eastern European build gave an impression of strength. Part of his youthful appearance came from his full head of wavy brown hair. He combed it back and kept it, and its companion thick mustache, neatly trimmed through monthly trips to a hairdresser.

He was dressed professionally—a step up from most regular county workers—but not elegantly. He had a fancy suit but rarely broke it out for use in his current job. Today's outfit was more the norm now—tan wrinkle-free cotton pants, a pressed blue dress shirt, and a dose of color from a yellow and green polka dot tie. He wore a light rain jacket, an essential tool in the drizzly Pacific Northwest. Irv had learned to dress somewhat conservatively. He had discovered through practice that he wanted to preserve tolerance for the unconventional ways he did his work, not for matters of outward appearance.

Irv groaned as he pulled himself out of his car seat—he might look young, but could feel the aches of old age coming on. The sheriff, a much younger man than Irv but scruffier and pudgier, stuck out both his badge and his beer belly as he turned from his police car and strode toward him. He hitched up his pants and spit on the ground when Irv got close.

Irv remembered another reason he wasn't happy about being here—the odd and sometimes cranky public servants on the scene. It was hard enough to put up with them even after a good night's sleep, and a very difficult chore without. Oh well, at least it wasn't a call from inside Seattle city limits, where attitude might come with an extra dose of hubris or confrontation. His friend Johnny would embrace encounters with folks like these as part of the great adventure of life, but Irv couldn't quite get there—unless Johnny was around to point it out and lead him to embrace it.

"Hey, we've been waiting for you. What's the hold-up? Think you got more important things to do than deal with some corpse out here in the hicks?"

"Yeah, like getting some sleep. Keep your shirt on, Sheriff—the budget cuts haven't been any kinder to my department than yours. I am covering a hundred square miles with my caseload right now, and folks just aren't cooperating by dying less."

Irv drifted closer to the officer, though not near enough to risk smelling the sheriff's breath and discovering what he ate last night. He pulled a pack of cigarettes out of his inside coat pocket, slipped out a butt, and lit it. Irv didn't really smoke—other than an occasional cigar at a campfire or to stay awake on an overnight drive—but kept a pack on hand for situations just like this. It was frequently a relationship flattener when he had to get folks comfortable, and quickly, with an urban government bureaucrat. It helped that his pleasant face, highlighted by a friendly smile, made most people feel comfortable, especially when backed up by his soft voice and gentle demeanor.

Irv lit up a cigarette, took a drag, and blew the smoke up and out toward the sky and the haze of the Northwest dawn, sighing. "Ahhh, that's better."

"Whoa, cowboy. Don't you know that's illegal? You are within thirty feet of a personal residence, and smoking isn't allowed. Hate to write you up a ticket."

"Go ahead. They won't let me light up in my county car, so this is about my only choice."

"Guess I can cut you a break this early. Got one for me?"

Irv slipped his hand inside his jacket, pulled out the pack, and offered it to the officer. His trick had worked again. He got busy on leveraging whatever trust a cancer stick would get him. "So what's the story here? All I got was that there was an emergency call about some corpse that looked a bit off. Somebody thought it was something that public health ought to take a look at rather than the homicide unit."

"Yeah, that was me. I was having a pretty uneventful night, staking out in the usual spots for drunk drivers, when a call came in from a neighbor. She heard a commotion out in the back field, maybe a bear or coyotes going after her chickens. When she went to check it out with her two dogs, they beat a fast track to the old Jones cabin here. They were sniffing and bobbing around and whining like all get out on the front porch. She took a look in and saw the body on the floor with a bunch of rats dining away on its face. Scared her to all bejesus and she made a 911 call. That's when I came in."

Irv turned away from the sheriff and assessed his surroundings. The dawn light was beginning to brighten the sky with a reddish hue, and he could now make out the path of the neighbor's journey across her field to the front porch of the cabin. Her house was about fifty yards away, with a thigh-high, rotting cedar fence between the two properties. It wouldn't have prevented anyone but a cripple from going from one property to the other, or any self-respecting dog from easily leaping over it.

"So what made you think you needed me?"

"Well, rats was enough to get me going. I don't mind 'em so much in my basement, but not on my corpses." The sheriff grinned at Irv, revealing two gaps in the teeth behind his crooked smile. A little cosmetic dentistry might have evened them out nicely and made him into a somewhat good-looking man. But Irv doubted that this was much of a priority in the sheriff's world.

"I seen worse though. Shooed 'em away with my flashlight and a few boots to the door and then came on in. The odor was something, and not the usual putrid smell of a rotting corpse. More like the stink that comes from a phosphorus mine, but not exactly neither. Never smelled nothing like it. But it was the pus and the holes that really got my attention."

"Thought you said the rats were nibbling away at our friend in here. What's the big deal with some holes? That's generally what happens at a corpse buffet table."

"Sure. Told you I've seen a lot of these in my time. But not like this. When I shone my light at the face, I could see that the rats had only recently been at it, and had been chewing away on the ear and forehead that was pressed against the floor. The other side of the face was unnibbled. But worse on the eye, if you ask me."

"How so?"

"Big, silver-dollar-size holes all across the neck, cheekbone, and forehead. Crusted red holes swimming into the skull and cones jumping out at you from the edges. Looked like they were once ridges of pus. The fluid was hard now and had a dark shade of green to it. Never seen nothing like it—or smelled either.

"I called the boys out from the fire department and the ambulance service. They thought the same thing. No sign of anything suggesting anyone else was even here, other than some tire tracks out on the edge of the road. Hard to suspect foul play without any sign of a suspect. So, our guess is he was done in by some nasty shit floating around under your jurisdiction, not ours."

"Fair enough." Irv thought this was not really the case. *Fair enough* would be a couple more hours of sleep, or maybe even a few days off to cope with the other crap in his life. He could also feel a growing tug away from fairness and toward curiosity. It did sound like something out of the ordinary, and way better than the monotony of investigating rabid dogs or botulated food.

"Your buddies inside?"

"Yeah. This shit creeped me out, and I wanted no part of being around that. Those two must've been watching too much *CSI* on the tube."

"Or they are a couple of dumb-asses. Sheriff, it was nice sharing a smoke with you and finding a public servant with a decent head on his shoulders. How about we start by getting your buddies to get the hell out of there before I have to put 'em in quarantine? I need to take a closer look, but I can tell you that this doesn't sound like anything I've ever seen before either."

Irv thought to himself that he actually *had* seen a lot of this—just maybe not exactly the same. He'd seen too much of it. And it was getting to him, too. He walked up to the cabin and looked through the windows. Seeing the inside of the cabin, he was sure of that. But duty called.

Chapter Two

Early Irv Tinsley

Irving Tinsley was born in Albuquerque, New Mexico, the second son of Rudy and Linda Tinsley. Rudy and Linda had moved to the American Southwest from Pittsburgh, going west to find a better place as their parents had done a generation before. But they were not escaping the economic and social brutality of Eastern Europe in the early nineteenth century as their parents had done. They were searching for the American dream, which seemed so achievable in the boom of the American post-WWII years.

On the surface, it was a job that had been the lure. Rudy took a new position at Sandia Laboratories, a fledgling research lab exploring weapons and flight technologies that could put America above its Russian enemies in the Cold War. Rudy had a degree in engineering from Pitt and had worked on missile technologies during the war. He also had a new bride with a son in the oven, a need for cash, and an even greater need for space from his in-laws.

His Jewish birthright was a non-starter with the Lithuanian reform church roots of his new wife's family, just as she was an unwelcome addition to his. It was one thing for his father and mother to abandon the agricultural traditions of the family in the new world and have Rudy's dad become a tradesman—a tinsmith and how they got their family name on Ellis Island—in America. It was quite another to become as one with a shiksa. Rudy and Linda resolved this conflict by finding a new place to build their hopes for their coming family.

Albuquerque was far away and different than anywhere they had ever lived. There was space, lots of it. And brown, oh so brown. Rudy never imagined that there could be so many shades of brown. Light brown. Dark brown. Tan. Orange-brown. Glossy white-brown—yes, even white was a new brown in the Land of Enchantment.

The people of Albuquerque were friendly enough. But Rudy and Linda found it hard to establish a social network anything close to the one they both had in Pennsylvania. Twenty years of social history in close immigrant neighborhoods was no match for an instant parachuting among people they had never known, let alone people in a strange and distant place.

It was a very Catholic land, with ties to the deeply religious and cloistered cultural roots of early Spanish explorers and settlers. They were not openly prejudicial toward Hebrews and Lithuanian reform church-goers, but they did not exactly embrace different belief systems like theirs.

The enemy was all around these first settlers of the new world, and they drew strength from religion and family. Converting the heathen was one thing; folding them into their social circles was quite another. So they kept these circles tight, even while being cordial to outsiders. Centuries later, Rudy and Linda found that history lived on. They needed to find a sense of belonging to their new home in other ways.

Rudy rarely dwelled on this. He just didn't have the time. Their firstborn son, Michael, came a couple of months before their move west. It wasn't very long before Irv himself was on his way, followed by sisters Jackie, Susan, and Beth. They were showing those Catholics a thing or two.

Rudy's work took up much of his time, even more than his now large family. He couldn't talk about it, state secrets and all, and spent most days holed up in his lab, weekends included. It drew a decent salary, and the cost of living was low enough in Albuquerque to get financially comfortable quickly. They purchased a spacious suburban home in the fledgling northeast section of the city, which rose far above the Old Town sitting next to the Rio Grande ten miles away and a thousand feet above. The land tilted upward from the Rio Grande Valley, until it went almost straight up as it met the three-thousand-foot face of the Sandia Mountains.

Linda found herself with lots of time on her hands. The regular tasks of raising five children took great effort, but this was the 1960s, when you put your kids on a school bus in the morning, welcomed them back in the afternoon, and then sent them off to play in the streets and sandlots till dinnertime. With a husband who left early in the morning for work and returned in the evening for late dinner, she found abundant alone time, which she filled with books, serviced by a new and well-stocked library five blocks from their house. She worked her way through the alphabet—reading everything she could from A to Z.

It was her second son, Irv, who became her closest companion. Perhaps it was the six months he was sent home from school because of suspected meningitis, or perhaps it was just natural for the second son to bond with Mom. Most likely it was his great curiosity about the ways of the world, a passion tickled not by experience but by the written word, and fanned by his mom.

Whatever the reason, Irv soon became the second and only other member of Linda's book club. By the time he was a teenager, Linda was into the H's. They swapped books and reviews each week, exploring together the secrets within the Sandia Hills Library Association. These were Irv's fondest childhood memories. He frequently passed on activities with his schoolmates and neighbors so he could enjoy being with Mom and her reading list.

Irv took it hard when Linda got sick in 1974. He was fourteen and she was into the P's. Linda had read some books on cancer during her foray through the C's, but there was not a lot to know back then. Books on cancer were short and without much depth. That it was breast cancer only added to the mystery, messing as it did with female body parts.

The time between diagnosis and treatment was short. And there was not much bigger a gap between treatment and a painful death. Looking back, Irv now knew there was little to be done when it was discovered. A small tumor that had begun in the soft mass of her breast had metastasized and spread to her lymph nodes well before she ever noticed the lump.

Michael, Jackie, Susan, Beth, and Rudy did what they could to make things better for Linda. Rudy took a six-month leave of absence from his job to care for her. He didn't need it all. Linda died only four months and a week after her diagnosis. She was put to rest in a small cemetery abutting the Sandia National Forest, with a view to buttes and mesas to the west.

Dad and Irv's siblings took her death hard. For Irv, it was the end of the world. Mother and son had continued their reading game through the early parts of her struggle, but after a couple of months, her pain became unbearable and her only comfort was morphine. She would hold her son's hand and talk about different books. Soon, it was Irv doing all the talking. Linda was weak but would smile, nod her head, or sometimes whisper words of encouragement to her loving son.

The end came just after dawn on a Saturday morning. Irv awoke from his sleep in the chair next to his mom's bed to hear a loud gasp. The noise shook his sleep cobwebs off, and he quickly moved in close to her, asking her if there was anything he could do. She peered into his green eyes and said, "Yes, dear. Live life, don't just read about it. Find what it is that makes you happy and go do that. It is all we can hope for." With that, she fell back on her pillow, took two shallow breaths, and left this world.

Irv had been a loner before his mom's death. As a teenager with racing hormones and now the loss of his best friend, his introversion became extreme. He went to school and passed his courses with ease, not from any effort or class participation. Years of reading and learning with his mom had given him enough book smarts to get by academically without needing to exert himself beyond the bare minimum.

He found school to be a poor substitute for the learning he had done with Mom. But it was, he began to see, his way out. Out of the pain of his loneliness, out of Albuquerque—and into the broader world that awaited him.

Many was the evening that he sat by his mom's grave, with her and only her. He was sure that the buzz of a bee, the rustle of reeds, or the occasional wildlife noises were her private responses to him. The mesas and buttes to the west called out to him. *Come on out, Irv. See what it's all about. Out here.* He didn't know what it would be, or exactly where, but he would as soon as he got through high school. He would get out by going off to college.

Go west, young man.

Chapter Three

Irv's Investigation Begins

Irv drove his plain white county Ford Fiesta into a small parking lot adjacent to his office building. He snugged the car into a skinny parking space between the rear wall of the lot and an overflowing dumpster, then stepped out into the damp afternoon. It had been a long morning of tracking down leads in Kent, and he was feeling the effects of the early morning wake-up call. His tired state was secondary to his anxiousness to see if the requested lab tests were done. "STAT" and "Potential Public Health Emergency" still meant something in the usually slow pace of King County government.

The Seattle-King County Public Health Offices were located in the south part of downtown Seattle. It was a ten-block walk to the stadium district, a three-block walk to the thrones of city and county governments, and even a shorter trek to the new jail. He caught a glimpse of the new incarceration and rehabilitation facility every morning in his short walk from the parking lot to his office and couldn't resist the thought that at least some part of government was still growing.

His office cubicle was on the fourth floor, along with most of the other investigators. The county occupied the majority of this twenty-four-story building, not just public health but other indispensable functions like tax collections, road planning, and audit—things you didn't want the public to actually be around. Those you did were located in the building a few blocks away in the county council office building—where they could keep an eye on things and ramp up security. It was better that the types of things Irv did happened under a cloak of secrecy.

Not long ago, he had a separate office in the administrative suite on the upper floor. Now, he was somebody the current administration preferred not to see. For what he was working on today, that was maybe good thinking. The problem was that his isolation had far more to do with politics than any rational thinking about his role in the agency.

He ambled off the elevator and nodded to the security attendant at the small desk immediately adjacent to a glass barrier separating the hallway from the staff office space. He swiped his security card to get access to the inner sanctum of public health headquarters and meandered through wall-to-wall cubicles to get to his own small workspace in the rear of the building. At least it was close to the coffee machine and the small conference room. *Isn't life grand?*

Sitting in his one guest chair was a small, smartly dressed woman reading a file wrapped in a brown covering, with a large red "Priority" stamp dominating its cover. She looked up at Irv, peering over the edge of the report. "Well, you've stepped in it this time, Tinman."

"Had a feeling. I imagine those are my toxicology reports from this morning?"

"Yes indeed. And none too pretty."

Irv sat down on the edge of his desk, hovering over Ann as he took a sip of his coffee. "Give it to me, Ann. I've been up since four and am getting a bit cranky."

"A new strain of avian flu, or so it seems. Nothing like we've ever seen before though."

"Isn't that why they would call it mutated?" Irv thought to himself that it was always difficult to get these young administrator types to understand the basic science underlying their field work. Even if he wasn't a scientist himself, it was pretty easy to grasp that what made avian or swine or other animal flus so potentially dangerous was that they could undergo a variation in their genetic code, consequently threatening transmission from animals to humans in ways that went far beyond our centuries of built-in natural protections.

"Spare me the lectures, Irv. I may not be a highly educated man like you, but I have figured out a few things over the last year of working here." Ann Baker had come on board with the election of a new King County administrator, fresh from her graduation from the University of Washington Public Affairs program. Not so much a political appointee, but a favor nonetheless to a major campaign contributor to new King

County Executive Brett Halvorson. Her dad had some bucks and used it to help get her career off the ground.

"Remember, I was the one who staffed the Pandemic Flu Surveillance Task Force last year. I got plenty of lectures then from you and every epidemiologist employed by the State of Washington. You all made it very clear that it was all too technical for this little girl to understand. But you know some of it isn't that hard."

Irv remembered well the Task Force created by the State Legislature to plan for the potential spread of pandemic flu after it hit several Chinese villages. The politicians were all over it; a couple of reporters from the *Seattle Times* ran into the story while covering a Pan-Asian Economic Summit. Instead of writing about how America could sell more planes, wine, and computer software to developing China, they suggested Chinese pig farmers were going to take down western civilization. Happening as it did during the state legislative session that winter, elected leaders decided to leap to action to protect the public. Yes, a study commission, that would do it.

Of course, all that happened years ago. Ann was referring to a group that was pulled together every few years to update the plan. But at least she thought she knew something about this. "So tell me more, miss smarty pants," he said.

"The basic results match up with what we saw coming from China in 2008, and before that from the Philippines in 2005. Encephalitic retroviral, leading to potential stage five pneumonia. Mutation on the N gene suggesting it was originally a bird-based flu that somehow leapt to our John Doe. But really nasty stuff—he probably drowned in his own juices. Literally drowned. And make that Juan Doe. We weren't able to match fingerprints or DNA to any known person in this country, but the residue from his clothes and fingers suggested he had been working with crops. Alfalfa, apples, and wheat. With a big splash of potato. We found a small note in what we think was Spanish inside his sock, and that has us figuring he was a migrant worker up from Mexico or even further south."

"What the hell was he doing in some shithole in Kent?" The county was not exactly the alfalfa, apples, and wheat breadbasket of the world— more mushrooms, cranberries, and other moldy foodstuffs.

"That I can't help you with. You are just gonna have to do some more work, Agent Tinsley." She was prodding him, undoubtedly aware that his hold on his job was tenuous. She actually liked him, but knew he was damaged political goods and that she should keep her distance. Still, he was fun to tease.

"What's new about that?" *Nothing*, Irv thought. What did she think he had been doing all day? He was not surprised by the speculation that the victim was probably an illegal. That much he had guessed at the scene by the strong hint of potato juices. The distinct mosh on the victim's clothing wafted the unique aroma of french fry processing plants located in eastern Washington. Not all workers were illegals, or Mexican. But the victim was a short man, about five-foot-six, and thin. Irv's experience was that this was far more common for visitors from the south than white-bred American chubbies.

What he didn't know was why the victim was in this shack in Kent, or why he would have arrived in a vehicle sporting brand-new RX-425 tires. The sheriff had pointed out the tracks and impressed Irv with his knowledge of radial tire tracks. The tires were the kind made exclusively for hybrid SUVs—not exactly the usual transport mode for itinerant farmworkers.

"Any other cases reported?" Irv asked. This was the thousand-dollar question. If there were more, then there was reason to believe the spread from animal to human could have some implications for the public's health and not just some unfortunate foreign worker. And it would set in course the quest for the answer to the million-dollar question—was it spreading from animal to man, or had it mutated further to spread from person to person as well?

"There are a couple of suspicious reports in eastern Washington that we are checking out. But unconfirmed for now." The state government cutbacks from the Great Recession had hit rural county public health departments particularly hard. They were barebones operations in the best of times. Now, there was one county health officer and a small staff for groups of three, four, or even five counties. A lot of ground and disease to cover, especially when major public health threats made their appearance.

"Okay, so we've got a nasty possible pneumonia-related death, an animal transmission, and suspicions of other victims. Doesn't yet make it AIDS or SARS though. What's so freaking unique that you are sitting in my little part of the world waiting for me?"

"That's just it. You are to head upstairs to the director's office. He wants to talk to you personally about this case. Anybody in the leadership chain wanting to talk to you, let alone the Grand Poobah, must be pretty freakin' desperate. Get your ass up there." With that, she tossed the brown folder on his coffee-stained desk protector, winked at him, and strode back to her private office.

Now that is pretty freaking unique, Irv thought. *I haven't been upstairs since I talked to that reporter about E. coli and the risks in our ethnic restaurants.* That was too much for the politically correct "we are the world" yuppies who had settled in Seattle during the tech boom. They lived in software bunkers that afforded them protection during the day, and at night they came out swinging as world adventurers. Who was he to suggest that their favorite eating establishments actually cook and check their food for safety?

He chuckled to himself as he recalled the shitstorm his comments had created for his boss. *Can't blame the director for not wanting to talk to me or ever see me again.* But going rogue, as it was now called, had solved that public health problem. Something inside tugged at him. He wasn't so sure that he would be able to say the same on this one, whatever it was. It seemed very big, maybe too big for anyone to control.

Chapter Four

Go West, Young Irv

Young Irv Tinsley made his move west a month after high school graduation, intent on leaving Albuquerque as soon as possible. He had applied to several colleges in California as his escape plan and been accepted at UCLA.

Dad supported the move. It was what Irv wanted, but he also thought the distance between them would be good for their relationship. It wasn't that they didn't get along. But Linda's death had created a sadness between them—for one who remembered all the time they once spent together and the other who regretted how much he hadn't. Perhaps the thousand miles between Albuquerque and Los Angeles would ease the pain.

College life in the 1970s had changed from what it was the decade before. The freedom, fun, and independence of the 1960s created a strange set of expectations. Mind-altering substances, loose love, and rejection of authority were always part of the college formula, but back then it was presumed that incoming freshmen would become social change agents too.

The Vietnam War was over now, and this new generation of students dismissed much of the social consciousness of the 60s' rabble-rousers. College became more about setting one's life up with good grades, graduate school, or a job. The days of revolution and change from the outside had faded, at least for the moment.

Whatever these trends, they had little effect on Irv. He was marching to his own drum—an escapism from Albuquerque. He wanted to find himself and would do this through some fuzzy notion of "doing." It was inspired as much by guilt as by the joy of discovery. Mom's words haunted him. "Live it." Try he would, even if he didn't really know what that meant.

So, he tried anything and everything. Easy enough were the broad choices of a liberal arts courseload. But books and classes were secondary avocations for Irv. Tops on his list of trying was a myriad of personal adventures—into urban Los Angeles, out into the California agricultural belt and deserts, to the beaches. Surfing became an odd fascination for a lad from Albuquerque. Maybe it was all of the water after years of dry dirt, or maybe it was the blonde beauties who hung out on the beaches in numbers.

His Los Angeles life was grounded by a group of friends he met in college who became his surrogate family. Only rarely did he return to Albuquerque to see his dad or siblings—usually once a year around the Christmas and Hannukah holidays. He would be back in LA in time to celebrate the New Year with his new family.

The bond with this circle of friends was mostly the accident of fate that had put them together in a freshman dorm at UCLA. Most were from California, and the bulk from Los Angeles. When they brought him home for dinners or holidays, he learned how other families came together, or not, differently from his. He saw nothing that made him long for this in his own life. Family was what it was, he would say—you are born to your relations and then you live and die with newfound strangers.

In his junior year, Irv set a course toward even grander adventures. Why stop with Los Angeles and California? There was a whole world to be experienced. He began hitchhiking to faraway stretches of the United States. Sometimes with a friend, sometimes alone. Irv would take out his atlas, identify some distant location, note the general direction and roads leading to it, and then hit the road. A thumb, backpack, and his curiosity provided most of the fuel for his journey.

One day, he decided on a trip to the Pacific Northwest. Truth be told, he had been aiming at Vancouver, British Columbia, and Canada. Several forays into Mexico had given him an international johnson, and he thought Canada would be a relatively easy addition to his travel résumé before he could trek to lands really far away, places he couldn't reach by thumb alone.

But unlike most of his other adventures, this one ended in a very different location than those he had pinned on his map. He was on the entry ramp to northbound I-5 in Los Angeles, waving his thumb, when a Volkswagen van stopped to pick him up.

"Where you going?" offered up a young man in the passenger seat. He had long, blond hair tied back into a ponytail and used his hands when he talked.

"Vancouver," replied Irv.

"Well, this is your lucky day. We are headed back to Seattle and can drop you off on the way."

"That would be great. But how? I need to go a lot farther than Seattle." Irv was retracing the map in his mind as he spoke, remembering some serious space between Seattle and Vancouver on the atlas.

"Oh, that Vancouver. I thought you meant the one near Portland. This highway runs right through it. But let's face it—there isn't much reason to head there unless you got some action waiting for you. Do you?"

Irv couldn't quite place this addition to his recollection of the map, but it didn't matter. He had found a ride that would take him a thousand miles closer to his destination. The man seemed friendly enough, even warm. It looked a far more comfortable ride than many of the trucks and cars and strange drivers that had serviced his trips in the past.

He slid open the side panel of the van and pushed into the vacant back, nestling in on the floor beside piles of food wrappers, boots, and all sorts of other road supplies.

"Welcome aboard, partner. The Sea Lion Express is headed north, and you are our first customer of the day." Irv looked at the driver of the van, who was greeting him not just with words but a smile that started in the Pacific Ocean and ended somewhere in the Badlands of North Dakota. Even though he was sitting with a steering wheel in his lap, Irv could see that he was a tall man, well over six feet and probably closer to six-foot-five. He had flaming red hair, a large Roman nose, and a scraggly beard of red and gold. He looked to be more lion than man. A young lion, maybe a few years older than Irv, but not much.

"Appreciate the ride. I will go as far as you boys can take me."

"Sure enough. I am John. My friends call me Johnny, and the draft board called me John Gibson. Take your pick. This is Seth, though he typically goes by the name of Red Freak."

"I guess there's some story behind that," Irv suggested.

"You better believe it, and we got a lot of time to tell it," Seth replied.

"What is sending you up to Canada, friend?" asked John.

"I got something to find up there—damned if I have any idea what it is though. Just got to be back by finals."

The driver eyeballed Irv top to bottom, smiling as he did so. It seemed his dark eyes were looking through Irv with some weird form of X-ray vision. But it was a genuine and warm stare, nothing to be scared about. "What's your name?"

"Irv."

John Gibson continued to take him in with his stare like a cup of coffee on a chilly morning. "Well then, Irving, let's get this trip started—you've got to be back in what, a couple of weeks?"

"A month, John. More or less. And I prefer Irv."

John peered back as he put the van in gear and started to roll up the ramp toward the busy interstate. "A man after my own sense of time. Irv. And call me Johnny."

Chapter Five

Irv Meets with the Director

Irv was standing outside of Director Phil Welch's office on the twenty-third floor of Seattle-King County Public Health Headquarters. He was talking with a gray-haired woman sitting at the desk just outside the office. "He'll be right with you—he's with a couple of councilmen and the mayor's policy aide down in the conference room. But I know he wants to see you very soon."

Irv nodded to the elderly woman at the small desk. Rose was Director Welch's assistant, as she had been for the last three of Welch's predecessors. She and Irv had worked closely together during the time of the last director, and they had forged a friendship. Irv was on the outs now, though, and she was cautious about being too chummy toward him in this public setting.

A long tenure in the director's post was five years; most never got that close . . . usually from the politics of some health problem gone wrong—and probably what this meeting was about. Rarely, in Irv's experience, did one come up to the public health throne of power on the twenty-fourth floor to talk about health. Usually it was more about politics, newspaper stories, or money.

"Surprised he wants to see me at all. Last time didn't go so well for me or him." Irv settled into the cheap office chair outside Rose's office space and against the outside window of the director's office.

Rose chuckled, after peering around to make sure there were no witnesses. "Yes, that was a bit of a dust-up, wasn't it?" She kept typing away on her computer keyboard even as she spoke. "You might want to try to restrain yourself a little bit this time. He seems pretty worked up about this one."

"Any idea what—" Irv stopped mid-sentence as he saw Director Phil Welch begin to turn the corner down the hall and take the dozen or so steps remaining to his office corner. Irv took one fast glance at Rose, who was now entirely focused on her keyboard, and shifted his attention fully to Director Welch.

The director was dressed smartly in a whalebone sport coat, blue tie, khaki pants, and a striped blue and red tie. Still, there were too many wrinkles, too loose a fitting on his tie, and fabric just a notch below the finest threads to carry off a slick look. Underneath the costume, Phil Welch was a laboratory assistant and a bureaucrat. He had ambitions, but looking the part was not natural to him. "Irv. It's been awhile. Let's go in my office." He turned back to look at Rose. "Any messages?"

"Just some more from DC, wanting to know if you've made any progress."

"Great. At least it's now dinnertime there, and maybe they will give me a few hours to make some." With that, he strode into his office, shutting the door behind him and settling into the overstuffed vinyl chair behind his large oak desk. Irv had already plopped down in one of the two seats facing the director's desk and sat waiting for the first volley.

"Okay. Tell me what we know."

"Not a whole lot, Director." Irv guessed this had to do with the investigation of the Kent corpse. "A yet-to-be identified corpse, with some exceptionally large fissures on the neck and face. Nothing like I've seen in person before, but similar to the nodules I've seen in pictures of victims of other really nasty outbreaks. Just got the reports back from the lab, and it looks like our victim might have a new strain of mutated bird flu. Nothing direct yet on where and how he got it, and no autopsy yet. But you must know all of this already."

"Yes I do. What else you got—you've been on this all day."

"Not much. I've been trying to figure out what our victim was doing there. From talking to the neighbors, this property has been vacant for a couple of years. If he was squatting there, there were no signs of food, bedding, or anything that says that this had been going on very long. If at all. No car, and no way in other than by county road, unless he walked across about ten miles of state forest."

"How do you think he got there?"

"My guess is by car, and somebody dropped him off. There were some SUV tire tracks that seemed suspicious. At the most he had been dead for a day or two, and I can't imagine that he wasn't already really sick by the time he got to the cabin. No way he hiked down a two-mile road or across a forest in that condition."

"Maybe some of his fellow workers—I understand we think he was an illegal, maybe a migrant farm worker. Not too surprising that they wouldn't want to take him to a hospital or otherwise draw attention to themselves."

"Could be. And it could be that they knew about this place from some of their jobbing trips. There is a large strawberry farm a couple of miles away where they might have worked."

"Makes sense. Probably the best we are going to be able to guess on this one, unless someone saw something. It sounds like no one did."

"Couldn't find anyone who did. Interviewed everybody living on that road and most of the people on the state road that it butted into. The cabin is tucked back behind some pretty thick trees and blackberry vines and not very visible. Not that there were many other places on that road to begin with—and even less traffic in and out."

"Let's focus on isolating the source of the flu transmission. Stay on top of the lab boys. They've shared all of the preliminary reports with me, and it sounds like that is the key issue on this one. I'll have Tracy work the statewide angle and see if we can find any other cases. With some luck, this will be a one-time thing and related to some sick chicken that he was sleeping with."

Tracy was the director's special assistant. She was an eager and bright professional who had gotten this job through her political connections within the local Republican Party. Although clever enough with the written and spoken word, she was no public health expert by any stretch of the imagination. Loyalty to the director was her primary talent, with rumors that her service came with benefits. Her assignment to this case meant something.

"I thought that there were some reports from the other side of the mountain?"

"Nothing confirmed yet. Tracy is on it now, and she'll let you know if we find some connection."

"You know, I've got some connections out there still." There were dozens of county health inspectors across the state, though not as many as before, as federal and state budget shortfalls pressed down on the already thin budgets.

"Let her work that angle, Irv. I need you to stay focused on the strain. The boys from the CDC will be out here soon, and I want you to be ready to show them all they need to know. And please, please—no talking to the press. The last thing we need is for this to raise a panic in the community. Your friends in the media would love it to no end, but it won't do us any good at all."

Irv didn't really have any friends in the press corps, and knew that this was a shot at the E. coli story that he had dropped a few months ago. He had leaked it to get higher-ups like Director Welch to pay attention to what he thought was a serious public threat, one that they were ready to sweep under the rug. He didn't regret it, even after the disciplinary complaint dropped in his file. But Irv felt like there was no need to involve the media in this case. It seemed like there was plenty of concern for this potential health problem, and it was far too complicated a threat to explain to reporters anyway.

All of which begged the question of why he was here in the director's office. Welch already knew everything about the case, except his interviews at the scene and whatever else he had found during his morning investigation at the corpse site.

"I'd like to take another look at the cabin and see if there is anything I missed."

"Probably not worth your time. The CDC asked us to bottle up the scene, and we've got the whole road closed off now to make sure no one gets in or out."

"How about the victim? I'd like to know the results of the autopsy."

"The feds are asserting jurisdiction on that too, and I am inclined to let them take it over. You can try and get some of the results from them, but you know how that usually goes." The director kept his gaze intently on Irv, trying to read his thoughts. Irv felt it too, wondering what this meeting was really about.

"I want you to focus on the flu strain. We will let you know if there are other victims. Or if there is something relevant in the autopsy. Get that strain and start checking to see if we can get any handle on its origins and path. And let me say again—no media. That's an order. Do I make myself clear?"

"Yes, Director, I got it. No reporters. Just do my job, the way it is drawn up on the job description. We've had this discussion before."

"Good, Irv. If you find something out, let me know, whatever the time of day or night. We've got some exposure on this with the election coming up this fall. Everybody and anybody running for public office will want to bite our asses if we don't do this by the book." The director stood up, marking the end of the meeting.

"By the book it is." Irv took his cue, nodded his assent to Director Welch, and strode out of the office. He shared a glance with Rose, who was still banging away on keys but peering over the rims of her glasses as he walked by.

Something about this case had unsettled Irv from the beginning. This meeting did nothing to stop the queasy feeling in his gut. *Follow the strain?* That was what the lab boys were for. Why wasn't he the one looking for other victims—that contract tracing was the real public health sleuthing needed on this one. Instead, a political hack was tracking down the other potential disease vectors. *Stay away from the body, stay away from the cabin. And don't talk to the press.*

Irv muttered to himself as he walked down the hall. "If I didn't know better, I'd think that Welch was trying to take me off the case, without really doing so." Stick to doing your job or else—that message was clear. Too bad the director didn't know that job security was not at the top of Irv's list of personal priorities. Sure, he was struggling to find himself and needed the work and money, but not enough to want to buckle to the whims of bureaucrats like Director Welch in the face of a real public health emergency.

Irv had every intention of sticking to the parameters of the job description for a public health investigator. No media, and there was that language about limiting access to his findings for the purpose of public control of messages. But the other parts were even clearer—as lead investigator for this case, his job was to find out what the real threat to the public was. How could he maneuver through the major roadblocks laid out by the director to do so?

Striding down the hallway to the elevator and his office cubicle, he noted the conference room to the right of the main elevators. This was likely to be the venue for his next disciplinary hearing, months into the future. "Just doing my job, sir." He smiled. That he would.

Chapter Six

Early Nancy Jones

Nancy Jones gazed out the large kitchen window of her small home in Ballard. Her location was Sunset Hill, to be exact, a neighborhood in the northwest part of the city of Seattle. The stores, restaurants, and nightlife of downtown Ballard were about a mile south and a few blocks to the east. Once a sleepy fishing village populated by Scandinavians, Ballard was undergoing rapid transformation. It was gentrifying quickly; almost every day a new sign went up in front of a small rambler, noting the death of a longtime resident and the plan to replace the small and funky home with a multi-floor condo complex.

Nancy's home was spacious but not massive—three bedrooms, two bathrooms, a good-sized study, living room, kitchen, and daylight basement. Guests would regularly stay with her in the third bedroom. The centerpiece of the home was a sprawling deck attached to the back of the house and open to most of the rooms of the house. It made for an easy transition to this outdoor space, and one that revealed, skies permitting, a spectacular view across Puget Sound.

The Olympic Mountains rising above and across the water were framed by the large kitchen window from the table—when they were visible. The snowy peaks were hidden behind a layer of gray clouds this morning. Since it wasn't raining, Seattle weather people would call this a partly sunny day. Nancy had grown up in New England and knew well enough that this was overcast to most of the rest of the world.

Clouds, rain or not, Seattle had become a hotbed of in-migration. Nancy was one of those, though having moved here over twenty-five years ago hardly made her a newcomer. She came a few years before Seattle became a principal base for the Information Age economy.

The Theory of IRV

Companies like Microsoft and Amazon arose and soon attracted thousands of young workers. Many became millionaires in short order. They brought with them a different point of view and the resources to remake the region in their image.

Some, like Nancy, found ways to live, work, and prosper with the newcomers. Others, including many of her neighbors, battled them. It was more Cold War than outright conflict. The stoic politeness of the natives carried a distant friendliness toward the newbies. Privately, they wished them to be gone and would secretly do all they could to hold them off from full integration into their community.

Nancy was open to change and understood, even as others forgot, that she was a migrant to the Pacific Northwest. Of course they all were, save for the Native Americans, who had largely been priced out of living in the city, unless it was under one of the many bridges in homeless camps.

It was also Nancy's business to welcome and understand the newcomers—they were likely to be voters and some of them clients. Her field was politics, and specifically campaign politics. She consulted with people who wanted to win or hold on to elective office—local, state, or federal positions. She would take clients running for the PTA, she mused, but they generally did not want to pay very much.

She had just celebrated her fifty-fifth birthday and was now prone to reflecting on the circumstances that brought her to the Pacific Northwest. She had grown up on the East Coast in Boston. More specifically, she'd been raised at Cambridge, where her father was a professor at Harvard Medical School. She was an honors graduate from this university and moved through the undergraduate program and the Harvard School of Government in record time.

The faculty of the school was made up of a political who's who of clinical faculty and guest lecturers who were leaders in the government and political world over the previous generation. Her grandfather, and then father, were among those, and that opened doors for her. She had known many of these movers and shakers over the course of her life—even sat on the laps of some as an infant. A few mentored Nancy as she set out on her career.

It began with an internship with a political consulting firm in DC. Early on, the firm assigned her to campaign consulting, dispatching her with a senior partner to help candidates running for office in congressional districts across the nation. They were mostly Democratic candidates, though the firm tried to remain bipartisan by working with several Republican clients as well. Back then politics was not as tribal, and moving across party lines was a common strategy among consulting firms. They could maintain their business no matter which party was in power.

The senior partners who accompanied Nancy on these early assignments were the fronts of the campaign work. They would take the lead with the candidate, setting the strategy and identifying tactics. Nancy, and any paid staff or volunteers, would then implement the campaign. The senior partner would come back for the party on election night—if it looked like a winning campaign or if the candidate had longer-term prospects.

Nancy had a knack for the work and was soon hired as a new associate. By her second year, she had ten candidates for whom she was, in practical terms, the lead consultant. By her fourth year, she was a de facto partner managing over twenty-five campaigns across the country. The people part came naturally to her, despite her introversion. She was smart and could translate their desires into winning campaign strategies. These were people who above all wanted to win, and Nancy was a natural at bringing this to them.

Much of her success came from what the Harvard program described as "good political instincts." That meant she was good at discerning what bullshit to listen to—and what not to. Most politicians had big egos, and this got in the way of their judgments, certainly about themselves. But that was no excuse for miscalculations of the abilities of others—this was where fatal mistakes were usually made. Nancy built her reputation as a winner by forcing realistic analysis of opponents by her clients, all while feeding their voracious egos.

Five years in, she was a success. The firm offered her a partnership: the first woman in its thirty-year history. She was making good money and enjoying life in Washington, DC. The nation's capital was undergoing its own transformation, as young professionals began to make it a full-time home rather than a waystation for temporary residents. This growth was fed by people like Nancy who had made politics bigger and more regular. Every group in America now seemed to have a need for a lobbyist and influence.

But Nancy was restless. She had an itch to do more. Part of it was very personal. It irked her that she felt like a second-class partner at the firm, able to share in the work but not all of the glory and trappings. It was no longer a shock when a female candidate won a campaign. This progress was important, but also highlighted how much further things needed to go to achieve real fairness—and power. The men at her firm, and across the nation's capital, believed the fences had come down, and it was now a meritocratic society. Nancy knew this was not even close to true; it remained the rare exception when a female candidate, or a professional like herself, rose to full success.

Her own orientation was an issue too. She had never openly come out, but she was aware of the rumors. Any woman who wasn't married or blatantly flaunting a field of male suitors was likely to be a prospect for the gay rumor mill. In Nancy's case, it was true, but really, whose business was it?

She found many were attracted to her good looks then and was dismayed that almost all flirtations came from men. She was a striking woman in her youth, near six feet tall with sandy blonde hair, long legs, high cheekbones, and twinkly Irish green eyes. Her introversion came off as a humble shyness to suitors, and not quiet rejection born of inclination and gender.

She had been assigned to a woman client running for congress in a northern Seattle district. The client lost the campaign, but Nancy learned that she was gay. Her client introduced her to how comfortable it could be to be gay in Seattle, which made a big and positive impression and got her thinking about a move. She thought Seattle had enough going on politically to build a base of operation. More importantly, it looked like one could get things done there that really mattered to people. This was the biggest force tugging at her then—her desire to make a difference.

Politics was not what rocked Nancy's world, though she was good at it, and even loved it. But it was just a means to an end: social progress. This had been drilled into her at an early age; perhaps it was even imprinted on her DNA.

Grandpops and Dad were among the leading policy experts of their respective eras, always pressing American society to be and do better. It was the family calling. Both had seen their own dreams for progress run aground by a political world resistant to change. They encouraged Nancy to confront this failing by getting into politics. Someone in the family needed to get better at this if their policy views were ever to take flight.

It was too late for them, and they had little appetite for politics anyway. Perhaps Nancy could grab the flag and finally carry their policy ideas for greater good over the finish line.

She had sat through numerous family discussions about health care and the need for fundamental change in how it was financed and delivered to the American people. Grandpa and Dad were among the leading experts of their time in this field. Both felt that this area was America's greatest policy failure, and both were frustrated by the lack of progress over their career. They had seen health care grow over their lifetimes from something close to witchcraft to now diagnosis and treatments out of science fiction books. If only the nation could harness a rational way to spread these new technological benefits fairly and effectively—but it couldn't.

Nancy accepted their arguments intellectually. Her love for her father and grandfather and the soundness of their reasoning made it impossible not to adopt this as one of her policy causes. Emotionally though, it was Grandpa's death that had sealed the deal.

Officially, he had died from pneumonia, but the real reason was an infection he had acquired while hospitalized for a bad case of the flu. Nancy's dad made sure she knew this—and gave her a copy of Ivan Illich's book on the iatrogenic failure of hospitals to make sure she understood that this was not a rare occurrence.

Her personal attraction to health care was grafted on to her professional expertise too. Because of her interest in the issue, she accidentally discovered health care was a leading issue for voters decades before polls revealed this to be so.

Even with this, Nancy wasn't solely obsessed with health care. It was one of a number of issues that pressed her to want real solutions for society. Housing, the role of women, all these wars, hunger, civil rights—these were just as wanting as health care to her.

Her frustration was that few of these issues saw major progress, even as she had gotten scores of people elected based on them. The issues were good enough to run on as candidates, and she believed in her heart that her clients still genuinely cared about the issues once they won their races. But they did not care enough to overcome the political inertia they then encountered in Washington, DC, Congress, or state government to actually solve any problems.

It was for all these reasons that she decided to take the leap to Seattle. She started her political consulting firm with several candidates that Speaker of the House Tom Foley from Spokane referred to her. Her sister would take care of the bookkeeping and other managerial needs of the business, and Nancy would do the client recruitment and consulting.

Nancy reflected on all that had happened since. It was initially tough to break into the Washington State political world, but she had built a unique practice by specializing in women candidates. Virtually no one was doing this, and she found a healthy appetite among wealthy and frustrated women in the Pacific Northwest.

Her expertise was also unique. Nancy was surprised by how old-school political consultants were in the Evergreen State. It made the old men's club in DC seem like youthful frat parties. In addition to bringing the new dynamic of women candidates to the political market, she opened up the campaign playbook in Washington State by introducing radically new strategies and tactics.

Nancy had learned some of these new tricks of the trade at school but, even more, was quick to adapt to radical new technological possibilities. There was this thing called the Internet, which seemed to have major implications for politics. Then there were personal computers that allowed for mass accumulations and management of data; new communications technology. The fax machine was an innovation early in her career, yet now it was a dinosaur. Surely everything she did would need replacing. She didn't know exactly what these changes might be or exactly how to move with them, but she was open to testing and folding these into her practice.

She also found a love life in Seattle. She had no long-term partner, but enough companionship to feed her soul. It was no big deal to be gay in Seattle, even in the political world. The ease around what she once counted as her guilty East Coast pleasure helped make this a home she would not soon leave.

Nancy noodled over all of these things this morning. She was happy, and a bit nostalgic. She had aged reasonably well, with a few wrinkles across her pretty face and streaks of gray through her blonde hair. She'd gained a few too many pounds around the midsection. But she was doing better than most, she figured.

She thought about Pops and Dad. Would they be proud of what she had accomplished? She looked at their portraits on the piano in the den adjacent to the kitchen. *Probably not yet*, she concluded. For all her wins, she questioned whether it was enough—for her mentors, or herself. How much real social progress could she claim?

Yes, it was possible to think bolder at the Washington State level, and she had helped pass many important laws. But major change was a second cousin here, just as it was in DC. She also realized that some problems called for national solutions. For all she had accomplished at the state level, the nation's capital must move back into her portfolio if she was to help achieve real social progress.

It troubled her this Wednesday morning that this was most definitively the case with health care. Washington State had dabbled in major state-based innovations throughout her time there, and even passed a comprehensive health care reform package in 1992. Her experience with this told her that while local progress could be made, much of health care policy, including especially the money that defined its nature, was national. Case in point—the Washington State health reform package was repealed the next legislative session.

She thought about her grandfather and dad. Their storytelling at the dinner table seemed like only yesterday, and so long ago. She watched the marine layer of clouds break up to reveal the snow-capped peaks of the Olympic Mountains. Their spirits were with her, so close and yet so far away. She would honor their careers in a new way. Anything could thrive here—why not rational health care policy for the nation?

Chapter Seven

Irv Forms an Investigation Plan

For most of the afternoon, in his small cubicle, Irv puzzled over how to proceed with an investigation that wasn't supposed to be. But there was only so much he could do from his office space. He doodled on a pad of paper, hoping his fingers might unlock subconscious answers to the problem at hand. After fifteen minutes of trying, he concluded that all he had was one ugly picture.

He ripped it up and pondered other methods of discovery. He decided the best that he could muster from this location was the web. He began to surf keywords to see what his Google app might uncover. It was one of the features that he loved about the web. It fit with what he had learned about the power of randomness in his biostatistics course in his graduate degree program—variability is our friend if we open our consciousness to learn from it. Not that many of his professors cottoned to such notions—they were more likely to drum him out of the program for such unconventional thinking. He found it best—then and now—to keep some of these worldviews to himself.

He also understood that the top line results from his search words were paid advertisements, so he focused on the later links uncovered. He found lots of interesting information from this random keyword search, on topics ranging from rat traps to potato processing to SUV tires to Kent to immigrants and farming. Nothing was really clicking in terms of next steps for his investigation though.

Irv also knew that he was now in his usual afternoon swoon, made worse by having been woken in the middle of the night. Or maybe the way forward was not yet cosmically ready to be discovered.

He was tempted to just leave, but knew that he needed to remain in the office a while longer to get the next set of lab results from the epidemiologists in the department. The county's integrated electronic record system had proven to be a financial boondoggle—millions of dollars—but most of the important information related to his job was transmitted across the department by paper, not by computer, including public health threat information. It irked Irv that he frequently had to be in his office to get the paper results of tests that were at the core of solving many of his public health troubleshooting problems. The traffic was a bitch and the parking fees horrific.

He drifted further from the immediate task at hand while he waited. He found a modeling amplifier that might be just the trick for advancing his electric guitar skills. It would be nice to get home and play a few licks. This was when he did some of his best thinking, as he considered big questions, and it was far more likely to bear fruit than his afternoon attempts.

The test reports were dropped off by a runner at quarter to four, earlier than Irv expected, and he immediately dug into the reports. He found nothing really new. The reports contained allusions to similarities to other mutated flu strains, but not exactly like the known threats now being reported by worldwide surveillance systems managed by the World Health Organization. Irv knew that mutated flu strains were actually down across the world, but that trouble was expected as the year moved on. Since the SARS threat, politicians had insisted on classifying the threats the way TSA did for airline terrorist threats. Washington was now yellow, moving to green, somewhere between a Seattle Seahawks and Oregon Duck road uniform.

Irv was satisfied that he had waited for the report. It was a necessary chore, even if it didn't tell him much. But the problem was the angle into his investigation that the director had provided him. It was probably only Welch needing to give him something to dig into, given that Irv was the first investigator to arrive at the scene and now had a legal duty to file a final report on the investigation. Irv knew he had to get outside of the boundaries of this limited instruction to find some real answers. First he had to demonstrate he was all over the test results—and that had now been accomplished.

Irv packed up a few papers and took them home. He poured a snifter of bourbon and played guitar for a couple of hours. He watched the *Daily Show* for a little comic relief. It amused him that this was one of the best sources of impartial news in this crazy new world of public information. Then he went to bed. When faced with particularly challenging problems, Irv found a good method was to think about things with his face pushed into a pillow. This was sometimes where and when the subconscious was most likely to make contact with the infinite variability of the universe, and bigger answers.

When he awoke the next morning and sipped coffee around his morning stretching routine, things started to come together for him. They didn't coalesce into any clear answers or even a detailed plan, but created a sense that his way forward was getting closer. He just had to stay the course and do it, technically, "by the book." Or at least "a book," somewhere to be found.

The tests did note the presence of potato derivatives. It was probably just a throwaway line by some hyperactive epidemiologist in the lab, but there it was, stated in the report. His instructions were to follow the flu strain. Well, until he had some data that said otherwise, this would seem to reasonably include the potato derivatives.

That Washington's agricultural testing facility was located in Moses Lake, midway across the state, was now a helpful coincidence. There was an active public health department in Grant County, where Moses Lake was located, and it was run by a classmate from his Masters in Health Administration days, Ken Wisterly. Ken was a good friend and the only classmate to go into the public health world upon graduation from the MHA Program. Today was Friday, which would offer a couple of days before Irv would have to clock in at the office again on Monday. If the Eastern Washington connection to whatever this was existed, Ken was likely to know something about it. Who was Irv to say no to taking a road trip for the weekend and perhaps finding such information?

Chapter Eight

Early Irv Moves to Seattle

A month became two, and two became four. Irv was still in Seattle and not at UCLA for the resumption of classes. Before all was said and done, Irv had taken an incomplete for that school quarter and resumed his college career by cobbling together a collection of independent study classes for which attendance didn't matter much. He memorized the textbooks for the classes and hitchhiked back to Los Angeles for finals. This approach kept him in school and on track to graduate. He used his book smarts to substitute for his lack of physical presence. Pass-Fail grading didn't hurt, either.

Irv didn't care all that much about the degree and graduating; that was for his dad, and perhaps so he could make some money to fund his adventures. His dad didn't even know that he had essentially moved to Seattle—not that they spoke very often.

Irv was content, for now. He had found himself in Seattle, or at least a big part of him. Johnny, it turned out, was a soulmate. Like Irv, he was focused on a life of adventures. Johnny was smart, but far more from learning about life out in the real world than from books and classrooms. Johnny even seemed to have built a life plan around his adventuring, and Irv admired him for that.

The trip up the West Coast in the van had been more than enough to suck Irv into the vortex of John Gibson's life force. The normal three-day journey up from California became eight when Johnny, Red Freak, and Irv took a detour to Crater Lake National Park in Oregon. They played around in the blow zone of the ancient volcano for several days, and then resumed the final leg of their journey to Washington State and Seattle.

Irv, Johnny, and Red Freak found much to discuss over the course of their trip: the failing of American foreign policy in applying post-WWII thinking to Asia; the heresy of using blue as the color base for institutionalized religion; the sexual proclivities of Northwest frogs; why we should read our books right to left as the Hebrews do; how the Mormons probably had it right with multiple wives, so long as they didn't take marriage seriously. Ah, some good pot and fertile young minds.

Irv felt something powerful strike him when he first saw the Emerald City pop over the horizon through the windshield of the van. It was one of those rare Northwest days—no rain or clouds and instead deep blue skies framing close to a 360-degree panorama of mountains, water, and trees. Yes, there was some basis in reality for the song that declared the "bluest skies are in Seattle."

Irv was even taken by the downtown skyline, compact and condensed into a small slice of land between water and freeways. It was so different from the spreading mess in LA or the flattened bubble of oozing suburbia of Albuquerque. This seemed like a land that held mysteries and also the possibility of being understood.

Just beyond downtown to the north, the odd orb that was the Space Needle rose like a hovering spaceship against one of the city's prominent hills. But the real wow for him was the Olympic Mountains pushing up in the west across the body of water called Puget Sound. They were snow-clad, jagged, foreboding, and friendly all at the same time.

He shivered. This was what was in his mind's eye those evenings crying by his mom's grave. He had started to question whether this place even existed after so many disappointments over his many adventures. He had ideas about different places, but when he went to them, there was something missing. They were likable enough, just not that magical place he had expected. Denver was one of the biggest disappointments—he had thought this would be his land of milk and honey. But when he got there and took a look around, he gathered up his disappointment like a bag of dirty clothes. The place was nice and pretty enough, but not "it."

How about Reno? New Orleans? Minneapolis? Sacramento? None were to be. He had stopped even looking, thinking it a foolish childhood quest. He still enjoyed his travels and loved the experiences within each destination. But he had started to believe his place on earth was to search, like the Israelites wandering in the desert for forty years. Fair enough, he thought—he enjoyed the process and would accept his fate.

Then, literally out of the blue, here it was before him. He tingled with excitement from his toes to his groin, torso and fingers, and all the way to the top of his long, curly brown hair. His first glimpse of Seattle made him feel warm—and it was cold outside.

It greatly helped that Johnny became Irv's best friend in this wonderful place. They found adventure after adventure to bond their relationship—in north Seattle, across the state and long-distance adventuring into Canada and the adjacent northern states. Yes, even the long delayed trip up to Vancouver. The two young men found a bond that went way beyond the expediency of the moment, or the new blends of pot propagating in the backyard of his new home.

This home was also part of what made Seattle special for Irv. It was in the dark basement of this home that he spent his first night in Seattle—a house Johnny shared with a group of other people in North Seattle. It was a big home, close to the University of Washington. Once a personal residence for professors, it was now a rental property. Its occupants were now students and working folk mixed together.

There was Steve, a roasting savant for a small coffee company—baking beans to perfection by day, and drumming up a storm at night. Tina, a PhD microbiologist, worked at a bike shop in the evening and spent her mornings experimenting with hydroponics in the backyard. Zeke, a woodworker from North Carolina, made cabinets while investing his small paycheck in old boats and cars that he would refurbish, slowly but surely. The driveway now held five of Zeke's projects, shaded from the sun and the rain by a large cherry tree and several blue tarps.

And there was Mary Beth, a brown-haired beauty who had moved to the University District after growing up a bit north of Seattle in the town of Edmonds. Mary Beth on paper was the least worldly of the household, but she had things that transcended résumés, exotic backgrounds, and experiences: blue eyes that could calm a stampeding herd of buffalo, a tight, athletic body that got bees a buzzing like they had just found their honeycomb, and an air about her that engulfed the white on rice.

The house as an entity was a mind-blowing discovery for Irv. The strangers, who came together to create a spontaneous family based on who was there at the moment, were far closer than his dorm mates from college. People came and went as they pleased because they wanted to, and frequently brought friends and acquaintances home for a meal, a several-month sleepover on a couch, or a conversation over freshly brewed coffee. It was different from anything Irv had experienced before, and he loved it.

It was Mary Beth who put the cherry on the sundae. The two had begun to chat regularly in the early mornings near the end of his first month in Seattle. She was an early riser, not wishing to disturb her sleep over boyfriend, an international study visitor from Guatemala named Jorge. Irv was not by nature interested in getting up that early in the morning, but had learned how to come to fast attention when he recognized Mary Beth's soft tread on the ceiling of his downstairs hovel. He had a fancy for her, and this time slot was the only one open for him to stare into her blue eyes without competition—or admire her perky ass when she turned away.

He had started to sense that the attraction was mutual. Mary Beth would stop floating around the kitchen when he came upstairs and would sit at the kitchen table. She would place her pretty bottom down on a kitchen chair across from Irv, look into his eyes, and occasionally ask him to get something from the fridge. When he did, she would survey him from top to bottom, with a way stop around his groin.

"So, finals next week?" She pushed the question between them like a rainbow looking for a rainstorm.

"Yup. It'll take me a few days to get back to LA. I really should get on the road tomorrow sometime."

"It's been nice having you around here, college boy." She winked as she teased him about his status in the world, something they regularly joked about. He was a college boy; she was a bakery assistant. Neither really thought of themselves in the way that most of the rest of the world did, though.

"Ditto. This is one of my favorite places ever. Don't even mind the rain, though I could handle a few more sunny days."

"What's so cool about it? Those other places you've been sound really exotic," she said, leaning in, hoping for something that would help her see what cards he was holding.

"But hard to match two mountain ranges squeezing a sliver of land between all this water. And somehow pushing back the suburbanization of America from the 1960s and 1970s and making what I feel here." It was true enough—North Seattle was a throwback to a different America, populated by an odd combination of working-class families, counterculture hippies who had found refuge in this corner of the globe to continue their version of the 1960s, and really smart people who used the time forced indoors by the rain to read books, go to movies, and talk about the world.

"Uh-huh. I've never lived anywhere else. But I love it here." She peeked down into her cup of coffee, stirring it with her disappointment that her offering was dismissed by an interesting comment. It was not what she was hoping to hear.

Irv picked up on the disappointment, somewhere between his temporal lobe and left testicle. He realized he had missed his mark with his answer. Over the last week he had been trying to read Mary Beth, not with his book skills but with his growing understanding of how to feel things—a fast application of his time together with Johnny. It wasn't just taking a new talent out for a spin—he was applying it with some urgency as the days got shorter toward his need to depart for LA.

He leaned in closer to her, peering into her eyes. "And it has some other things, too, that I have never found anywhere else."

"Do tell," she volleyed back.

"Hard to describe from where I sit today. But Jorge probably has a pretty good idea of what I think is here."

She smiled at him. "Maybe. But then, Jorge is about to move out, so maybe he doesn't know as much as you think."

"Do tell. When did this happen?"

"Oh, about thirty seconds or so ago. He will find out as soon as he gets up. Depending, of course, on what you say next." She pushed her soft face even closer to his, so close that he could smell the peppermint toothpaste on her breath. Her lips pushed out at Irv, with a mouth that he wanted to smother with his own.

"How about you just leave him a note? And you and I take a walk around Greenlake? There are some things that I want to tell you about. May take a while—don't think I'll be able to make it to LA for my finals. Bummer."

"Deal. Let's get out of here." She jotted a ten-word note on a pad of paper and folded it over and placed it on the table. She stood up, extending her hand so Irv would help her up. "I got a few things that I want to tell you too."

Chapter Nine

1932: Patrick Jones and the CCMC

Patrick Jones held up the bright red book and examined it in the light of his desk lamp. It wasn't just his work product—dozens of others had worked on it over its five-year run from 1927. He played a big part in its completion, though, and for this he felt a deep pride in its publication. It was a thing of beauty, a guidebook for further improving the nation he loved. That it was about health care still amused him; he knew so little about this field when his opportunity arose. He never imagined that the health care system's failures would embrace his destiny.

Mom and Dad had instilled in him a belief he owed the United States more than his own personal success, or theirs. They had emigrated to the United States from Ireland at the turn of the century, escaping starvation and serfdom to the English. They, and their generations before them, had tilled the soil for their own survival. The hard times of crop and weather cycles were theirs to bear, while good times meant that the crown demanded even more from them.

When another famine descended upon Ireland, escaping to the Americas seemed like their only option. They jumped when an opportunity arose for passage on a steamship departing for New York City. They packed their meager belongings into a potato sack, bade their farewells to family and friends, and ran to the shipyard and boarded. After many days of rough seas and sickness, they awoke from a night of broken sleep to see the Statue of Liberty welcoming them to a new world.

Scared as they were, they felt joy and a sense of belonging bubble within as the dawn light reflected off of Lady Liberty. His parents now hoped for economic opportunity in the form of jobs that could allow them to start a family. They believed these would not only be found, but would come as part of a new social compact where they contribute not in bondage and fealty to a faraway king or queen, but as lord and master to themselves, their family, and their neighbors.

But life in lower Manhattan was not easy for the Jones and their six children. Manual labor was the only way to make enough to survive, the types of jobs that no one else wanted, other than fellow immigrants. Nor was being Irish a welcoming proposition to most Americans. Parents and kids learned new forms of bigotry and oppression, choking these down as necessary in order to survive. Through it all, Patrick's parents hung on to their dream, not for themselves as much for their children and their families to come.

Patrick was the first born, in 1901, and faced the greatest pressure to contribute among his siblings. He was supposed to lead the way for the next Jones generation; Mom and Dad insisted on this. Childhood games gave way to working for needed family income by his tenth birthday. He found steady work building the railways that would bring people and goods to New York City. He would dig through the night shift and then hustle home in time to attend high school. His parents saw his education as the way out and up for the family, and they made sure he took his studies seriously, no matter how tired he might be from his physically strenuous job.

They also instilled in Patrick their belief in a duty to their newfound home. It was part of his charge to be a good citizen, they told him over and over again. Any country that would throw off the chains of English bondage and welcome them to its shores deserved no less—even if it was to fight and perhaps die for his home on the field of battle.

This proposition came with World War I in 1914. Patrick was most willing to do his duty, but an errant hockey puck had destroyed most of his sight in one eye, making him ineligible for service. He felt guilt as he watched his friends and classmates, most second-generation immigrant sons like him from Europe, return to their former continent to fight for their new country. Many went to the killing fields of Belgium and Germany, never to be seen again.

He learned that many of them had not died in battle but as the result of disease—some from the regular maladies of the time, but most from the scourge of the Great Spanish Flu. Fear of it was not confined to

Europe; New York City itself was forced into quarantine as the flu broke through the local population, killing thousands. Its most virulent time would see bodies stacked up on sidewalks like cordwood, waiting for officials to remove them in a way that would not spread the disease further.

The sacrifice of his friends and classmates only deepened Patrick's resolve to contribute to his new home, and he promised to put this duty above career and money. This determination, and his keen mind and personal charm, led to a scholarship offer to attend college at Columbia.

Living at home with Mom and Dad, and still able to hold on to his rail job, Patrick proved to be a first-rate scholar. His classes on jurisprudence were his favorite, and he found a friend in their professor, Ezekiel Reed. Professor Reed saw great potential in the boy and encouraged him to apply to law school and make it his career. Better yet, he arranged for an interview with the dean of the law school at Georgetown Law in Washington, DC.

Patrick was accepted, and moved to the nation's capital in 1923. The loss of income for the family and the distance between them and their firstborn son were hard on Mom and Dad, but they had been through so much worse. Besides, it was the fulfillment of their dream born on the deck of a ship in New York Harbor just a couple of decades ago.

Patrick took to law school like all his educational endeavors. His grades put him in the top quartile of his classmates, and he was quick with his feet and tongue in oral classroom debates. As he moved into his second year, he came to understand that the practice of law was far removed from the interesting philosophical and existential questions of the classroom. Several classmates took summer jobs managing mundane legal transactions, with a special few finding clerkships with the major firms in New York or Boston. Patrick had the grades, work ethic, and interpersonal skills to be among them, but not the passion to make this his career path.

He hoped for more, a meaningful way to contribute, and these clerkships seemed to be more about serving the economic masters of society than the people. It was a different form of tyranny than what his parents had escaped, but tyranny nonetheless. Nor did the regular transactions of the business of law—contracts, wills, divorces, and such—

appeal to him. He would do these jobs if this was what had to be, but he hoped for another option.

Georgetown Law was little more than a stone's throw from the United States Capitol, and Patrick began to explore the government campus just down the street. It began with the revelation in a constitutional law class that while law school focused on court-made law, most of society was practically governed by statutes passed by legislative bodies. The nation's statutory law was being created right around the corner, and Patrick began to sit in the Senate and House galleries and watch this happen.

It wasn't easy to figure out what was going on from the galleries. The legislative process then was largely shielded from the public eye, and action to pass bills was cloaked in tradition, rhetoric, and complicated bill language. It was not impenetrable to Patrick, though, and with the help of the security guards watching over the galleries, he soon began to pick up on the process.

One guard of Irish descent took a liking to Patrick. When Patrick told him of his need to find work to pay for school and to send money back to his family, the guard introduced him to the Senate Committee administrator. A non-partisan staff member, his job was to find people to staff the committees through which Congress did much of its work. There were no permanent openings, but there was a need for a temporary and part-time staff member to the Senate Labor committee.

Patrick took the job, intrigued by the conceptual opportunity and greatly needing the money. The committee's primary work was to deal with issues surrounding the growth of union power across America. Unions were pushing their collective voice and trying to assert their rights in Congress. Corporations and vested interests were trying to squash their efforts, and did so by killing legislation before movements ever got started, usually in committees.

It took staff to help with this process, and Patrick became the junior member of their team. Most of his duties were mundane, from fetching food and drink to making written notes of meetings. Other staff passed off what they did not want to do to him—including an assortment of bills relating to health care.

Back then, health care was not much of a thing. It existed, but hospitals were mostly places where people without resources went to die. Most of the care was provided by barely trained physician practitioners, who frequently bartered for services rendered. Things were beginning to change, and there was some talk about health care becoming an important new field, but that potential was something beyond the imagination of Patrick or, really, anyone in Congress.

He did ruminate over his experience in 1918 with the Great Flu. Thankfully, that pandemic had run its course, but not before killing over 650,000 Americans and perhaps as many as 50 million across the globe. He wondered whether this was just God's judgment upon mankind, or whether there was something more that could have been done to stop it, maybe by Congress, or at least an institution that saw health care as part of their governing responsibility to the American people. Wasn't this included in the phrase "life, liberty, and property"? How could it not be?

Philosophical optimism aside, Patrick initially thought the committee a dead-end assignment, and looked at the health care matters assigned to him as a chore—one that provided him a perch from which to watch Congress operate, and money to boot, so a chore worth doing.

He was a good worker, and did his job, including meeting with those seeking to make changes in the health care system and who wanted Congress to be part of their solution. He was honest with them about their lack of prospects, but this didn't do much to quell their enthusiasm; they continued to seek action from Congress or, oddly enough, him. He became more curious about health care through these visits and thought more critically about the picture these visitors painted for him.

As graduation day got nearer, the problem of money became more acute. The nation was beginning to reel from an economic downturn, the prosperity of the postwar years a now distant memory. Patrick would be graduating just as the business cycle was turning downward. He had also met a young woman by the name of Ann. They got married in the summer between his second and third years of school. Ann shared his Irish roots, including parents who had moved to America to escape poverty. Neither they nor her job as a perfume counter girl at a downtown department store would pay the family bills. And, as in any good Irish Catholic family, more mouths to feed were around the corner. Ann was expecting their first child in June, around the time of Patrick's graduation.

His temporary committee job was set to end in May, right before graduation, and it would not parlay into something more permanent within Congress. The declining economy was beginning to send a message of discontent to the elected. More and more constituents were becoming unemployed and poor and demanding relief. Congress was not ready to do much about that but did cut back on its own staff as a symbolic gesture of empathy to those who needed a response far more meaningful.

Patrick was preparing to take a job at a small law firm in Maryland, with a solo general practitioner who needed someone to provide him basic legal support. It was too late for Patrick to make a play for the jobs in New York City, and he was now grateful for any lead toward a paying job. He was referred to the Maryland prospect by a classmate who had grown up around the corner from this attorney. The job did not offer much in the form of pay, and almost nothing to Patrick's greater ambitions, but it was a paying job, and he needed one, and soon.

Just before he took it, a different possibility arose—one that changed his life.

It came from his acquaintance with a gentleman from Philadelphia who had been visiting with him because of Patrick's committee work. Rufus Rorem shared with Patrick that he was involved with a group of academics and other leaders seeking to solve the problems with the American health system. He and his colleagues saw the promise of health care innovations being developed, but questioned how these national assets would be made available to America and its citizens within the current system.

Patrick thought it at first to be a silly proposition. He soon learned from Dr. Rorem that it was a most serious endeavor. It was so serious that it had found favor among some large and well-endowed national philanthropies. Several were willing to commit major dollars to fund an organized and comprehensive study of the problem. It was to be a multiyear effort, and since their ultimate purpose was to generate policy recommendations, some of which might require action by Congress to implement, they were making visits to DC to test the waters and curry future favor. They were especially keen toward senators, who controlled much of the agenda on Capitol Hill.

Most senators were up to their necks with other issues and priorities and knew nothing about health care. They had little inclination to learn or do more. Rather than outright rejecting folks who had major financial backing, they would refer them to the committee of jurisdiction. That was Patrick's committee, and since no one there really cared about these issues, Patrick was it.

Patrick met Dr. Rorem, and some of his colleagues, several times. He began to appreciate their point of view, even if he didn't completely understand their arguments or assertions. What they said made him question for the first time how health care did work, a question made practical by Ann being with child. Their visits to their physician provided few answers to the types of questions raised by his work visitors. He wondered, for example, why their doctor was adamant that the delivery happen at home; they had met other couples who were going to have their baby in a hospital.

When Dr. Rorem came to meet with him in April, Patrick informed him that it would be their last meeting, since his assignment was ending in a matter of days. Dr. Rorem was surprised, but quickly shifted the conversation to the work of the committee that was to formally begin early that summer. He told Patrick that the financial commitments promised were now in place for a five-year study, and they were in need of the right people to do the work. Dr. Rorem was an economist, one of several professional members of a research staff who would report to Staff Director I.S. Falk. He said that Dr. Falk had asked him to find other staff to help.

Dr. Rorem saw great potential in Patrick, including both his legal training at one of the nation's top law schools and his congressional experience. Patrick didn't quite get why he could be such an asset to the committee but was in no position to object. He welcomed Dr. Rorem's overtures and let him know that the timing was right for him and that he would be most appreciative of any good words that Dr. Rorem would put in for him.

Rorem wasted no time. On the spot, he offered Patrick a job as chief clerk to the fledgling Committee on the Costs of Medical Care. It didn't sound like much at first to Patrick, but it was a job, it sounded interesting, and a five-year job prospect sounded like gold given the economic times. He would have to move to Chicago, and the position didn't pay all that much—a little more than the law job in Maryland, though, and with far more intriguing career and social opportunities for young Patrick. Ann and Patrick moved up to Chicago in July 1927, with three-week-old son Christopher in tow.

Five years later, in October, the committee released its Final Report. Patrick had become a key contributor to this seminal report on the problems and solutions to America's health care system. Among its products was the bound report that Patrick now held in his hand.

Close to a hundred years later, the debate about health care continued to rage across the American continent, just as it had for many decades. Tragically, few if any of those making their arguments had any knowledge of the work of the committee or its recommendations. It had its influence nonetheless.

Chapter Ten

Irv Goes to Moses Lake

Irv drove to Moses Lake, two and a half hours away, on late Friday morning, the day after the discovery of the corpse in Kent. His classmate Ken was not only in town, but would put him up in his house over the weekend. He hoped that the trip would help his investigation, but if nothing else, it would be good to catch up with an old friend and re-tell old stories.

Irv was a bit vague about the reason for the trip in his call to Ken, only saying that he needed to explore some potato plant linkages for a case. Better for this to be an in-person conversation—he wondered who might be listening in on his phone calls. He was sure "they" were keeping an eye on his emails, even if why was not clear.

Irv found car trips to be a good time to think about big questions, and the several-hour trip this time did not disappoint. The drive reminded him of his many travels with Johnny, some of the most vibrant times of his life. There was so much out there to learn and experience, and the road was such a wonderful classroom to do it in.

Seattle's suburbia faded as he approached the mountain pass through the Cascades on I-90 and then quickly gave way to mountains, snow, and trees. On the eastern slope, the mountains shrank to rolling plains and coulees. He crossed the Columbia River in the center of the state, before steeply ascending a plateau leading to Moses Lake. He arrived about two in the afternoon. Knowing that Ken would be tied up with work meetings until dinnertime, he stopped off at the Washington State Agricultural Lab Center in the southwest part of town.

He entered the building and put on his King County Public Health badge. He knew how to work the bureaucracy of most systems; it was a core skill of his. He needed to demonstrate an indicia of public purpose and legitimacy, followed by a genuine interest in what folks were doing on the job. In many of these larger organizations, he preyed on the inability of leaders and managers to care about what went on below them. Irv regularly found devoted and smart staff who hadn't been asked an intelligent question about their work for years. It took little to get them talking about their work, and soon they would spill their guts like a town crier on speed.

With a few inquiries at the main desk, and then with referrals made by several workers, Irv hit a mother lode of information with Edward Stravinski. Ed was a field officer working on potato crop testing. His principal duty was to assure the state that the billions of potatoes being processed in facilities around Moses Lake each year were of sufficient potato-ness to carry the brand of "Washington State Potato Product." He would make routine surveys of the potatoes being brought to the processing facilities, run lab tests, and then make presentations to the Washington State Potato Commission, a group of political appointees who used their appointment for their public service résumés and more connections.

Ed was thrilled to have someone in his office interested in his work and curious about what he knew about potatoes—someone actually interested in his world of potato growing, processing, and distribution. Irv was genuinely interested, and Ed had much to share.

"As I was telling you, most of the potatoes are grown on fairly large farms across eastern Washington. Labor is a big issue and there aren't that many natives who want to do the work. So the companies regularly bring in workers from other countries. Sometimes legally, but just as often, by linking to illegal immigrant worker streams. The laws have regularly allowed this to happen with a wink and a nod, even as politicians, and even the potato farmers, rail against immigration as a national issue. Most of the workers in this region trace their roots to southern Mexico, and many have been here for over a generation. When more workers are needed, the word goes out and family members and community members from where they came find a way to get here. Some for just seasonal work who go home once the crops are in and processed; others who put down some roots in the community."

"So, by and large people are known here, if you can talk to the right people in these worker communities?" asked Irv.

"Yes," replied Ed. "And I know almost all of these key contacts in these communities from my work in the region. They trust me, I believe, as I have never done anything but treat them like the real human beings they are. I don't have an agenda against them, and I look the other way when I know that some of them are probably here beyond the permission of federal law. Give me a day or so and I will make the rounds and share this picture of your victim and see if he is from around here."

"Thanks. Most appreciated. I am also curious about whether there have been any reports of illness among them. Flu strains or even colds. Anything with more serious symptoms that might be spreading among the workers and their families. A little old-fashioned contact tracing."

"Will do." Ed had a lot of time on his hands since the bulk of the potato crop was in, and he was happy to stay busy doing something that someone cared about. It seemed important.

"You were also starting to tell me about this potato derivative that I got in my report."

"That's right. It's an interesting one. It is a masking agent that was once used to try to make inferior potatoes legitimate."

"I didn't know that was even a thing," noted Irv.

"Yeah. It goes back to post-World War II, when America became one of the major supplier of agricultural products across the world, since much of the rest of the world was so destroyed in that war. Some big growers started to introduce potatoes that were much cheaper to produce and dump them into international markets, and sometimes even in US. They had little nutritional value and also had a short shelf life. Many countries got pissed off once they figured out that they had tons of shitty potatoes on hand and pressured our country to do something about it. They set up some testing processes with standards. The derivative in your report is identical to an agent that the really slimy growers used to hide the defects in their product. They could spray their crops with it so it could pass inspection—though the underlying problems with the crop remained.

"It soon went out of use. Not so much because of international pressure, but the need for McDonald's to have a reliable source of potatoes for their trillions of french fries for the millions served on their sign. The masking agent created a mess when mixed with their secret frying oil.

Later on, more enlightened groups like our Potato Commission made sure that the masking agent was made useless by setting higher standards for what is a suitable potato. It really hasn't been a thing since the 1960s, and I was surprised to see it show up on your report."

Irv thanked Ed and left the building. As he got in his car and plugged in the address to Ken's home in his GPS, it occurred to him that this case was getting stranger indeed. He could feel that he was on to "something." Just what it was remained a mystery.

Chapter Eleven

The Committee on the Cost of Medical Care

The Committee on the Cost of Medical Care found its origins in the problems with health care in the United States in the 1920s. The opening of the Report notes that "Pain, sickness, and bereavement have shadowed mankind throughout the ages; today there is a vast amount of unnecessary sickness and many thousands of unnecessary deaths." It goes on to state that medical science had made tremendous advances over the past fifty years, and that the knowledge and resources were available to make even greater advances into the future. But people were already not getting the service and benefits they needed from what we knew and had in place—in large part because of the great cost that put health care beyond most people's reach and, in some parts of the country, because it was not even available.

Fifteen leaders convened in Washington, DC, in 1926, which triggered, with some twists and turns, a five-year voluntary program of research that began in 1928. The work was financially supported through $750,000 provided by some of the largest foundations of the time. Various trade associations participated in the endeavor, even if some of them were less than thrilled with the recommendations that might come from the study. Some ultimately even condemned the work product.

Patrick Jones had moved to Chicago to be a member of the staff for the committee in June of 1927, accepting Dr. Rorem's offer to serve as chief clerk. Most of his initial assignments were clerical in nature, such as taking minutes of official committee proceedings. His legal training proved to be excellent preparation for his duties—synthesis, clarity, and accuracy were key ingredients to the study process. Over time, his duties expanded, at first administratively and then into research.

Patrick was an eager staff member, willing to do whatever it took to contribute and earn his keep. It was sometimes challenging to balance his work commitment with the needs of a wife and new baby in a new home. But the paycheck took priority, and Ann was a strong partner who asserted command over the family needs. She managed a home that grew to include three more children over their five years in Chicago. She missed her family greatly, but Chicago was a friendly city, and their neighborhood included a number of recently arrived Irish families also trying to make a go of things in a new home.

The committee offices and the Jones' apartment were on the south side of Chicago, near the campus of the University of Chicago. The location was chosen primarily because the staff directors for the committee were tied to the University of Chicago, but Chicago itself provided a central location for committee members who traveled from across the nation to meetings. The chair of the committee was Dr. Ray Lyman Wilbur of Stanford University in California, for example.

Meetings of the committee were typically held in downtown Chicago at the Palmer Hotel. Many committee members traveled substantial distances to attend, and would spend a few days in the city, with the committee putting them up for the week at the hotel.

One of Patrick's principal early assignments was to make sure that the members of the committee arrived for the meeting and had what they needed. He would take the elevated train downtown and stay overnight in a small room in a lodging home near the hotel for most of the week so he could be of immediate service to committee members. Some members were just looking for company, and he got to know many of them well over the course of their years of meetings.

Staff leaders would join committee members at a lavish dinner the night before the start of the formal committee meeting. Dr. Rorem would almost always attend, and he went out of his way to make sure that Patrick was included in the dinner. Patrick was there to fulfill any last-minute needs, and in the normal course of events, would have sat outside the dining room waiting for an assignment. Instead, Dr. Rorem made sure that Patrick joined in the dinner and was seated next to key members of the committee.

Patrick appreciated Dr. Rorem taking him under his wing, and he learned a great deal from these dinners. Post-dinner cross-examination from Dr. Rorem made him realize that part of the reason for his inclusion was espionage—Dr. Rorem greatly wanted to know what the committee members were thinking. It was not unlike some of the posturing Patrick had observed within the Senate Labor Committee, and it was a revelation to him that politics was endemic to more human behavior than just that within government.

Early on, a research agenda was set for the committee. Much of the work for the next couple of years became organizing and completing the research so that the committee members would have the benefit of scientific study to inform their debates and, ultimately, their recommendations. The timelines for sub-products were staggered over a couple of years so that there would be ample material and time for debate. Over the first year, there were not many committee meetings, as the first studies needed time to conclude.

Patrick filled his available time over this first time period by volunteering to help the research staff. He began by examining various legal questions related to the research agenda, which got him noticed as a capable adjunct member of the research division of the Commission, and soon he was being assigned questions within the harder sciences and even mathematics.

Doing this work for the research staff earned him a regular invite to the policy martini klatches that Dr. Falk hosted each Friday evening. The research team would close down their offices at 4 p.m. each Friday and have drinks and dialogue in the committee's library. Typically, unless it was summer, there would be a fire blazing in the large stone fireplace in the center of the room, with Dr. Falk, Dr. Rorem, or some guest from the University of Chicago or elsewhere leading a dialogue over major policy questions of health care. While these discussions sometimes related to the committee's research agenda, that was not always the case. A fly on the wall, Patrick enjoyed these receptions and began to understand the complexity, depth, and importance of questions of health care policy, all while enjoying a pleasant buzz.

Early on in his service on staff, Patrick wondered whether he had made the right career choice. The health care issues were fascinating enough, and he had a chance to make a contribution to society through the committee's potential recommendations. But it was not the typical path for a lawyer, and he wondered how his classmates were faring with their more conventional legal positions.

Whatever doubts he had were stomped down in October of his first year with the committee. The stock market crashed one Tuesday, sending the nation into a panic over the economy. What's more, Patrick was in New York City on this day, delivering some materials to a committee member who was from Columbia University. He had been walking through Wall Street and watched in horror as a man jumped from his tenth-floor office, landing with a sickening and mushy thud on the hood of an automobile just ten feet from him.

It was no time to take anything for granted, and it was then that Patrick decided to make himself not just a valuable but indispensable member of the overall staff of the committee, even if it wasn't all he was capable of as an attorney. But it was best and safest for Ann and Christopher and his family in New York, who were struggling to make it as work and income dried up everywhere in the nation.

It was not like helping to staff the committee was an unwelcome chore for Patrick. The issues were interesting, there was always plenty to do, and the people were fascinating. By year two, the committee met more frequently to review the results of the research agenda, and it became Patrick's job to help publish committee agendas and make sure that the principal agreements and disagreements were accurately recorded.

Patrick proved most capable at discerning the different views and positions of the committee members. It was much like law school and the competing sides of appellate court cases, with a little less of old English tradition and Latin, and more science and math. The key factions among the committee members soon became clear to him, with the help of Dr. Rorem—there were those who saw a major role for government in ordering a private health care system, and those who did not.

This fault line was at the core of the committee's debates, and never fully resolved, as evidenced by the inclusion of Minority Reports in the committee's Final Report. In later years, Patrick realized that he had early on lived the fault line of American health policy, one that had never been reconciled. He thought this provided a unique experience that gave him special insight into the system and its failings.

The committee's divisions over this fault line were heated; they would prove to be explosive after the publication of its Final Report in 1932, which included conclusions, recommendations, background information, and disagreements, published in a shiny red book printed by the University of Chicago Press. The five essential recommendations adopted by the committee were:

1. Group Practice. Medical service should be provided through organized groups of practitioners, including physicians, dentists, nurses, pharmacists, and other associated personnel, rather than solo practitioners. These groups should be organized around complete home, office, and hospital care in a way that maintained high standards and developed or preserved a personal relation between patients and caregivers.
2. Public Health. Basic public health services should be extended to all, whether through governmental or non-governmental agencies, and these health departments should be staffed by trained health officers.
3. National Health Coverage. The costs of medical care should be placed on a group payment basis, through insurance, use of taxation, or both methods.
4. Community-Centered Care. Medical services should be better coordinated, and study, evaluation, and coordination should be an important function undertaken by every state and local community.
5. Professional Training. The education and training of health professionals should be improved for physicians, dentists, pharmacists, nurses, midwives, and hospital or clinic administrators.

All of these five recommendations were accompanied by extensive discussion and analysis in the Final Report.

Recommendation 1 was one of the dividing lines of opinion for the committee. It was calling for group practice of medicine at a time when almost all physician care was provided by solo practitioners. Group practice was a novelty, and in its infancy in but a few communities across the nation. Representatives of the American Medical Association were hostile toward this idea, in large part because it threatened to be a first step to one of their most feared developments—the corporate practice of medicine that would wrench control and benefits from the practicing physician. The AMA, and most physicians, also felt that any form of price competition by providers was unprofessional and unacceptable.

Even more controversial was Recommendation 3, which was one of the first American calls for some form of national health "insurance." While the Report emphasized the notion of prepayment more than necessarily "insurance," it recommended that all Americans have the opportunity to be covered through some social method. On this issue, the AMA and most physicians feared a slippery slope to socialism in medicine as had developed in several European nations, even if it started on a voluntary basis. Some committee members branded it as a communist proposal, and strenuously objected to its inclusion in the final report.

Recommendations 2, 4, and 5 received less criticism but were also crucial in their own right. The clarion call for a strong public health role was novel, in both its purported role and the notion that creating and protecting health was a primary function of not just the American health care system, but the government. Recommendation 4's notion of organizing around the community seemed obvious, but more revolutionary was its hidden implication that health care should actually be organized around community life rather than the workplace, government jurisdictions, or other alternatives.

Recommendation 5 was probably the most accepted recommendation, extending a view that had already been asserted by the Flexner Report of 1910. This landmark study had called for a major change at America's medical schools—a movement that had begun with the American Medical Association. The Report called for higher admission and graduation standards, curriculums, and training methods that relied on mainstream science and elimination of what it found to be poor medical schools. It shaped American medical education for the future, but also greatly constricted the number of graduating physicians. The CCMC Report was reminding policymakers that many more practitioners were needed, capably trained consistent with the Flexner Report recommendations, and that this need extended beyond just physicians.

One of the ways that the committee was able to bring conclusion to its charge, given the extensive disagreement, was to allow the inclusion of Minority Reports. This provided the cover for some committee members to approve of the more controversial recommendations; opposing views would be expressed in the Final Report. Two extensive Minority Reports were filed, from physicians who strenuously objected to the inclusion of Recommendations 1 and 3. Two other committee members rejected the Final Report as not going far enough in finding answers to the problems it was intended to solve.

Patrick tracked these major divisions as chief clerk, and tried to bring some cohesion to frequently contentious committee meetings. He dutifully recorded opposing views in the minutes, without his own bias, and tried to carry this neutral tone through the recording of the committee proceedings included in the Final Report.

There was no doubt in his own mind as to who was right in this debate, however. He thought the committee recommendations were not only rational but the type of change that had to happen in American health policy going forward. Five years of research and observation had made him a keen witness of American health care and its defects. He felt the CCMC Report should become the blueprint for policy change in the American health care system.

Above all else, he thought, was the need for a systematic response to health care's prospects and failings. After all, there was one conclusion that every committee member agreed with—the basic problem was not about *the* American health care system, but the lack of one. Something needed to be formed, or it would continue to accrue in its largely unguided way.

It was also time for Patrick to find his next job. No matter what the Recommendations, the committee job had run its course in 1932, and he needed a new way to put bread on the family table. He hoped something would open up around the next steps with the Report, but was not sure what it was. All he needed was a chance, he thought, just like the committee Recommendations.

Patrick would find his, but the Committee Report would not, for the most part.

Chapter Twelve

Early Johnny

John "Johnny" Gibson was born in 1950 to Paul and Joanne Gibson, who now resided in Hoboken, New Jersey, a suburban town across the river from Manhattan. It was a stormy summer night when he came into the world, and a Friday the thirteenth to boot. To anyone paying attention, it was clear there was some serious juju rolling in.

From afar, Paul and Joanne looked to be a typical post-WWII American couple. Paul was a second-generation son, his parents from Scotland, and he was destined to be part of the American war effort as a tank driver. He had met Joanne in London during a leave from the European battlefront. She was in high school, but that was a time when people grew up fast. No one knew how long they could expect to live with death all around them. They got married one crazy weekend, and Paul was off to the front the Monday after.

Paul was on his way home to New York City, with a new bride in tow, grateful to have survived the war. He remembered his pledge one frightful night of combat to never take life for granted and live it to its fullest should he make it out of there alive. He felt this was something he owed not just to the God he prayed to that night, but his many buddies who lay in graves in battlefields across the European continent.

Joanne was excited to be going to America. The bombings in London had soured her view of home, and the newspaper reports about the United States sparked an eagerness to learn more about this place, at this time. It was a sophisticated palate she brought to this ambition. Both her parents were on the faculty at Oxford, and her dad a professor in world history. Many a night she sat next to him on the couch as he told her stories of civilizations and places gone by. She would imagine herself walking down the streets of these places back in time, wondering what it would be like and how she would feel. Then a bomb would explode, shaking her back to reality.

Now she had such an opportunity—to experience the wonders of New York City, the most cosmopolitan city in the world. And maybe the only one still standing across the globe after many years of devastation from war.

Her new husband made this adventure even better. Many of her friends had looked for an American, almost any American, so they could escape a destroyed London. Joanne was more picky, and felt incredibly lucky to have found Paul. He wasn't your ordinary American GI—most were good-looking, but he was also outgoing, smart, and witty—a life partner worth having. He was tall as a corn stalk too, with flaming red hair beginning to grow out from his GI cut that made him shimmer like the amber waves of grain in a strong wind.

They settled into a room with his parents on the east side of Manhattan, just below Harlem. The place was nothing too fancy, but a good location from which to explore the city. It was a few blocks to Central Park and just a bit longer walk to midtown. They would spend a good deal of their time out and about. They didn't have much money and appreciated that his parents made room for them when they first came home; still, they wanted not just a place to base their adventures, but some privacy.

One of Paul's tank buddies got him a job interview with the New York City subway, and he was hired—first repairing cars at the main depot and then as a driver. It was a lot simpler than driving a tank, and no one was shooting at him—most of the time, anyway. He loved his job rolling across the city, above and below the city streets, with new people moving in and out of the cars at every stop.

Joanne got a job at New York University in the History Department through one of her father's colleagues. It was a secretarial post, but close enough to the wonders of learning to satisfy her great curiosity. She loved attending lectures, and receptions for foreign dignitaries. In the summer when school was out, she would wander the city, sometimes figuring out which subway car Paul was driving and spending the day as a passenger with him.

America was bustling, working to fill the demands of a rebuilding world. New York City was the hub of it, and opportunity was everywhere. Paul and Joanne were able to save enough money to get an apartment of their own in the Chelsea area, which deepened their happy life together in the city in their own apartment.

It was more than a little surprise when Joanne told Paul that she had missed her period in late 1949. They weren't trying to have children, and hadn't really planned on doing so either. They were just enjoying life. They treated the news of Johnny's conception as their next adventure, and embraced it fully.

Complications in childbirth meant that Johnny would be an only child. He never knew things any other way, and loved the attention from his mom, dad, and the rest of the extended family. Paul and Joanne thought it their essential duty to orient him to the wonders of the world, and they had such a fascinating place to do so in their backyard. Every weekend was a new adventure; every summer a chance to travel out of the city and show their son the world.

Johnny shot up like a beanpole and was over six feet tall by junior high. He had inherited his dad's shock of red hair and large feet. There was nothing but cheery optimism to gather from the genes of his parents, and he was an extrovert, pleasant and happy as a child and even as a teenager. He was a good athlete and played on the football and baseball teams at his city high school. An avid reader, he loved English studies and gobbled up the books he was assigned—math and sciences, not so much.

New York City was changing though, and in some ways, not for the better. The inner cities of America were becoming a dumping place for the ills of society, and New York was one of the poster children for urban decline. There were still many wonderful places across the city, but these became more exclusive. Without a lot of money, those who were left in the city were left to deal with the crime and violence that absorbed many city neighborhoods in the mid-1960s.

Paul and Joanne stuck it out as long as they could. They felt Johnny would learn from his experiences in the changing city. One armed robbery later, with Paul having been shot in the chest during a late night robbery in a pharmacy, they changed their minds. The pharmacist had been killed during the robbery, and Paul was the last customer of the night. He lay on the ground bleeding out until he was found the next morning. He survived, but a moment in time had passed for him and his family.

They decided to join the urban flight to the suburbs growing around the city. Many were moving to Long Island to the east. But Paul and Joanne found better deals and a more adventurous opportunity to the west, in New Jersey, where they bought a small but attractive home near a subway line, so it was a simple commute for Paul to his work. It was also close enough to Rutgers University, where Joanne found a new job and a way to stay connected to an academic environment.

Johnny settled into his new life as a suburban kid at fifteen, making friends, now starring on the sports teams among the lesser natural athletic talent in his suburban enclave, and excelling at school. He had learned well from his parents to embrace the moment, and he did so. All three found ways to keep life exciting and positive in suburbia, even as others across the nation were finding that the grass was not always greener.

It was an easy trip into the city to experience what it had to offer. Greenwich Village was a favorite of Johnny's, and he would spend many a Saturday night enjoying music and the interesting cast of characters in small bars and cafés. He discovered a music scene in the New Jersey suburbs too, and began to frequent some of the clubs in Newark and other cities. In the summer, he would hitchhike to the Jersey Shore, where he would search for great music and camp out on the beach.

The sour in his big apple came as he got close to graduation. Neither he or his parents were big on the planning side of life. Normally, Johnny was content to let things happen, and so were they. They found it was not easy to do as a young man graduating from high school in 1968—there was a war in Vietnam going on, and a draft looking for warriors.

Paul was a vehement critic of the Vietnam War. He was proud of his service in WWII, but he had seen the horrors of war up close and personal. That was a necessary war, he believed, with his company's liberation of a Nazi slave camp justifying his thinking. This war in Southeast Asia was pure horse shit—politicians fighting ghosts—and he was not going to let his son be a part of it. He openly talked about moving to Canada with his family if his son was drafted.

Paul thought the best way to avoid military service was for his son to go to college. Johnny wasn't so excited by the notion of going to school—he had been observing the academic world through his mom for years and desired more real-world experience. No, he was ready to go out and test the world. He dreamed about heading out west.

Paul and Joanne convinced him to hold off on that for a few years, for his own safety. He knew that it was a serious conversation—they had rarely shared fears and the need for security during his life. He resisted, as many a teenager would.

What convinced him was seeing his neighbor Ronnie return from the war. Ronnie was a few years older than Johnny, but brought him into the pickup football games he played with his friends. Johnny was the runt in the group, but such a good athlete that he was adopted into the sports gang. Ronnie became an older brother to him, and they would sit after games talking about guy things into the evening hours.

Ronnie's dad was a mechanic, his mom a housewife, and his destiny was to be a working-class kid from suburban New Jersey, not a college man. He had neither the inclination nor the grades to go to college, and was drafted on his eighteenth birthday and signed up for the Marines. Johnny was at first impressed when Ronnie would visit home in his smart-looking uniform; they found time to continue their curbside chats about life.

Then, he was gone for a while. All Johnny knew from talking to Ronnie's dad was that he was stationed somewhere in Vietnam near a place called Da Nang. Johnny looked it up on a map and followed newspaper stories about the war. He knew it was a hotspot where battles were being fought.

Two years in, Ronnie returned home. He had been wounded—a land mine had blown off his legs. Johnny went to see him the day he came home. It was a horrifying image. Yes, it was a shock to see his athletic brother in a wheelchair, and a surprise to process his long hair and beard. It was like a physically different person in front of him.

Worse, far worse, was that Ronnie's spark of life was gone. He had little to say. He was disoriented; his mom shared that he had gotten hooked on heroin. Johnny didn't know what to do. He weakly hugged his friend and said goodbye, crying as he crossed the street back to his own house.

That night, he shared this experience with his parents. They consoled him and convinced him to apply for college, and they filled out applications the next day. His mom made sure he got an offer to attend Rutgers. They could afford that with the employee discount, and with him living at home.

Johnny enjoyed college—like everything else in his family's lives, it was an opportunity for some unique experience and learning. Most exciting for him were the new people he met. While many of his classmates shared his greater New York City homeland, there were also students from around the country. They interested him, especially the women.

For the most part, though, he felt like his life was on hold during his four years at Rutgers. He yearned to pick up and move, but couldn't—he had made a pact with his parents and he would honor it. He would get a monthly calendar every new year and cross off the dates each evening. Someday he would have his freedom to travel. He would dream of western vistas as he nodded off to sleep each night.

In his last year of school, Johnny had begun to date one woman more seriously; his love life up to then consisted of one-night stands with women he met in bars. Kristen Peterson stood out for him in a couple of ways—for one, she was a blonde, and a buxom one at that. She was tall, not as tall as his now six-foot-five frame, but big for a woman. Scandinavian heritage, maybe even a distant relative of Leif Ericsson, or so Johnny suggested to his friends. She told him all the girls were like her where she came from. He told her she was a goddess among the serfs of New Jersey.

Kristen was from Seattle. That clinched it for Johnny. On graduation, the pair got a drive-away car—intended for someone relocating to Seattle who needed somebody to drive their car there—and moved to the Pacific Northwest. His parents were sad to see him go, but knew that his departure had been delayed as long as possible already. They gave him a camera and asked him to send pictures.

Two weeks later, Johnny found himself in Seattle, after a wondrous drive across the country. He had no idea what he was going to do now that he was here. It was thrilling, though—that was the point. It was a dark and drizzly northwest day. Yet he was happy, even happier than before.

Chapter Thirteen

Irv Tours Moses Lake with Ken

"Who knew that we'd find such good food around here," Irv said while taking a bite off a slice of pizza. "This is really tasty." Garlic and basil pierced the air of the small pizzeria located in the old downtown of Moses Lake.

"Glad you like it. There are a number of pretty decent spots to eat in this town. Might not be the prettiest place in the world, but it's not bad. Lots of recreational things to do brings a lot of out-of-towners, and the economy is really good with the agricultural processing. Last twenty years have seen a lot of computer-related businesses set up shop too—land and buildings are a lot cheaper than in western Washington." Ken Wisterly was proud to brag about his adopted home. He had moved here twenty years ago after a stint as an assistant administrator in Snohomish County Public Health, the large county north of Seattle that housed the city of Everett.

It was Saturday night. Irv had arrived at Ken's house at 4:30 the evening before, after his meeting with Ed Stravinski. He had waited in his car in Ken's driveway until his friend got home a few ticks after five. They caught up on life stories and the whereabouts of MHA classmates for much of the evening over cocktails. After a light dinner of salad and tacos, Irv outlined as much as he could the work challenge that brought him to Moses Lake.

Ken was intrigued by Irv's tale and told him that he had heard rumors of flu problems among the agricultural worker community, but that these reports had proven unfounded. He needed to be in the office on Saturday morning to take care of a few administrative matters and promised Irv to review the environmental assessment reports again.

On Saturday afternoon, Ken drove Irv around town and into some of the outlying rural communities surrounding Moses Lake. Irv found it helpful to get the lay of the land. He and Ken were comfortable with each other, partly because of the shared career path but also because they were always good with each other. During the tour, Ken shared that his review of the written reports on local disease surveillance were exactly what he told Irv last night—nothing really remarkable or threatening.

With that confirmed, Irv tried to get a better understanding of the community. "I was really struck by the size of the city. Always thought of it as a small rural community, but there is a lot of geography to it."

"That's what a lot of people say when they come out for a visit. It is the biggest city between Spokane and Seattle, and being right off the freeway has made it a convenient location for all sorts of residential and business purposes," Ken noted. "Way bigger as you saw than some of the towns out beyond the city. Those towns are part of my territory as public health officer, and it doesn't take much to know most of the folks living out here in the more rural areas. Moses Lake itself is a bit bigger. I know a lot of people after twenty years, but I can still get lost in the crowd too."

"Nice. A little anonymity is a good thing when you are the guy on call for every infectious disease known to man. And the water and air and just about everything that people care greatly about when things go wrong. That is one thing I like about being in Seattle—it is so large now that I can easily get lost in the crowd," said Irv. "Did you get a chance to look at the lab reports I gave you last night?"

"Yes, I did spend a little time at the office taking a gander at them." Like Irv, Ken was administratively and not scientifically trained, but after decades of reading reports from public health workers, he knew his way around the science pretty well. "To tell you the truth, they didn't make a lot of sense to me."

"What do you mean?"

"Well, first, the flu strain is just too normal," Ken replied. "It is a nasty strain, for sure. But it is so close to the SARS virus in its genetic details that it just doesn't seem likely that it is a natural mutation. When we were on high alert back then, I had to attend many a state briefing on the virus, and I remember well the CDC experts sharing with us that any mutation of regular flu bugs through birds or animals should demonstrate a major and almost random molecular leap from what we see. Having the SARS virus come back again so close to the original version just doesn't seem possible.

"Second, those potato derivatives are more than a bit odd. Now, I get that the crops around here can hang in the air like balloons when they are being picked, moved, and especially processed around this town. It would take a serious dose of any crop, in almost direct contact, to somehow graft enough of its essence to show up in a lab report. But there it was in your report, clear as day. I just don't get it."

"Huh. Interesting. Maybe I should think better of my boss and his direction for me to stick with the lab reports on this one. My gut still tells me that he was mostly trying to get me off the case, though." Irv reflected on his uncomfortable meeting with Director Welch a couple of days ago. "We should learn a bit more about this from my guy at State Ag Lab. He called me this morning and asked if we could get together tomorrow. He said that he'd done some more digging into the derivative and wanted to do some more this afternoon before telling me more. He was kind of like you, though—things just weren't making a whole lot of sense to him."

"I hope *somebody* can make some sense of this. Why don't you have him come by my house?"

"Thanks, Ken. That is what I told him and glad you are up for it. You both have been really helpful. I have to head back to Seattle sometime tomorrow so I can get to the office on Monday morning."

For the rest of Saturday, they just enjoyed each other's company, talking of the good old days.

Chapter Fourteen

Early Johnny Part 2

Life in Seattle was a grand adventure for Johnny, sometimes almost too grand. It was entirely different from his life on the East Coast, yet also the same in a bigger way. Johnny's parents had taught him to be a life learner and had massaged his curiosity so that he would always need a tickle of adventure to feel whole.

Kristen and he flopped in a garage apartment of a high school friend of hers on their arrival in late May. Kristen was a good host—showing off her favorite places in Seattle. Almost all qualified as cool on the hip meter for Johnny—Pike Place Market, the bars in Pioneer Square, Discovery Park, the Blue Moon Tavern, the Space Needle. When they could borrow a car or catch a ride, they would venture outside of the city, where she showed off the grand natural environs of the Pacific Northwest. There was water and mountains and hidden places to explore everywhere, and Johnny could not get his fill of them. The days were long in the summer, with light from the sun popping out around 4:30 in the morning and stretching to almost ten at night.

Fall's shortening daylight came with a realization they would need to pay for their fun. Kristen took a sales job at the local department store, a place called Nordstrom's. She was a distant cousin of a member of the Nordstrom family, and her dad helped parlay that into an entry-level job in the company. She liked the work, and the security of the paycheck, and began to settle into post-college life in her hometown.

Johnny was far more restless. He wanted to find his own way and turned down connections to potential jobs from Kristen's dad in favor of a job driving tourists around town. The tour vehicles were old WWII landing boats, the type used to land troops on beaches during D-Day. He got a kick thinking of his dad possibly landing side by side with his car-boat in France. Everyone was undoubtedly scared shitless, he thought. He took a picture of himself standing on the hood and sent it back east.

Johnny liked learning about the sites and the history of his tours. He made an excellent tour guide, embellishing the stories provided by the company with his own fabrications. Some nights, he would go to the library to find enough facts to keep his stories fresh, arguably in the spirit of the truth. Other nights, he would be out exploring the city in another way. He usually went by himself, as Kristen needed to get her sleep to be ready for her early morning start time at Nordstrom's.

He saved up enough money to buy a car. Seattle was a wonderful place, but it was the entire west that fascinated him. He yearned to get out to the mountain ranges before him to the east and west, and found hitchhiking an undependable way to get to trailheads in more remote locations. He found a well-used 1950 Studebaker and figured out how to get it running with an automobile self-help book from the library, duct tape, and a hanger.

It wasn't long before Johnny and Kristen went their separate ways. It wasn't that difficult a moment. Theirs was a romance of opportunity and convenience, not any deep love. Johnny had used Kristen to settle into a new locale just as she had used him back in New Jersey. She was now ready to settle in and make a regular home; Johnny was ready to sow new oats of discovery.

They split in late November of that year. She went to an apartment; he went to a room with a friend he had met during one of his bar-hopping nights. That attraction proved to be more a product of alcohol than any real chemistry, and Johnny was asked to leave before their first weekend together was over.

He didn't have enough money for anything resembling a home, apartment, or even motel room. His income from his tour boat job was mostly from tips, and this had dropped dramatically as the volume of tourists dwindled with the arrival of Seattle's winter. He had spent almost all of his savings on his car. The only solution was to make his car his home, and he began to live in it, parking in an alley next to the tour boat dock.

It was still an adventure, and Johnny was mostly happy. He did long for the comfort and friendships of home in his weaker moments, especially when he was alone at night in his car. The cold here wasn't like that of New York and New Jersey; the temperatures were higher. But, oh, they were so wet. He felt like he lived in a fish tank, regularly wiping condensation off the windows of his Studebaker to see outside, and wrapping blankets around himself for warmth from the biting dampness.

Privately, he would admit to himself that he was lonely. He missed his parents and his friends back east. It was hard to do more than pen an occasional postcard or place a collect phone call from a payphone. But he found time every week to do so, as he longed for some intimacy in his new life. It was also just so freaking dark in Seattle this time of year; the long days of summer had been replaced by short bursts of light in the afternoon, and even this was usually through gray clouds and fog. He began to understand why Seattle had such a high suicide rate—there were too many bridges in this town for winters like this.

After a few weeks of this lifestyle, and a dreary Christmas season where it rained buckets almost every day while he shivered in his car, Johnny concluded that a change was in order. He reviewed the bulletin board at a nearby food coop. He shopped there because they had food in bulk that allowed him to buy his meals fifty cents at a time for preparation in his car with a Bunsen burner camping stove. There were postings for apartments on the bulletin board outside the store that were certainly outside his income bracket. Of greater temptation were notices of people looking for roommates—more in line with his pocketbook—and other people were mostly what he was looking for anyway.

One day as he was looking at the board, a middle-aged woman approached him. She was medium height, with brown hair, glasses, and a friendly enough face. It was hard to make out her build under her layers of sweaters, vests, and a coat, but it was clear that she was not a Nordic goddess with Kristen's bloodlines. No, this woman looked more like someone he might meet in the lower east side of New York.

She introduced herself to him as Tina Nelson. She had noticed him reviewing the ads and asked whether he was looking for a room. Yes, he said. She suggested that they go next door to a coffee shop and talk about things. He asked whether she had to do some shopping first. "No, I was here just watching people at the bulletin board, looking for someone interesting who might fit with our housing opportunity," she said. "You, Johnny, caught my eye."

Johnny found her approach interesting, and accepted the cup of coffee. As they chatted, he began to appreciate her method of hooking up a living arrangement with someone else. Tina rented a large house in the University District with her life partner, Bob. She was a botanist who worked at a bike store in the District, and Bob was a professor of Natural Sciences at the University of Washington. They rented out rooms to others in their house, and, as she explained it, not really for the money but to build a network of interesting people. She said that she had a good feeling about Johnny and hoped he might come by for dinner to meet Bob.

Dinner sounded great to Johnny; it had been a while since his last real sit-down meal. Even more, he could feel that this match was good for him. It echoed with the sense of mystery and opportunity that he was seeking out west, and it invigorated him that he was already breaking out of his December depression with this chance meeting.

He and Bob hit it off. Really, Johnny could hit it off with almost anyone, but with Bob it was extra easy. Both Tina and Bob were transplants from back East; he from Baltimore and she from a farming town in North Carolina. As it was for Johnny, the West was calling, and they answered. They had arrived in Seattle about fifteen years ago, just a few months apart, and had met at a group dance at a music festival. It was love at first hop, and they had settled in together as partners in their adopted home.

Johnny stayed at his new home that night, sleeping on the sofa on the back porch. It was closed in and far warmer than the Studebaker. Warmer and drier yet was the second-floor bedroom that became his the next day. It had a futon and an old dresser: Johnny's first pieces of furniture. Possessions interested him little. Relations—and his friendship with Tina and Bob and the many fellow roommates who came and went from their home—these were treasured.

Of particular note on that score was his roommate down the hall, Mary Beth Collins. She had been living in the home for about a year when he plopped into its midst, and he met her his second night there, inadvertently walking in on her in the bathroom while she was on the toilet.

It was an awkward beginning, but a fast friendship. She was pretty and shy. Introducing himself while she held a sheet of toilet paper was a great icebreaker. They reintroduced themselves at dinner that night, and talked in the living room into the deep hours of the night.

Opposites attracted. She, an introverted West Coast girl, was raised in the suburbs and sheltered from much of life by her parents. He, an extroverted New Yorker, was exposed to everything and anything by his adventurous parents. They were united by circumstance, both working on escape plans from the perceived shackles of their previous lives.

Mary Beth was nothing like anybody Johnny had ever met. She was a looker, and in his bar-hopping days, he would have tried hard to get in her pants. He wasn't bad-looking himself and was all sorts of East Coast exotic. Yet he knew, and he sensed she did too, that this was not a sexual relationship of any sort. They were to be friends—close friends—without romantic intrusion.

For a couple of years, they developed this friendship, in between Johnny's adventures. The Studebaker had broken down, and he had taken to riding a bike around Seattle. His out-of-town adventures were forged mostly through hitchhiking or ride-sharing arrangements from the bulletin board at the food coop. That was a good spot, he thought, and he regularly sought good fortune from the cards pinned to it.

Every once in a while, Johnny felt a romantic urge for Mary Beth. These were usually quelled by a hookup at one of the bars with some young blonde thing. Satisfied, he realized his urges were more about horniness and that he should preserve Mary Beth as a friend. He understood this with even greater clarity one day when a new roommate arrived. Actually, Johnny was the one who brought him home, picking him up as he hitchhiked his way up from California. Irv Tinsley was his name.

Mary Beth was shacking up with some South American dude at the time. From the moment Johnny introduced Irv to Mary Beth, Johnny could see that the closeness he had found with Mary Beth on their first encounter was more than being matched by Irv, and vice versa. There was something else to it too—the temperature in the room notched up about twenty-five degrees the moment they touched hands.

This made Johnny happy. He really liked both of them.

Chapter Fifteen

A Discovery in Moses Lake

Ed Stravinski stopped by Ken's small rambler in the northeastern part of Moses Lake around one in the afternoon. After introductions and a few pleasantries, the three men sat at the table in Ken's kitchen, discussing the problem at hand.

"As I told you the other day, I confirmed that the potato derivative you shared with me was the masking agent that went out of use in this country ages ago. It is spot-on to the samples we have in our storage labs. Now, how it could get on someone who wasn't even born when it was last in use, that is a mystery." Ed had spent most of his Saturday morning sleuthing through potato reports.

"It is possible that there are large amounts of this masking agent still around. It isn't the easiest thing to dispose of, and would have cost a lot to do so in a way that met federal standards. Most of these types of additives would have been applied in rural areas where land is cheap and available, so my guess would be that most of the companies just stuck the remaining inventory in steel barrels out in the country somewhere."

"What if there was a spill of some of these barrels?" asked Ken. "Would that be enough to end up on a lab report? I was telling Irv yesterday that it seemed to me that one would have to be in contact with a lot of this stuff for there to be enough to show up on our lab reports."

"That would do it," shared Ed. "But I don't think that was what happened in this case." He smiled as he offered this assessment to Irv and Ken.

"Tell us more." They both spoke in unison.

"Turns out that there was a fair amount of data and analysis around the use of this masking agent. The feds did a pretty thorough job of looking at this stuff years ago, and while they now tend to look the other way at many of these things, state labs like us have access to their historic data. I spent a while yesterday morning reviewing it and found something pretty interesting. The masking agent was applied to crops in an aerosol version of the liquid chemical, and any significant quantity would leave a trace and detectable amount in the atmosphere. It had a bit of a shelf life too—roughly a week of potato pollution in the atmosphere."

"So, we might be able to identify where this stuff was used, if it happened in the last week?" asked Irv.

"That is what I am telling you. And I can tell you where it was used because that is what I spent yesterday afternoon doing. I took our atmospheric testing truck around town and hit the payload after about an hour of driving. I could only get so close to the location, though." Ed pulled a map out of his back pocket, unfolded it, and pointed to an area circled with a Magic Marker. "It was right here," he said while drilling his forefinger onto the spot on the map.

"That's right next to the airport," said Ken.

"Yes, it is. It is a rather large lot with a big metal storage facility. Fenced in with barbed wire and the front gate was locked with some pretty serious hardware. No way to really get close to the building without raising some major attention. But it is a stone's throw from the runways. I dropped into the airport management office and asked around, but no one there seemed to know much about the facility."

"You would think that anything going on there would get a lot of attention," noted Irv. "There can't be that much going on at your airport."

"You would be wrong about that, Irv. We actually have a pretty large and busy airport. Goes back to WWII, when the armed forces developed the airport and used it as a training base for B-17 bomber crews. It was safe from attack, with plenty of room to teach and crash if need be. There were also a fair number of federal facilities and even workers around the area going back to the construction of Grand Coulee Dam.

"After the war, the runways and facilities provided a great place to land and park really large planes. It was also convenient and cheap, and the airline industry started to use the airport for training their pilots as the commercial air industry took flight, no pun intended. The great irony was that over time, the major user of the airport for training was Japan Air. There are now so many training flights for them that we have a Japanese restaurant in the airport concourse. So, it is a pretty large airport, with a lot going on, and pretty easy for anyone to go about their business without notice."

The three of them continued their conversation in the car; they all agreed that it would be helpful to take a ride to see the location. Irv drove. It was as Ed and Ken described—a large airport. The specific location was a generally nondescript square lot the size of two football fields in all directions. It was well secured and there were wires running along the fence that were probably part of an electronic security system.

"I don't know where this leaves you," said Ed as they peered through Irv's car window at the steel building in the middle of the lot.

"I don't either," replied Irv, "but I am way further along than I was two days ago. As the saying goes, you two may not have cleared up the mystery, but you've really helped make the mystery clearer. Can't thank you enough."

"What's next?" asked Ken.

"Been pondering that. If there is some hanky-panky going on here around this masking agent that showed up on my corpse, my guess is that it wouldn't happen during the daylight. It is pretty easy to blend in around here, but wouldn't you also want the cover of darkness to make sure what you were doing wasn't too obvious?"

"Makes sense," replied Ken.

"I've got a night available to see if I get lucky. Don't really have to be in the office in Seattle until late morning, and I can blast out of here at daylight and still be there in time. How about if I drop you boys back at Ken's so I can grab some supplies and come back for a good old-fashioned public health stakeout?" Irv thought this was about the only choice he had. He put aside what the next step would be if "something" didn't happen this one night, but he was on a roll and believed it would.

Chapter Sixteen

1933: The CCMC Report Gets Buried

Patrick Jones replaced his copy of the Final Report of the Committee on the Cost of Medical Care on the bookshelf next to his office desk. He centered it at eye level, between a small trophy he had earned on the debate team in college and his framed diploma from Georgetown Law School. He took pride in his contributions to the Committee Report and dreamed that it would serve as a blueprint for building a new and more effective health care system in America—which, he had learned over the last five years, was essential.

Unfortunately, the Final Report was mostly relegated to other bookshelves rather than becoming a blueprint for action. Perhaps its greatest contribution was its influence on those who worked on it, like Patrick. Many of the staff and committee members had become disciples of change from their experience with the committee and brought these ideas to new career pursuits.

The Report did mark its arrival with a bang. First came the criticism of it, especially from the medical establishment. The American Medical Association, not happy with the Minority Report as its only statement of opposition to Recommendations 1 and 3, adopted a resolution at its annual meeting discrediting the committee and its Report. This was a symbolic blow to the advocates of the Report, especially since the CCMC effort had initially organized around the AMA Annual Meeting in 1927.

This thumbs-down would have been easier to swallow if the Report had stimulated major policy change. The opportunity was there to be had. Just as the committee was wrapping up its Report, America had elected Franklin Delano Roosevelt President of the United States. With

America in the grips of the Great Depression, Roosevelt had promised a "New Deal" for Americans and was intent on fulfilling this promise.

In his first 100 days, he blitzed into law a number of new work programs aimed at providing jobs for America's many unemployed. Next came the start of building a real safety net for them. Among the central ideas was to provide government-based security to workers through unemployment insurance and pensions. To get the ball rolling, Roosevelt created an Economic Security Conference.

This Conference became the process for crafting the legislation now known as Social Security, which was enacted in 1935. Among the questions before it in the early days was whether this economic security would include assistance to Americans for the cost of their medical care. The Report of the committee, and Recommendation 3, would make an excellent starting point for this consideration, thought Patrick and other advocates of the Report.

The AMA's condemnation of the Report was used to discredit the notion. What's more, several physicians were engaged in the Economic Security Conference and hammered away at the very principle of national health coverage. Parts of the Report were cited and used in the study process, but it proved unusable as a base policy statement as Congress contemplated how to implement Social Security.

The idea behind Recommendation 3, if not it or the overall Report, still had a chance for inclusion, even into early 1935. This chance was lost largely thanks to the AMA's organized political opposition to any vestiges of Recommendations 1 and 3 being part of Social Security. Individual physicians had strong connections with elected members of Congress, who listened to their warnings of including medical care in what already was a revolutionary package of benefits to the American worker. Better to leave it alone, they said.

Allegations of socialism were part of this opposition, and the Bolshevik Revolution in Russia had sensitized many lawmakers to such notions and labels. Ultimately, medical assistance was not included in the 1935 law. Some believe that a consolation prize that the committee could take credit for was the inclusion of grants to states for public health, and the beginning of funding for what became the National Institutes of Health. But not a notion of national health coverage for all

Americans—an idea that has since held American health policy and politics captive for decades.

Patrick Jones, chief clerk of the committee and Grandpops to Nancy Jones, stayed in Chicago for one year after the committee closed its doors. When not looking for work, he joined with Dr. Falk and Dr. Rorem to link the Committee Report to the ongoing policy debates. Unlike them, he did not have the assets to do this on a voluntary basis. He needed a job, and soon. He also began to fathom the great political challenges facing the Report and thought it likely that he must carry forward its ideas elsewhere.

Jobs of any type were few and far between then—it was the Great Depression and millions of Americans were without work. With a young family, now of four, in tow, Patrick needed to find employment and worried that he would need to leave his family to accept a manual labor job within the public works jobs programs started by Roosevelt.

His work with the committee spurred a different opportunity. Over his five years with the committee, he had met many individuals who were thinking critically about the future of American health policy. Many were members of the committee itself, and Patrick's role as chief clerk and handler of their personal needs while in Chicago had led to familiarity and even friendships.

One member who took a particular shine to Patrick was Professor Lindsey Edwards, a tenured faculty member at the Harvard Medical School. Professor Edwards was a surgeon and one of the few physicians on the committee who strongly supported Recommendations 1 and 3. Dr. Edwards fought the criticism of the AMA and most of his colleagues, but to no avail. He could see that the Report was not going anywhere soon in terms of congressional action.

Wanting the ideas to sustain, he devised his own plan for keeping the CCMC's policy ideas alive—to add them into the medical care curriculum at Harvard Medical School, where he could more easily infuse his viewpoints upon potential new disciples. Other medical schools across the country might follow suit, as they had adopted other components of Harvard's innovative medical training program based on the recommendations of the Flexner Report.

Professor Edwards got approval from the dean of the Medical School, a friend, to move forward with his plan, though he did not describe the full conspiracy. Rather, it was sold on the notion that new physicians should be trained in public policy so that they could assert their natural leadership positions within the community and nation. Implementation was dependent on funding, though, and Professor Edwards arranged for this through a generous grant from a major regional philanthropy housed in Boston. All that was left was to find someone to do the work, and he offered this position to Patrick.

Patrick was flattered, and in need. He promptly accepted, and weeks later, he and Ann packed the children up and moved to Boston.

Patrick was in place as an adjunct professor in the Harvard Medical School by the fall semester of 1933. Professor Edwards made this appointment work through Patrick's possession of a juris doctorate from Georgetown and his extensive experience with American health policy. His job was to teach an elective course on American health policy and otherwise assist Professor Edwards in building a health policy educational track within the Harvard Medical School.

Patrick quickly realized that this was not going to be as easy as it sounded. Professor Edward's passion for change was not something shared by many of his colleagues in Harvard, faculty or students. Philosophically, the faculty were much like the rank and file members of the AMA, even if they might have a more liberal academic background and inclination for social reform.

Nor were medical students that eager to explore these bigger social policy questions. It was the prestige and career of becoming a Harvard-trained physician that had brought them to the Medical School, and their interest was medical theory and its clinical applications. Most found health policy an uninteresting distraction. About the only idea that found interest among them was a session on how to get involved with one's local medical society, as this volunteerism offered prestige and support for their career advancement.

Nonetheless, there was plenty for Patrick to do in his new position. For one, Professor Edwards wanted him to keep his eye on the national health policy debate. He especially wanted to be ready for any opportunities for them to step in and influence this debate. Patrick made several trips to DC in his first year at Harvard to make sure that his connections were in place.

Another assignment was to research key health policy topics for possible submission of articles to medical journals. Almost all of such articles in the field were clinical in nature. An explosion of scientific discovery had stimulated a need for the filtering and sharing of new knowledge, and most practicing physicians subscribed to these journals. Professor Edwards thought that pushing policy articles into the journals might be another way to inject a more liberal view into the physician world.

Edwards had the requisite connections to be considered as an author, and was able to secure publication of a policy article on medical training in early 1934; he and Patrick collaborated on the article. They successfully published a couple of other policy articles the next year and then accepted an offer to write a quarterly series for a prominent journal. Patrick was the principal researcher for the early articles, and soon his role grew to editing the professor's drafts. By 1936, Patrick had become the primary author of the articles, even if he did so as a ghostwriter with the professor's name on them.

The job stimulated Patrick's mind and paid for a comfortable existence for his family in Cambridge, Massachusetts. The Great Depression had worn on, and recovery was slow. But Patrick had survived this difficult time and become a leading expert on national health policy without major academic credentials or broad notoriety, but practically, as one of the more experienced and thoughtful observers of American health policy across the nation.

He still hoped that FDR would turn his attention and agenda back to medical care. The New Deal had brought radical new thinking to a host of issues faced by Americans, and many found their base upon a strong role for government in aiding Americans to secure basic life, liberty, and security. Health care couldn't be that far behind these other sectors in some form of action.

It was not to be. Subsequent efforts to add medical care to the New Deal failed. Organized medicine continued to exert its might, and leading politicians had enough on their plate, giving them cover to avoid this issue.

Then, in December of 1941, Pearl Harbor triggered entry into the Second World War, putting an end to any possibility of national health insurance or other health care legislation. America had new priorities now, and even an ardent health reformer like Patrick could see that.

Chapter Seventeen

Young Irv and Johnny Look to the Future

Irv skipped his graduation from UCLA. He celebrated instead with a hike in the Olympic Mountains with Johnny. Through the rain and slick trails, Irv processed the odd circumstances that had brought him to this point in his life and wondered what might come next.

The last two years had been the most satisfying of his short time on the earth. He had successfully turned his remaining degree work at UCLA into a correspondence school, allowing him time to pursue other passions. It was a breeze for him to complete his undergraduate work, and he spent far more of his time enjoying his new home. Nor did he feel any need to move on too quickly, and spread his last year of school over two, taking the minimum number of credits until UCLA told him it was time to graduate or get off the pot.

This timeline left oodles of time for adventuring. And Johnny was all too ready to accompany him, or more likely, to lead the expedition.

Along the way, Irv got a part-time job in a coffee and tea warehouse, the one where his roommate Steve the drummer roasted beans. The coffee company always had a need for manual laborers to toss around coffee bags, grind coffee for shipment to restaurants, and make deliveries. It didn't pay much, but it got him a check and another group of interesting people to hang around with during the day.

It also came with free caffeine—as much as one could ingest day to day, through drinking, eating espresso-chocolate coffee bean samples, or any other way to get a jolt. By far the most effective was grinding coffee for restaurants. It was hard to unwrap and bend the five-pound bags of coffee spilling from the industrial grinder. The juicy oils of hundreds of pounds of coffee beans over an afternoon on Irv's bare hands left him with the energy to try to leap over the Space Needle.

He used this energy to explore Seattle most evenings and nights. He especially liked to do so with Mary Beth. She had been promoted to hostess at her bakery's new restaurant and worked evenings till about eleven at night. Irv would spend his hours after work on one adventure after another, many with Johnny. But, unless adventure took them on some nature hike in the woods or a road trip over a weekend, he would be sitting on a bicycle rack outside the Black Cub Bakery at 10:45 p.m. when she got off work.

Mary Beth and he would continue their adventures well into the night. They would maybe catch a movie at some classic film venue. Or they would listen to music at one of the many funky bars in the University District—some 1960s throwback bands and other experimenters searching for a new sound—searches that sparked the grunge movement and Subpop Records in a few years to come.

Sometimes they would just go back to the basement room they now shared. They spent hours gazing into each other's eyes, laughing at each other's jokes, and sharing dreams of what life would hold for them in years to come. And, yes, they had sex—a lot of sex.

She was all that he wanted, without ever knowing that he was looking for it. Much as he enjoyed his adventuring with Johnny, Irv missed Mary Beth to the tips of his body whenever he was away. He learned there was a reason people yearned for homes that really mattered to them, and it pained him to be away from her.

The times had also been a-changing. Nixon was long gone, as was the Vietnam War. A former peanut farmer was in the White House, and America was now obsessed with getting gas—and jobs. The gas lines and rationing days were not that big a deal for Irv, as his commuting mostly involved his thumb or an old ten-speed bike that he had bought from a Deadhead across the street. Once in a while he took the bus, though the wet stink of crowded commuters made him a bit nauseous.

Irv's job was okay too. The coffee business was going strong, and his book smarts had gotten him into the shipping department for a few more dollars, though with expectations for regular attendance. He had said yes to the offer, partly because he found himself wanting to stay in town with Mary on a regular basis, and partly in that getting a steady paying gig seemed important as a hard recession hit the Northwest in the early days of the 1980s.

Irv's dad was no longer paying his way through school and life—though he did now at least know that Irv was in the Pacific Northwest and not LA. Dad didn't seem to care all that much. His responsibilities at work had grown, and he was now a senior manager in the Experimental Research Division of Sandia Labs. He had met a younger coworker at a company retreat, and they had found reason to continue their conversation outside of the workplace, though most of it took place in the company cafeteria. She was also a devoted worker bee for the company and soon his dad's new wife. Irv got an invite to the small wedding, but couldn't gather the energy in his thumbs to make the trip down for the ceremony.

His college buddies had also moved on. Irv graduated two years behind them due to the incompletes he took from his Northwest journey. By then, most had found entry into the workforce down in California, which was humming along economically, unlike the Pacific Northwest. Some were in the entertainment business, others in hospital management, and still others in offshore oil exploration. Their friendships faded with the loss of proximity. People were moving on with their lives, Irv observed. *It happens to us all*, he thought.

Irv was feeling many parts of his past fray like a rotting string of rope: school, Dad's money, college friends, even his yen for hitchhiking across the world. The release was oddly liberating—and frightening. He had found a new place, one that washed good feelings over him like a chocolate fountain. He had friends and fellow adventurers to share his experiences and ideas with, and a never-ending stream of comers and goers in the group house in the University District. Johnny was a close confidant and friend, someone he could get deep with as he worked through ideas about the world and life.

But more than anything, he was in love, and she was in love with him. Every day sparkled with Mary Beth, certainly when they were together, but also in eager anticipation of being together again when they were apart. Hanging on to her and that feeling became his major addiction—and the resettling of his previous life pieces and the recession got him thinking more and more about what he would need to do to keep it.

"Those beans hot yet?" Irv asked Johnny from across the firepit. They had stopped to camp in the Enchanted Valley, a pristine valley in the heart of the Olympic National Park. They were midway from their entry point of the waterfront town of Dosewallips on the eastern flank of the Olympics and Lake Crescent Lodge to the west, and only an hour or so to the Pacific Coast. It had been a solid two days of hiking for them already, and it was slow going in the muddy trails of the flooding streams of one of the wettest spots in the world.

"Just about. Bean burrito coming up in about five minutes. Got anything left in that pipe of yours while we are waiting?" Johnny raised his eyebrows as he spoke, a sure sign that he was ready to expound on some new philosophical twist he had worked through during the long day of hiking—with a little THC bump to help the story along.

"Sure enough." Irv pulled his small wood pipe out of his backpack's top storage section, swiping a small slug off the zipper as he pressed his hand in to find it. The damp smell of cedar logs filled the air, and a bloom of smoke billowed from the wet wood popping in the firepit. He lit the pipe and passed it on to Johnny, who dropped the wooden spoon in the bean pan and took a deep suck.

Johnny held the smoke in his lungs for about thirty seconds and then blew it to the sky. He smiled and looked around the campsite, soaking in all that was teasing his senses for a minute or two. Then, slowly, he shifted his eyes to Irv. "This is what it's all about, hey, buddy? Just us and nature—survive or thrive. It is up to us, and what we can adapt to."

"You mean like how we adapted to that tornado in east Texas? Or the flash flood that almost blew us off the mountain in Zion?" Irv was a bit more wary of the natural state around them than Johnny and was quick to remind him that mind over matter only worked when the matter wasn't a shitstorm far beyond your capabilities to control. Johnny had never met an obstacle that he couldn't overcome with wits and action.

"Sure. Partner, we did get out of those predicaments, didn't we?" He chuckled to himself. "I will admit to wondering a bit, at least when that twister picked up that barn across the pasture and tossed it half a mile away."

"Remember, you were the one who wanted to wait out the storm in that flying fortress!" Irv liked to remind Johnny that he was not infallible. And maybe just a little bit lucky.

"No doubt. And I recall that you were the one who thought we had scrambled up out of the way of the water on that ledge in Zion. Instead of some wet toes where I took us, we would have been the Flying Wallendas of Zion Canyon as we flew over the wall to our death."

Irv chuckled back. Johnny wasn't just lucky; he did seem to have a good instinct for survival.

"But it's time to set our sights on some adventures outside of nature. The nature of man." Johnny was getting to the point of his quiet contemplation while hiking the last few days.

"Is that nature good or bad? We never have settled that debate, try as we might," Irv replied. This had been a regular source of conversation during their journeys. Or when they settled into a night of drinking at a bar.

"That's just it—I don't think we know yet. And the only way to find out is to get into that nature of man even more."

"More? We are plenty into it already." Irv's natural tendency, with too many painful memories of the frailty of man, was to avoid too much human contact.

"But not like we have tackled nature. Think about it—we wondered about bears—and spent a month in Glacier National Park. We wondered about the ocean—and took the ferry to Ketchikan. We've hung out in almost every major park in the American West and a few in the East and Canada to boot. Surviving, yes, but learning about nature and ourselves at the same time." He pulled the pan of beans off the fire, and the two began to assemble tortillas, beans, and other limited trimmings on their aluminum plates.

"It's been great, don't get me wrong," Johnny continued. "And I don't want to stop either. But, you know, this world is now as much about man as it is about nature. For every mountain and every park, there are dozens of cities and towns. Even countries. With human dramas playing themselves out every day and every week. We've got to get out there and learn about that too . . . that's what I've been thinking."

Irv was a bit wary of this new topic, but up for the debate. "So let's say we do. How would we? Camouflage our way into different places and make-believe we are someone's brother Johnny or grandson Irv?"

"That's just it—we can't experience this without diving deeper. Becoming a part of it. We just can't do the idle visitor thing that we've been doing."

"You've lost me. Why not?"

"Because while we might not know the nature of man yet, we do know that it is deep and complicated. We've got to be like a Zen master and embrace it in all ways to find its meaning."

"And how are you going to do that, pray tell?"

"Change things up. Dig into life for a while in some different way. Get a family. Get a new home. Get a job."

"Holy crap—you eat some mushrooms on the trail? You've never wanted to work more than a few days at a time. Remember, make enough to survive, and not a dollar more? Johnny's Economic Theorem 1."

"Good theorem. Just time to apply it differently. And it's not about the money—it is about the experience. Think about it—so much of human life happens at the workplace, for most of us, more than our family time. Or our leisure time. It is where American life happens—and we won't know the nature of man till we find a way to experience that."

"So, you got a way to do that? How can you do more than experience one workplace? Maybe it's a good one, maybe it's a bad one. Maybe it shows you the nature of man is good, or maybe bad. In that one place. And it will take you years to figure that out in that one case."

"Ah, but there is another way—to find out a whole lot more, and faster." Johnny leaned over his plate and took an enormous bite of his burrito, slopping the overload onto his plate. He chomped it slowly while looking at Irv, letting his swallows provide a pause to build excitement over his revelation.

Irv had seen this before, and typically was pretty impressed with what Johnny had come up with. But this was a little bit different, prying at his instincts for less, not more, human contact. "Okay, Mr. Burrito—give it up . . ."

"It's like this. I am going to become a politician. Run for office and get to know people. It would give me a great place to check the angle out on lots of stories—they should be providing me their stories every day. That is the job. And I hear it pays okay too—so who knows what I could afford to do to get deeper with a little capital to invest. I'll be like Lenin—

figuring out the mind of the working man and able to run some grand experiments to adapt the world to them."

Irv gaped in astonishment. Johnny had regularly surprised him before, but not like this. "Holy shit. You are going to become *the man*?"

"No—I am going to become Lenin. Without the freaky beard, of course."

"Let's hope you don't become Trotsky."

"Why—what happened to him?"

"He found his way to South American, hiding from the freaks that Lenin empowered. Stalin in particular. They finally found him and shot him in the head. He vegged away in a hospital for months, unable to form a sentence. And then just faded away. From dark to blackness."

Johnny took in the possibility of a different role. He smiled again and raised his plastic cup filled with brandy to the air. "Then, yes, to Lenin it is! I am just not ready to get shot in the head."

Irv laughed, bested again. He raised his own glass. "To Lenin," he shouted to the forest and the mountains and the life that was to form around this new plan.

Chapter Eighteen

Irv Stakes Out the Airport

Irv was a light sleeper who had learned how to function with sporadic rest. He regularly awoke in the middle of the night and, after many a restless night, concluded it made more sense not to fight it. He would get up and catch up on his work or personal projects, and find some other time to get his sleep. Many a night he was cranking out emails at 3 a.m. He learned it was best to wait till daylight to actually send them so he wouldn't seem too crazy to the addressees.

In the late afternoon, he napped at Ken's house for a couple of hours, then bid his thanks and farewell to his classmate. He stopped at a mini-mart to pick up supplies: an extra-large coffee, some snacks, and two large bottles of water; one he poured out so he could use it as a pee jar. He drove by the lot adjacent to the airport and circled it, looking for the best spot to set up a hidden camp, and found a small patch of a parking spot partly protected by small trees. There was something that resembled a home a hundred yards away, and a parked car would not look entirely out of place.

Darkness came soon and provided the full cover that he needed. The black night was broken by the occasional blinking lights of large jets landing or taking off—most landing and then taxiing off to some distant location on the other side of the airport. Minutes became hours, and Irv was starting to doubt that luck was on his side. He began to consider different next steps; there was not much else to do in the front seat of his car.

It was at about 4 a.m. that his fortunes turned. Headlights suddenly appeared down the road near the airport entrance, and a large truck, about fourteen feet long, stopped in front of the locked gate. An imposing figure got out of the truck and unlocked the gate, swung it open to let the truck enter, and then swung it shut, staying behind to guard the entranceway. The truck pulled up to the entranceway of the storage facility, an automatic door opened, and the truck drove into the building with the steel door shutting behind it. About fifteen minutes later, three plain white paneled vans also drove up to the gate and, after brief dialogue with the guard, drove into the lot and then the storage facility.

Irv took as many pictures as he could of the vehicles. He regretted that he only had a cheap pair of binoculars to try to get a better look; it was all he could find on a Sunday evening in Moses Lake. As near as he could tell, all of the vehicles were plain to the point of boring, without any clear markings. Even their license plates were covered over; Irv speculated that this was a temporary condition, as it would draw suspicion once they were on well-traveled roadways.

There was no way for him to get closer. The fence was between him and the building, as was the guard at the only entrance to the lot. He had no choice but to wait. About an hour later, the steel door of the facility opened, and all four vehicles left the building and made their way through the exit. The large truck was last, stopping to let the guard back in after he padlocked the front gate.

Irv started up his car. Since all the vehicles were leaving in sequence, he could only follow the last vehicle, which turned out to be the truck that Irv suspected was now empty. A mile down the road, the truck turned in to a secured entrance to the airport. There was a guard on duty, and the truck stopped at the security booth and then continued on into the expansive airport grounds, beyond Irv's sight, even with binoculars.

Irv could go no further without better papers. Being a public health investigator would not be enough in post-9/11 America to violate airport security. He stopped his car and parked on the side of the road, thinking about what he had just seen, and what to do next.

He looked at the pictures on his phone and made a few notes on his notepad. Then he started his car up and turned on to the road leading to I-90 and Seattle. *Yup*, he thought, *the mystery is getting clearer, even if it remains not clear at all. All I can do for now is head to Seattle and the start of my workweek.*

Chapter Nineteen

Post-WWII: The Age of More in Health Care

World War II was underway. The nation had mobilized for global war, and Congress's primary interest was harvesting national resources toward victory. Health care was one of those resources, and the only objective was to make sure it was available to support the war effort. Patrick Jones was ready to help in any way he could.

Inadvertently, within this "win the war" context, Congress created an incentive for employer-provided health coverage that remains a major cause of health system fragmentation to this day. A labor shortage was created by the significant number of workers going into military service. Competition for the remaining workers was great, and there was worry that the shortage might dramatically raise wages, inflation, and the costs of war. So, Congress froze wages and salaries.

But they did not freeze benefits—and business began to attract workers through these, including health insurance. In 1943, the Internal Revenue Service went further and exempted employer health coverage benefits from taxation, and the horse was completely out of the barn, galloping toward work-based health coverage. It was a monstrous financial incentive for employers to reward workers with health benefits rather than pay.

This was all, at best, an afterthought when it happened. The top of mind objective was to figure out how to win the war, and health care had a more direct place in that story—as did Patrick.

Patrick's childhood eye injury, which exempted him from service in WWI, continued to make him ineligible for military service. He volunteered to help organize Boston's civil preparedness for a potential invasion. He was thankful for this—it made him feel closer to the war effort than his experience of WWI. Nor could he satisfy his patriotic urges through his children—his oldest son, Christopher, was only thirteen when the war started, too young for service. By 1945, Chris was on the cusp of a draft call-up when the atomic bomb brought an abrupt end to the war.

Patrick was able to lead civil preparedness and continue in his post at Harvard, due to the University's support of his volunteerism. The truth was, Harvard was fearful of an invasion and found comfort in having one of theirs working to make sure it didn't happen.

His work duties at the school changed dramatically. It was a time to shift Harvard's training approach to the war effort, not to pursue new health policy. Many faculty and administrators were off to war, creating gaps in management and leadership, and Patrick was asked to take on this reorganization.

Any and every able-bodied medical student had been called to service to be part of America's battlefield Medical Corps. Casualty rates were high, particularly in the Pacific Theater, where the Red Cross was a primary target for snipers. New students were needed to take their place, and their education had to be fast-tracked so they could get to the battlefield in short order.

While the military had their own training program for corpsmen, there was also a need for battlefield physicians with a higher degree of competency. The nation's medical schools were asked to help with this, and they retooled their training programs to expedite battlefield training.

Patrick's assignment was to make this happen at Harvard. He welcomed this opportunity as he had others before. When researching the advances in battlefield medicine during and after the First World War, he uncovered a series of medical discoveries from across the globe from the pre-war years. Waves of new medical thought were flourishing, and there were provocative potential applications of these new theories into medical practice for patients. These could save lives on the battlefield and beyond, Patrick realized.

One example of this was the acceptance of the germ theory of disease. This theory was not all that new, finding its roots in the mid-1800s and the work of medical heroes like Joseph Lister, Louis Pasteur, and

Robert Koch. Before then, the prevailing view was that diseases like cholera and the Black Death were products of poisonous vapors coming from rotting matter—the Miasma Theory of Disease. It was through this matter that disease was transmitted among people, not from humans to humans. Germ Theory explained the transmission as the spread of microorganisms—bacteria, viruses, protists, fungi, prions, or viroids.

The idea, though, was slow to take root, especially in America. One breakthrough moment was in WWI, when a vaccine was developed for typhoid. Ten million doses were used on troops on the western front, and there was a tenfold decrease in the number of cases. On the other hand, ignorance of the bigger application of the Germ Theory of Disease was a major cause for the spread of the Spanish Flu, a pandemic that killed between 50 and 100 million people worldwide. A major source of transmission was military bases, where close living quarters stimulated a horrific spread of the disease. A repeat of this would be devastating to the allied war effort.

WWII also provided another reason to better understand how to respond to the Germ Theory of Disease. The Japanese began to use biological agents during their occupation of Manchuria, and military leaders needed medical professionals to build a defense to their possible use elsewhere.

Another paradigm-shattering discovery with implications for Harvard's medical curriculum was anesthesia. Again, this was something discovered and first used in the mid-1800s, but it took quite a while for it to become a recognized and standard tool of health care. The grim reality of WWII and advanced weaponry pressed for its fast adaptation to be of use to casualties on the battlefield.

Patrick's job was to discern which of these innovations, and others, were most worthy and adaptable to battlefield use. Then he had to work them into Harvard's training program. Medical practice evolved dramatically during the conflagration of the Second World War, and Patrick was a key player in this advance.

Peacetime brought a return to the older and slower days of medical training. Many wanted to more forcefully inject these and other new technologies into medical practice and medical school curriculum. Harvard was at the forefront of the discernment process around such new medical knowledge, and Patrick continued his leadership role at Harvard in doing so, despite his lack of formal medical training.

Professor Edwards had suffered a stroke in 1944. Though still on the faculty, he was unable to perform any significant duties, and Patrick for all intents and purposes assumed most of them for him. Until Professor Edward's death in 1950, Patrick did this while remaining in his original adjunct faculty member position. Then he was offered a tenured faculty position as Director of Policy for Harvard Medical School, and remained in this role until his retirement in 1963.

This position offered a forum for Patrick to continue his work to shape American health policy in postwar America. It pleased him that he was finally getting some recognition for doing this, mostly because it gave him new power to express his views. He became more assertive in his policy recommendations, within Harvard and in national health policy circles. Many of the ideas he pushed were drawn from the report and recommendations of the CCMC.

It angered him that American policy leaders continued to reject the committee's call for national health coverage in Recommendation 3. There was another moment in time where that seemed possible again after the war. President Harry Truman had proposed a national health insurance program, but organized opposition from the business and medical communities had beaten it down.

Patrick could see the politics of the idea had only gotten more difficult. The Cold War had brought communism sharply into focus as the new enemy of the United States, and anything that could be brushed with that label was a policy non-starter. The AMA had not changed its tune, and there was no chance to get this idea on a better track until the communist scare abated. McCarthyism made that even harder, and for many years such talk was not just controversial but even career limiting.

There were other opportunities to advance American health policy, though, and Patrick was aggressive in using his newfound role and power to shape and help this next age of health care advance in the United States. The country was now doing well financially, its economy the only one standing after the war and now with the confidence to leverage its vast resources on a global basis. This financial capital enabled Congress to invest more in providing health care to the American people, and that it did.

Patrick came to call this era of American health policy the Age of More. More business, more markets, more money, and more for America's health care system. Health care was now a public good, something that should be provided to as many Americans as possible—short of doing so through socialist means, of course. But certainly the government could help stimulate and build more—and if need be, more quietly, try to control health care through laws affecting this supply.

For example, anesthesia had opened up a range of new treatment possibilities. These surgical interventions needed to be done in hospitals for safety reasons, and, as the Committee on the Cost of Medical Care found in 1932, there was a great shortage of such facilities. The shortage was especially acute in rural America. In 1954, Congress passed the Hill-Burton Act, which provided construction grants for new hospitals. Thousands of new hospitals were built with these grants in the decades to come.

This supply subsidy was accompanied by strings that would help achieve other health policy objectives. To be eligible, new hospitals had to be owned by the community through formation of a not-for-profit organization. What's more, they had to commit to using their assets for the community's benefit, including providing some level of free care to those in need for perpetuity. It was a back door way of providing economic security to uninsured Americans in the Age of More.

"More" was also to be the ethic underlying America's approach to its health care labor force. New and more and better trained practitioners were needed, from physicians to dentists to nurses and more. Congress began to pass measures providing major new funding support for this initiative. Some of the funding went to students in the form of tuition support or scholarships; other funding went to schools and hospitals. Again, strings were attached that would give the government a way into the regulation of these students and organizations as they provided "more" to the nation.

There was also policy that triggered far more insured Americans, primarily the IRS's tax-free treatment of health benefits and business's use of this incentive, rather than wages, to pay their employees. The notion that health care could provide positive benefits to its recipients also took hold, and new private entities were created in droves to fill this market need.

One large movement that helped trigger this growth in health coverage were Blue Cross and Blue Shield plans—health prepayment programs operated usually on a statewide level through the leadership of hospitals and physicians respectively. These became an accepted new social model of coverage, legally and operationally distinct from what was provided by traditional indemnity insurers. American policy encouraged this development by passing new laws governing their structure and requirements, such as new ways of calculating necessary financial reserves for the plans since they were owned and operated by providers.

Much of this policy happened at the state level rather than the federal, but it signified a national movement promoting health insurance nonetheless. That "more" was created is indisputable. About 9 percent of American had some form of health insurance in 1940; by 1950, half of Americans were covered.

Patrick became a national leader in devising and advancing this new government thinking for health care in the postwar years. He was active at the federal level, where his contacts and experience proved invaluable. He also became a leader in the formation of the Massachusetts Blue Cross Plan, and advised the hospital community on how to ensure that this program was built on sound public policy for the state.

It made him feel good to see health policies that he was working on become law and part of the underlying fabric of the American medical system. Much of his earlier career had seen unrequited efforts to make system-wide health policy. He so wanted to contribute to meaningful change, as his parents had instilled such values in him decades ago.

On occasion, Patrick would open up his copy of the Committee on Medical Care on the bookcase next to his office desk. He would peruse its recommendations and contemplate the difference between then and now. The committee began its work in 1927, recognizing that there was great benefit in better distributing health care to the American people. Patrick reflected that then no one had any idea of the amazing discoveries to come and how dramatically health care would transform itself in terms of this potential betterment over the course of the century. The technology advances were staggering, so much so that the causes of death in America were changing.

American policy needed to adapt to this new reality, and Patrick thought the Age of More was progress in that respect. He did not second-guess the "more" he had helped create; no, it was good. He did acknowledge that it should be adapted to make sure that its application was more finely tuned. For example, if the causes of death for Americans were changing, shouldn't the nation's investment in health care change with it to make sure attention was focused on these new or emerging priority needs?

Patrick's frustration around the lack of national health coverage did not go away. This primary recommendation of the committee was a fundamental matter of fairness, and Patrick regularly reminded policy makers and students that the rationale for it was also rooted in American values of life, liberty, and property. Fifty percent was better than 9 percent, but it was still no better than flipping a coin in terms of one's odds of having health coverage. It had also accentuated the gap between the haves and have-nots across America.

An even bigger problem to him was that the health system remained dysfunctional. It was hardly a functioning system at all. He recalled vividly how all of the members of the committee agreed on one central proposition in 1932: that it wasn't that the American health care system had to improve, but that there was no real American health system in place. Now, as they had worried then, a system was in place through necessity and the passage of time. But it wasn't rational, and it wasn't efficient. It was fragmented and disjointed, and the "more" resources were added, the more complicated and disjointed it became.

Somehow, this now had to be put into some rational order. It was for him, beyond fairness, the larger value reason why some form of national health coverage was necessary. Without it, there could be no effective rationalization of the American health system. Too much time and effort were being applied to filling the gaps in fairness, or at least for those with political favor. This energy would be better deployed in creating and managing a more effective overall health system for all.

For all its good, Patrick feared that the Age of More had only made this proposition more difficult, and without bold action, the health care system might be beyond the point of no return unless there was some way to bring all Americans into the system in a way that would allow for some unification in system thinking.

In the 1960s, as Patrick neared retirement, one more chance to achieve this new change arrived. It gave him hope that it would finally bring the committee's universal coverage thinking into reality.

Ultimately, though, it was just another nod to the Age of More. The moment shifted to creating a new health care coverage program for the elderly and a few other groups of needy Americans, a program called Medicare. It was the good of More and an injection of more of the bad at the same time: fragmentation and dysfunction of the American health care system.

Chapter Twenty

The Formal Investigation Is Closed

Irv made good time on his drive from Moses Lake to Seattle Public Health headquarters through the late night and into early Monday morning. Traffic was light through the mountain passes, and he only hit a mild backup when he got to the beginning of major population centers just east of Issaquah on the western slopes of the Cascades. He was in a county car, so he took the risk of using the express lanes driving solo and made steady progress all the way to downtown Seattle by avoiding the long delays in the regular traffic lanes.

He was tired from his nighttime stakeout. He kept the driver's-side window rolled down halfway for the trip and let the cool air rush through his body. He also stayed awake by working the problem at hand in his mind—what to do about what he had learned in Moses Lake, and more immediately, what to tell Director Welch when he undoubtedly was asked for an update at the office.

The obvious next step was to track the vehicles at the airport site, but this would be difficult to do without license plate numbers. Perhaps there was a way to get a shot of the vehicles from traffic cameras once they presumably uncovered the plates to resume their journey to god knows where. That was the problem—he had no idea where they were going. There was just too much ground to cover. Unless there was a camera on the one or two roads leading to the highway from the Moses Lake airport—if they went that way. If, if, if.

Irv did know where the truck went—back to the airport. Maybe there was a way to get some data about it from the gate it entered. There must be some record of it coming and going. Maybe via a sticker on the van window? Or a card used by one of the people inside of the truck?

He also guessed that the truck had come from the airport to meet up with the minivans. Otherwise, what was the point of their location right outside the airport? And it must somehow be connected to the cargo of a flight coming into Moses Lake. It could have been one of those red lights he saw landing in the night. It also could have come in during the daytime and held until the cover of night. Again, there were too many possibilities.

The many questions rushed at him like the mountain air through his open window. He should be able to get access to many government records given his security clearance as a public health investigator. Might he scare more into existence by dropping epidemic threats? Would this bring unwarranted attention to what he was doing? What was really going on in the big picture? Dead bodies. Potato derivatives. Storage facilities in Moses Lake. None of it made much sense by itself.

The only sure thing was that he had to get to his office to take his next steps. He also had to be careful not to disclose too much to Welch. Irv was far beyond the tips of his skis of tracking the lab results now and likely to lose his job if his weekend activities were fully uncovered.

Doing the right thing would have been so much easier under the previous director. That was an understatement. Where the previous director had hired him and become a mentor and partner, Welch was an opportunist and bureaucrat. They had no relationship, and Irv didn't trust him.

Nor did this situation come with any easy answers. Oddly, Irv was having a tough time seeing any public health emergency related to it. Perhaps there was something evil going on, but not a public health type of evil. If there was one, Irv would be duty bound to share what he had learned, and this would be his protection—the danger to the public would transcend his misgivings about other workers and what the government might do with this information. But it wasn't. Still, it seemed like there was something really important that needed to be found, and if not by him, who?

He couldn't outright lie to the director. A deeply held tenet for Irv was to tell the truth, something he resolved as a teenager during his mom's cancer ordeal. So much of what was wrong with that experience involved lies from the medical care system—to her, to him, to the whole family. Some had good intent underneath, but still, in the end, they were hurtful. He would not live by a code that perpetuated the scourge of dishonesty.

This principle was on occasion challenged. The health insurance disclosure statements that asked about smoking or drug use, were one example. He would find a way to phrase his answers in a way that was technically truthful but shaded the response enough to distract from its plain meaning. This would have to be a similar response, so long as the director asked questions in the right way. Or the way Irv responded to questions if they weren't asked the right way.

Up to the twenty-fourth floor he went, coffee cup in hand. He felt it best to go straight to the mouth of the beast and set up a time to meet with Welch that morning. There was Rose, as usual, guarding the entranceway to the director's office. "Go right in," she said. "He is expecting you."

Irv was surprised that the director was already in the office and apparently waiting for him. On entering Director Welch's office, Irv saw that there were three people sitting at the small table situated by the window: Director Welch, special assistant Tracy Atkinson, and someone Irv had never met, a tall fellow with a handlebar mustache and a fancy suit.

"Good morning, Irv. Glad you could make it in." There was a sarcastic note in the director's greeting to him; he demanded punctuality in others, even if it was not something that he lived by. "You know Tracy, of course. This is Sam Bridgewater. He is on assignment from the feds to help us with our investigation."

Irv shook hands with Bridgewater. He tried to look into his eyes and get a read on who he really was, a skill he had learned from Johnny, but Bridgewater averted his gaze, as if experienced in preserving personal secrets. It creeped Irv out. He needed to know more to assess what he was now up against, but his instincts were that things were getting worse, not better. "Part of the CDC, Sam?" Irv asked.

"No," Bridgewater responded, directly and with a frost in his voice that would chill a beer mug on a hot summer day. "I am a contractor assigned to this case by Secretary of HHS Ben Olsen. His office is taking jurisdiction on this matter, and he wanted me to lead the assessment to make sure it was handled appropriately."

Irv wondered whether this was more of the privatization bullshit that the national administration spoke about regularly. Surely they weren't foolish enough to believe this ideologically and politically driven clap-trap when it came to potential epidemics? For all the failures of government one might point to in making the case that it was inefficient and ineffective, public health surveillance and action were not among them.

The public health world had proved their mettle around SARS, AIDS, and Ebola in recent years. If these "private market reformers" were students of history, they would know that but for the professional public health response to the Great Flu Pandemic of 1918, millions more would likely have perished. A repeat of that disaster would be political suicide for any politician, and talking points would be quickly thrown aside in the face of bad outcomes. No, Brownie was not doing such a great job in response during Katrina. Everybody saw it, and he was soon out.

It occurred to Irv that maybe the higher-ups in DC already knew that there wasn't a real public health threat at play. This line of conjecture heightened his suspicion of Bridgewater even more, but didn't really change the strategy for meeting with the director that he had come up with during the drive.

"Well, whoever you are with, it is good to have you involved and helping," said Irv. He looked at the director and kept going. "I've got a bit of an update on the lab results. I've really stayed focused on that, as you asked." His look was not hostile but intended to convey subservient conformance with orders. "But maybe you can update me on what you've been finding first so I can make sure that what I have to share is relevant to where you are at with the overall investigation?" This was his strategy—go on the offensive by being ready to throw out all he knew about the actual lab reports, if only someone would provide context so his update could be responsive. Ideally, he would learn what they had without sharing much they didn't know already.

Tracy took the bait, wanting to impress the director and now someone from DC who might prove useful to her ambitions for advancement down the road. "Director Welch, I've been working the statewide angle on this all weekend." It was important for him to know just how hard she was working. "Our statewide surveillance is showing that there have been no more instances of this particular virus reported. It looks like this was an aberration, and since the gestation period for SARS-like viruses is around forty-eight hours, most likely we are out of the potential danger zone on this one. We will need to maintain our heightened surveillance for a few more days since we've seen a bit of an uptick in flu cases in a couple of counties. But we don't think there is any link to this case. We should be optimistic that it is a one-time situation."

Irv knew that part of this was not entirely accurate. Ken had access to the statewide surveillance reporting system and had checked it on Saturday morning. There was reference to the case in King County, but there were no reports of more than expected flu cases from anywhere in the state. It was certainly not the case in Grant County, but the statewide public health system was tracking it in all thirty-nine counties. More likely, Tracy had gotten this information from someone directing her how to communicate the incident. It must have been deemed more useful to spread a tale of "more flu" for whatever reason. The rest of her analysis was still close to accurate.

Bridgewater spoke up. "That's great news. And consistent with our national surveillance on this matter. We just don't think there is any reason for public alarm and would ask you to keep this matter confidential. I've asked Director Welch to release the body to our team so that we can do further testing. I assume that this is now in process?"

Director Welch nodded to affirm that he had acted on the federal orders. "Irv, anything to add from your point of view?" he asked.

This was all too easy, thought Irv. He didn't need to go on the offensive, as the purpose of this meeting seemed to be to make sure that little was happening to advance the investigation. The less said the better, and no one in the room was likely to challenge him on it.

"No, not a lot," said Irv. "You have the official lab results that were released last Thursday. The strain is very close to the SARS strain of the flu from the 1990s. My best guess is that our corpse is someone who was exposed to that, then survived, and otherwise died for unrelated reasons last week. The *how* of that would best be found through an autopsy, and it sounds like the feds will take the lead on that now."

Bridgewater nodded.

"Other than that, the only other interesting piece of information was the potato derivative noted on the report. I talked to a staffer for the state potato commission, and he said that this was the type of trace matter that could show up on someone working to process potatoes." This was true enough given his nuanced framing of Ed's analysis—for this meeting, anyway. "My guess is that our John Doe was a worker in the potato fields and got enough of the particulates on him to show on the lab report."

"Probably an illegal," interjected Bridgewater. Irv wasn't sure why this mattered, but kept his emotions in check so as to let this meeting naturally run its course to what seemed like a swift ending. "So, nothing else to add?"

"No, I was busy with some other things this past weekend, and that is about all I can say about the lab reports." Again, this was true enough, especially since there seemed to be no interest in a deeper probe. Sam Bridgewater would likely assume Irv was another lazy bureaucrat and there was no reason to delve into whether this was really where things ended for him.

"All right then," asserted Director Welch. "As you requested, Mr. Bridgewater, we are formally closing our investigation of this incident. We will release the body to you and your colleagues. Irv will draft a final report for our files and submit that to me for approval. As you requested, we will be placing the case under our 'not for public distribution' records. There will be no specific mention of this to our public information officers, and all that anyone will see who has official access to our records system will be that we investigated an incident in Kent. We will also, as you asked, suggest in the file footnote that the victim was most likely an illegal immigrant." Director Welch, like Tracy, was more than happy to do what was needed to curry favor from a bigshot from DC.

"Excellent. I suggest we consider the matter closed and let me take it from here," said Bridgewater. With that, the four stood up from the table, exchanged closing pleasantries, and moved on with their day.

Irv smiled at Rose on the way out. "See, nothing to it. And you thought things always get a bit out of hand when I am involved." Rose gave him a thumbs-up as he continued on down the hall. "Of course, they still might," he muttered under his breath, thinking that the whole episode stunk to high heaven.

Chapter Twenty-One

2020: A Patient Dump

Helen Neederdam awoke to the roar of diesel engines just outside of her apartment in Shelton, Washington, around 5 a.m. Shelton was in western Washington, about two hours from Seattle as a crow would fly. It was a rural town and most of its economy related to some form of government activity, now that the timber industry was a shadow of its former self. The vehicles she was hearing out her window were used to repair county and state roads, and workers would be on their way to their assigned sites by six in the morning.

What was unusual was the dryness in her throat, and the runny nose. At least, it was unusual for this time of year. She suffered from spring allergies, and alder trees across Mason County were a particular irritant. These trees flowered in March, however, many months ago.

No, this felt worse. She took the thermometer out from the drawer in her nightstand and put it in her mouth. Twenty seconds later, it beeped and she looked at the digital readout. 101 degrees. No doubt about it. She had a fever.

Her first instinct was to go to a doctor—not as much for whatever she had, but for fear of its impact on her other health conditions. She was a diabetic and had begun to experience health failures related to the disease. Chief among them were problems with her circulatory system. She had coronary artery disease and had one foot amputated after it swelled badly last fall.

One might have thought that she would have a regular physician, suffering from as many ailments as she did. But she did not. This wasn't even because she was among the millions of Americans who were uninsured. No, she had coverage through Medicare because of the extent of her disabilities from diabetes.

Helen had enrolled in a Medicare Advantage plan two years ago, enticed by the extra benefits offered to her. She didn't really understand Medicare that well, and didn't realize that she was choosing to reject the traditional program that would have offered a broader range of providers and services than those offered by a private, restricted health plan.

After signing up with a private plan, she had contacted her then primary care physician, a family physician whose practice was in downtown Shelton. When she told him of her new health plan, she discovered that the doctor's office was not included in the health plan's panel. They had been, but the plan had dropped them right after the open enrollment period for not agreeing to the provider agreement, which discounted their payment rates by 50 percent.

She had called the health plan to complain. After being put on hold in their telephone call center five times, she finally spoke with a representative. That didn't help at all. She could barely understand the young woman helping her; she had a heavy foreign accent and mostly told her that what she wanted wasn't possible. The only recourse was to file a complaint and request a waiver. The form was on the company's website.

Helen had a computer but didn't really know how to use it. Navigating the company's complicated website was even more difficult, even once she finally figured out how to get there on the Internet with a little help from one of her neighbors.

Her neighbor was not much more computer savvy than she was. Helen thought about asking her son Kevin for help. He would occasionally visit her, usually when he needed some cash to help make ends meet. He had promised to come over and help her, but hadn't done so. She knew that he would later in the month, after she received her monthly social security check and had some extra cash.

Helen decided to wait out her symptoms. She settled into bed with tea and a book and rested throughout the day. By six in the evening, she felt worse. Her temperature was now up to 102 degrees. She was having trouble breathing, nausea, and the pressure on her chest got worse when she lay flat and tried to sleep.

She figured it was time to do something more. In the past, she would have just driven to the emergency room at the hospital in Shelton; it was only about a three-minute drive from her apartment. They had always seen her there and usually helped ease whatever symptoms were making her life difficult. She was what they called a "frequent flyer"; five or more ER visits a year.

The last time she was there, a young woman at the desk in the emergency room told her that she was being enrolled in a special hospital program. She was supposed to call up the emergency room before driving to the hospital and walking in, using a special phone number on a large magnet they asked her to put on her refrigerator.

She called the telephone number before driving to the hospital. It was hard for her to talk given her shortness of breath, and she tried to explain her symptoms to the man on the other end of the line. He seemed less interested in that than the information on her most recent health insurance enrollment card.

The man told her that she was not eligible to be seen in the emergency room because of her change in insurance coverage. He explained that the hospital had just been acquired by a new owner, and they were not part of the health plan's network. He suggested she call the health plan instead, and register a complaint. He even gave her the phone number to call.

After ten minutes on hold, her call finally went through. It was another foreign accent, and her ill state made it even harder to understand what was being said. She kept explaining that she needed to see someone and had been turned away at her local hospital. The person offered her other options—hospitals in Belfair, Olympia, and then Portland, 150 miles away.

She wasn't sure her car could even make it ten miles down the road. It was in poor condition and almost out of gas. Kevin had taken all of the cash she had on hand at his last visit. All she really knew was that she was feeling even worse. By now it was 8:30 at night and her temperature was up to 103 degrees and she began to vomit.

What the hell, she thought. *I am going to the emergency room anyway.* She hobbled down to her car, drove the short distance to the hospital, and parked in the closest parking lot to the emergency room. It took her about ten minutes to make it the 100 yards to the ER entrance on her crutches.

The Theory of Irv

It was the same emergency room she had visited many times before. But the desk had been moved to the other end of the waiting room. It was now packed with people, and there was a line of five people in front of her.

She waited for fifteen minutes, feeling worse by the minute. Finally, she got to the front of the line. The woman on duty asked for her insurance card, and asked her why she was at the ER. Helen handed over the card and began to tell the woman her health care problems, then realized that the woman was not really listening to her. The woman had entered the information on the card in her computer and was reading something on the screen.

"Ma'am, it says that you called up earlier tonight and were told that you are not eligible to come to the emergency room. Why are you here?"

"Because I have nowhere else to go," replied Helen.

"You could go to the hospital in Olympia, or in Belfair," replied the desk clerk.

"They are too far away. Over forty minutes. I don't think my car could go that far."

"Why not take a taxi?"

"Because I don't have the money to pay for it."

"Don't you have a credit card?"

"No. It was taken back by the bank last year. Something about my credit history."

The clerk looked at the screen some more. "It says you have a son in the area. Why don't you call him and have him give you a ride?"

"I would try, but he never answers when I call."

"I am sorry about that, ma'am, but do you think that is fair to our other patients? You can see we are quite busy."

"But I don't know what else to do."

"All right, all right. I will put you on the list, and you may sit down in the waiting room. I can't promise when we will get to you though."

Helen thought that this was progress. Most of all, she felt terrible and needed to get off her foot. The one remaining was throbbing in pain, noticeable even through her other symptoms. She shuffled the twenty feet to the only open chair in the waiting room and sat down.

Minutes became an hour, and she tried her best to patiently sit and wait in the stiff plastic chair. The waiting room was still busy, but now was not as crowded. A number of hospital staff dressed in blue gowns left the hospital through the ER exit at a little after eleven.

She was starting to feel even worse, especially the nausea. Surely somebody would see her. She went back up to the desk. There was a different woman who asked her name and went back to her computer screen to find some answers. She began to ask questions of Helen—the same questions she had answered before.

Helen was frustrated, sick, and unable to cope. Rather than argue, she thought it best to go out to her car and try to get to the hospital in Olympia, but she struggled to walk across the parking lot. She vomited as she got to her car, the greenish brown sludge from her mouth spreading underneath her left rear tire. She wiped her face with the sleeve of her coat and got in the driver's seat, pulled out of the parking lot, and took several turns before arriving on US Route 101. She took a left onto the four-lane highway, knowing that in about thirty minutes it would run right through Olympia and the next closest hospital.

Route 101 was a busy enough road during normal hours, but there was little traffic now that it was close to midnight. Helen was feeling worse, but thought she had no choice. *I have to get to the Olympia hospital.* She looked at her gauges—her fuel tank indicator was near the bottom.

Sometimes this was because the gauge on her 1968 Maverick got stuck. She began to rap on the outside of the gauge to see if it would show some life. It was a flash of an instant when she realized that the road had curved sharply to the left and merged to one lane in her direction. She was now almost off the road and could hear rocks and dirt spinning through her tires.

She just missed the guardrail on the right-hand side of the road. But it was too late to regain control of the car. It was now speeding up as it turned down a sharp embankment bordering the highway, careening toward a small valley of trees along the dark highway. Her car hit a Douglas fir in the trench head-on, smashing the front of the car back onto Helen's chest. It was unclear whether she died from the engine being shoved into her lap or from her head hitting the hard dashboard as it recoiled from the contact with the tree. Or maybe it was just that she had, finally, succumbed from food poisoning from the take-out food at the Chinese restaurant the night before.

Regardless, Helen Neederdam was now dead.

Chapter Twenty-Two

Young Johnny Builds His Political Résumé

True to his word, Johnny forged a career in politics. He moved to the little community of Duvall, living in a small rental cabin just outside of town. During the day, he got a job in the local grain and feed store to make ends meet, and then spent most evenings and nights getting to know folks at the two bars in town.

In short order, he had met enough people to plan his first political move. He decided to run for the local school board. The fact that he had no kids and knew little about schooling was no match for his enthusiasm and charm, and his new neighbors voted him in. He had his start, and he spent his first year breaking into life in east King County with a mix of evening school board meetings and continued visits to the bar.

By his second year in Duvall, he was ready to take his next leap. An important step was meeting and marrying a woman named Reena Grisham. They met at the grain and feed store, as she needed some grain for the horses kept on the family farm. Johnny offered to deliver the load and, before the night was over, spent the night in the barn with Reena and the horses.

She was tall, good-looking, and fond of Johnny. He was unlike anyone she had ever met, and at first it was just a fun way to spend her time. Johnny felt the same way—it was a pleasant way for him to find companionship and sex as he adapted to the distance between him and his best friends in Seattle. Soon, though, it became apparent that she had other things to offer, and him to her.

Reena came from wealth and had access to money—under the right conditions as it related to Johnny. For the right man, she was willing to convince her dad to invest in Johnny's need to build a political résumé. Dad was a former state senator and had political connections... and money. He was more than willing to help his daughter's new man, once she asked him, and he was convinced that it was more than a fleeting relationship. It had to be more than a fling—he insisted on matrimony. Johnny was intrigued by the possibilities, and found Reena to be a more than adequate companion.

Reena was eager to find a new husband, having been deserted by her first, six months after delivering their second child. It was too much responsibility for him to accept, and he bolted town with his secretary. The two moved across the country, dissolving all ties to her and her two young children.

Johnny was a major step up in all respects. He was good-looking, fun, and a decent man. He was even responsible when compared to her first husband. Johnny also had ambitions, though they were a bit off the beaten track of her experience. Reena was lonely, and she found all of these reasons to be enough to tie the knot with him. Most of all, she thought Johnny would be a good substitute father to her children. Love, if she was honest with herself, was probably not one of the reasons, but this was far down her list of requirements.

It was a match made more out of transactional needs than heaven, but neither was hung up over that. They really liked each other and saw the happiness and convenience of the match. Just a year and a half after moving to the east side of the county, Johnny now also had a wife and family.

Reena's dad and his cash helped Johnny accelerate his rise in the political world of east King County. This help was important, but not the most important factor. His greatest assets were those he brought to the endeavor. Cash and contacts opened a lot of doors, but Johnny smashed these in with his natural charm and persistence. He was soon noticed by political handlers looking for new blood to infuse into the stale and conservative politics of the region.

Seattle—the dominant city in King County—had long liberal traditions, but was politically controlled by local businessmen and old money. The rest of the large county, made up of many small but growing towns mixed among the water and trees leading up to the Cascade Mountains, was still finding its nature. It was a combination of second-

and third-generation homesteader families, mixed with social dropouts who found isolation in the backwoods. Now wealthier newcomers were beginning to spread east, away from the rising costs of housing in Seattle.

Johnny molded himself to the fabric of his new environs and its people. He was comfortable with homesteader, hermit, and yuppie alike, and they with him. He added a few new twists to applying his natural charm through political coaching.

He was appointed to the King County Council in 1983, filling the vacant seat of a mill owner who lost his life and office when he slipped and fell into one of the enormous bandsaws in his tree factory. The council was a full-time gig, with a decent salary, and Johnny let go of his day job at the feed and grain store in Duvall.

The King County Council post allowed him to focus full time on his chosen profession rather than also loading and delivering sacks of grain and stocking rakes. He learned that most of the councilman job was listening to the stories of the people across his district. It was a match made in heaven. After all, it was this that inspired him to choose politics as a career. He was a natural personalizer and soon became a rising political star in east King County.

The greater Seattle region continued to be a hotspot for relocation, including Johnny's region. Some newcomers came from the East Coast and even more from California as housing prices and taxes pushed folks north to the Emerald City by the thousands. Many found jobs with emerging technology companies. Computers were taking off in America, and a company called Microsoft provided career options for many newcomers, sprouting cottage industries that offered well-paid work. Many of the newcomers were attracted to the beauty and solitude of east King County and the Microsoft campus to the east of Seattle.

This growth in population created a new political opportunity for Johnny when a redistricting of congressional seats in 1983 reshaped the boundaries of Washington's districts in Congress. None of the incumbents lived within the newly shaped eighth congressional district, and Johnny, on the other hand, resided right in the middle of it on Reena's family ranch in eastern King County.

Johnny and Reena decided, with her dad's encouragement, that they should move to the family ranch and use this as the base for Johnny's run for a House seat in the next election. Most political observers scoffed at the notion and predicted his fast demise as a candidate—mostly because of his decision to run as an independent. The system was rigged to make elections a choice between Republican and Democratic candidates. Independents were seen as spoilers who tipped the election to one party by peeling off votes, not serious candidates.

This election was a bit different in that there was no incumbent, or history—it was a new congressional district. Nor did either party identify great candidates to run for the newly configured seat. It was at least open for competition.

Johnny showed his great interpersonal skills as a candidate. People liked him, and that was a fantastic place to start. He was also willing to work hard. The other candidates had more initial name recognition than he, but Johnny personally rang the doorbells and spoke to almost everyone who lived in the district.

He also met a woman named Nancy Jones through his former roommate, Mary Beth Collins. Nancy ran a small Seattle political consulting group that specialized in women candidates. Johnny charmed his way on to her client roster, with Reena's approval. Her dad had heard good things about Nancy, and Nancy didn't disappoint—she figured out how to get thousands of Eastside housewives to the ballot box to vote for Johnny in an upset win. Meet Congressman John Gibson.

Chapter Twenty-Three

Irv Investigates Anyway

Irv returned to his office cubicle after the meeting with Director Welch and Sam Bridgewater. He was irritated. No, make that angry. *Case closed* was the message. He had been around long enough to know when the fix was in, and this one stunk like a rabid skunk.

He needed this job, at least for now, but not enough to let something like this pass without doing something about it. He would also need to be careful. The case could not be fully closed until he, as the investigator assigned to it, said so, and he would be slow to draft the final report and send it to Director Welch. For now, he would consider the investigation to be under review—his—for as long as he could figure out how to maintain it.

This might not be long, but the bigger question was how? There was no apparent way forward, and he had to find one that could bear fruit and not be easily discovered by his boss. He spent the rest of the morning and early afternoon thinking about this challenge in his office.

Irv began by reviewing the ideas percolating in his mind while driving back to Seattle from Moses Lake. It was a struggle to think clearly though. He wasn't so much tired as frustrated. The meeting with the director had provided an adrenaline jolt far better than caffeine, but also made it hard for him to focus his newfound energy.

Why? For whatever his faults, Director Welch was a responsible public health officer, so Irv knew that there must be serious juice from the top pressuring him to bury this case. The information available was plausible enough to allow Director Welch to conclude there was no public threat at play. Even Irv's instincts were that this was not a public health threat of the ordinary, but something else. Welch could easily make a case for wresting the case from his troublemaking public health investigator who only got the case because he was on call when the body was discovered.

There was something far off about this case, though, and Irv couldn't rationalize it away so easily. Whatever had happened didn't really seem to have much to do with any pandemic or even flu. Or potatoes, for that matter. The presence of these possibilities seemed to be hiding whatever was really going on. What in the world could that be?

Irv mapped out several possibilities for keeping the investigation practically moving forward, even in the absence of a hypothesis. Or hard evidence. Little to nothing came from his search for cameras outside of the Moses Lake Airport that might identify a license plate or some other features on the white vans. There was only one camera on the roadway to the freeway from the airport, and no minivans in sight on the recording over the night. More likely, the vans took an alternate route away from the airport.

Similarly, the truck was a dead end. He tracked down a vehicle that entered the airport at that time, but it was a pool truck used for short deliveries. The record sheet was sufficiently garbled to prevent him from clearly identifying who signed it out, not that it was likely to be the right information anyway.

Irv called up Ed and Ken in Moses Lake—on his personal cell and theirs—and gave them a condensed report on where the investigation stood, leaving out the drama of the meeting with the director. He told them to be careful discussing this case with anyone since it seemed like political higher-ups were looking for someone to blame. It was true enough, he thought. He also asked Ed if he could quietly locate the airport pool truck and use his detector to check for the presence of the potato masking agent. Irv was sure that applying this was what was going on in the storage building near the airport.

Irv got the flight schedules for the twenty-four hours prior at Moses Lake Airport. He skipped over small planes, knowing that these would be even more difficult to trace, and focused instead on large cargo jets. There were twelve that landed over that night—from five different destinations: Memphis, Chicago, Dallas, Rapid City, LA, and Phoenix.

Irv was now running out of steam and packed up for an early departure. It was time to get home and catch up on his sleep—and let his subconscious take over the investigation. Putting his phone into its belt case, he stopped to review the photos he took the night before. Nothing seemed to pop from those, but he would download them on his personal computer at home so he could blow them up on his desktop screen and take a more thorough look.

There's got to be something I am missing, he thought. He had an itch in his gut that told him there was and that he just hadn't remembered it yet.

Chapter Twenty-Four

Early Mary Beth Collins

Mary Beth Collins was a local girl, born and raised in a small city north of Seattle called Edmonds, which was about a half-hour ride to downtown Seattle by car from her home—before the days of traffic gridlock on the interstate.

She was a third-generation Pacific Northwesterner. Grandpa Joshua Collins was a homesteader who settled on farmland west of Seattle, across the other side of Lake Washington. His father was a German migrant who had sought refuge from wars on the European continent by settling in western Pennsylvania. But Joshua found life hard in coal country too hard, and he ran off with his bride-to-be, Edith, when he was eighteen, seeking a better life in the still unsettled West.

Joshua and Edith did find life better in the Northwest, relatively speaking. The land was fertile, and drought was never a thought. They could grow enough fruit and vegetables on their land to feed their family, and supplemented this with salmon Joshua regularly caught in Lake Washington.

But farming was not all that profitable, and they were always on the brink of economic failure. The dark winters fed their depression, and cheap whiskey made Joshua a mean drunk. On particularly bad nights, he was prone to beating his wife, and sometimes the kids.

He would feel shame the next morning, but could not give up the bottle. Mary Beth had limited memories of Grandpa; he had died when she was only five. She overheard a conversation between her parents when she was a teenager and realized that he had killed himself. He had done so with a shotgun, she learned later.

Joshua and Edith raised three children, and lost two more in childbirth. Mary Beth's dad, Francis, was the youngest child, three years younger than his next closest sibling, a sister named Sarah. Oldest son Frank was a year older than Sarah. He had been drafted at the outset of WWII and died in combat on a small island in the Pacific called Peleliu.

Francis was too young to be drafted; he was barely sixteen when the Japanese surrendered. He joined the war effort by working at a shipyard on the Seattle shore of Lake Washington, ferrying to the job after school and putting in a twelve-hour shift. He found purpose in his work and preferred it to toiling on the family farm with his mom and sister.

After high school, he accepted a full-time job in the shipyard. Military craft were no longer needed, but there was a new appetite for boats for commercial and personal use, and the yard refitted its product for the burgeoning economy of postwar America.

Francis was a hard worker. He also had an aptitude for business. The owner of the family business admired these qualities, but it was Francis's courting of his daughter Mary that put him under his wing. They wed the year after the war and began to raise a family north of Seattle.

Three sons later, Francis and Mary brought Mary Beth into the world. Mary was happy; she wanted a girl badly after three sons. Francis looked at a girl child as a disappointing second choice. He had made a deal with their obstetrician that he would pay double for a son and nothing for a girl.

Mary Beth sensed her second-class status within the family. It wasn't that she wasn't loved by her mom and dad; there were just few expectations for her. It was assumed her brothers would go into the family business—by now Francis had become the president of the shipyard business—or go to college. Francis set up trusts for the brothers—they would advance within the company or contribute to society in other ways.

Mary Beth had no trust or career plan. Her lot was to find a husband, settle down, and produce grandkids. It mattered little that she, not her brothers, had inherited her dad's acumen for business and organization. No, her parents' dream was that she would produce grandsons, nothing more.

She had options, if that was to be the case. She was an attractive young woman, slim and athletic, about five-foot-four with blue eyes and light brown hair. Introverted but friendly, she always shared a smile with others. She was a bit of a late bloomer and was growing curves in all the right places when she graduated high school. Suitors would have been easy to find. She was not so interested in that, however. She had nothing against boys—she liked them a lot—there were just other priorities in her life.

Mary Beth took a job in the office at the shipyard, working for her dad. She also signed up for classes at a local community college: typing and speed reading. She lived at home and seemed cheerful enough to most. Quietly, she was struggling to find her way.

She found the office work at the shipyard to be the most interesting part of her days. Seated in the central office, she was able to observe how an organization like this ran. The managers who led the personnel, finance, purchasing, sales, and other functions were ready to share with her what they did and how they did it.

She also got to meet those who came to the office for meetings, since she served as the de facto receptionist for the company. She would set up clients, consultants, or other visitors in a conference room with coffee, and talk with them while they waited for their meetings. Mary Beth enjoyed learning what they did.

Her frustration peaked when she talked to her best friend from high school on the phone. She was attending the University of Washington and shared her experiences with Mary Beth. It was a life Mary Beth wanted, and she began to visit her friend at the University on weekends.

It was a ten-minute bus ride to get there. Her parents objected to her going, but couldn't stop her. Sometimes she would stay overnight in the dormitory so she could go to parties with her friend. Others were glad to have her around, especially the young men, who were enticed by her good looks. She was shy, but pleasant to talk with and curious about others.

More and more she pondered how to get closer to this university life, and began to hang out regularly in the community just beyond the university. The University District neighborhood was connected but separate, with many former or non-students living close to the school, not for its classes or structure or degrees, but for its ability to gather around a bohemian culture.

There were movies and taverns and concerts and informal gatherings of all sorts, open to whoever wanted to join in the fun. Some were local like Mary Beth, while others were from across the United States or the world with stories completely unlike hers. She soon formed a circle of friends in the University District and spent most of her free time there, much to her parents' chagrin.

By the summer, she had had enough of their complaints and announced she would be moving out. She would rent a room in an old Victorian home on a corner lot a half mile north of the University. Adjacent from a city park, it was once an estate for university professors.

She didn't tell her parents it was coed; that would have given them a collective stroke. They were angry enough as it was and threatened to cut off her tuition at the community college and take away her job at the family company. So be it, she told them. Grabbing a suitcase stuffed with a few personal possessions, she left that night.

Mary Beth needed to find a new job now that she was unemployed. When walking the main avenue in the District, she saw a "Help Wanted" sign at a bakery. They were looking for a waitress and could only pay minimum wage. She took the job.

When she wasn't working, life for Mary Beth soon revolved around the people coming and going at the group home. The prime tenants were a couple who were living together in the large upstairs suite. They were older and with more substantial employment. They made enough to pay the bulk of the rent and rented rooms to people they found interesting. Mary Beth had met the woman, Tina, at an experimental college class on yoga.

Roommates came and went over the five years that Mary Beth lived in the group home. The longest tenured roommate other than her was a man who moved in about a year after she did. He was from the East Coast—a tall and engaging man with fiery red hair and a long beard. Johnny Gibson was his name, and the two became fast friends.

Mary Beth loved her new life. She was learning, having fun, and setting a different course for her life. Still, she didn't have major ambitions. She enjoyed her newfound freedom but didn't have great confidence in her abilities to do more than be a bit player in the stories and success of others. She was content to live her life in this interesting home, with interesting people. She could have done much more, but had not the confidence to believe it was possible.

Nor did she have a plan, other than to not be what her parents wanted. For the time being, it was enough that she was content and on another path. When she did think about what she might want to do with her life, she would imagine a mid-level management position in a progressive business. She was fascinated with how organizations ran and had even taken a few experimental college classes on the theory of organizations. Maybe she could, someday, become part of one and contribute in a useful way.

Tina encouraged her to explore her interests. One night Tina told Mary Beth that someday she would run the company of her dreams. Mary Beth laughed. Imagine that. Sure, a woman. An introverted woman. Everyone knew that leadership positions were meant for extroverts, and usually men.

Tina tried to convince her that she had the potential to lead, but Mary Beth was having none of that. Tina saw it would require a different approach to crack Mary Beth's lack of confidence in herself, so she convinced her to volunteer at a local women's shelter, a group home for domestic abuse victims. The home didn't charge the women, and needed funds and an organization to maintain what they were doing; the demand for the service was far more than anyone thought.

Mary Beth helped organize a concert to support the shelter. It was a success, and others were impressed by her natural abilities to organize an event. They asked her to become one of the board members of the shelter when they formed a not-for-profit organization that would allow it to sustain and grow. She believed in the cause and took great pride in how she had uniquely contributed to it. Mary Beth started to believe a bit more in herself and her abilities.

Another opportunity soon arose at the bakery. She had been working there for several years, and the owners asked her to supplement her waitressing by helping with office functions. They were hoping to grow the company and needed some help. They knew she had been studying management at the community college, and part of their idea was to grow a not-for-profit cause through the bakery. They thought her experience with the women's shelter would be helpful.

Mary Beth greatly enjoyed her new duties and learning firsthand the complexities of starting up an organization. The not-for-profit issues were particularly fascinating, though many of the questions about this were beyond her or others in the bakery.

The owners were looking for consultants to provide advice. Mary Beth remembered meeting a woman who ran a consulting company back when she was at her dad's business. The woman had a range of clients, including political campaigns and not-for-profits. The mix fascinated Mary Beth then, as much as she understood it.

The woman was there to meet with Mary Beth's father, who was being encouraged to run for a local political office. She came to the shipyard to interview him on behalf of the local chamber of commerce. Her name was Nancy Jones; she had given Mary Beth her business card and encouraged her to give her a call.

Mary Beth dug through her belongings and found the business card. She placed a call to Nancy and asked her if she would be interested in helping the bakery in its business venture.

"Maybe," said Nancy. "But let's discuss it over lunch."

Chapter Twenty-Five

Evidence in a Sock

Irv jolted upright in his bed and looked at the clock across the room; it took a few seconds for his vision to clear enough so that he could read the dial. It was ten minutes past three—earlier than he would like, for sure.

His awakening was caused by a recollection of that which had been forgotten. The lab report had made an off-hand reference to a piece of paper in the sock of the corpse. With all the hubbub of the potential SARS-like infection, and his quest to figure out the bigger "what is really going on here," this factoid had remained under the radar. At least his.

There must be something on that piece of paper for it to have been inserted there, and maybe it would be something useful to his investigation. His first instinct was to go online from his home computer into the Public Health database and see if there was a photo of the piece of paper in the case files. This would have created a record of entry into the Director's Office—and potentially by who and for what. He wasn't so sure that Director Welch was really looking at these reports, but he couldn't chance it. Phil Welch thought he was off the case and onto new things, and it was best for Irv to preserve this impression.

He also wondered whether the photo would even be there. Things attendant to this case had a habit of disappearing, like the corpse and seemingly anyone who really wanted to get to the truth. This piece of paper, and whatever was on it, would likely be another MIA data point.

He did remember who authored the lab report: Maxine Flores. Max was someone he knew, liked, and trusted. She started at the department a year after he did, and they had lunched several times. Max was a breast cancer survivor, and he had reached out to her when this scourge had invaded his adult life. He now hoped she could be helpful again by telling him what was on the piece of paper found in the sock—or other useful information that might not be in the report.

Max was surprised to find Irv waiting outside her cubicle when she arrived at 7:45 a.m. "Hey, sport. Long time no see. I don't recall you being an early riser or, should I say, one to get into the office at this early hour. How is Mary Beth doing? And you?"

Irv smiled at Max. She knew him well enough. "We got through the worst of it, I hope. But not out of the woods yet, as you would know. I'd like to find some time to chat with you about that. Right now, I've got a deadline, and some questions about the lab report you prepared last week on that SARS-like incident. I was wondering if there were any details that were not part of the official report?"

Max could see that Irv was focused on a work task, and shifted her focus to last week's report. "I was a bit surprised by some things about that report, and I will feel better sharing whatever I got with you. This dude in a suit came by after I issued it and insisted on reviewing the full record—and he took some of it away with him, mumbling something about national security. Bridgestone, or something like that, was his name."

"I have met Mr. Bridgewater. What did he take?" asked Irv.

"All of the physical evidence. There were a few pieces of clothing and such that we use to cross-check our lab analysis and samples. He said that the CDC was taking possession of the body and that he needed everything that wasn't just our analysis."

"Did it include the piece of paper noted in the footnote of the report?" Irv's mind was ringing like a fire alarm.

"As a matter of fact, yes. Glad to see you are a thorough reader of my reports. Most wouldn't have noticed the reference. That federal guy did too, though. He told me that since he had possession of the paper, I should amend the report and delete mention of it. Said it in a way that was short of an order, but it sure seemed like a threat underneath it all. If you read a later version of the report, you won't even see the piece of paper mentioned."

"That matches my dealings with him too. Kind of why I am privately asking about this now. It would probably be smart for you to do everything he asks. And you won't want to say anything about me asking you about it. Here's what I really want to know though: was there anything on that paper?"

"Yes, and when I turned it over to Agent Vader or whoever he is, I took another look and memorized what was on it. It was a series of numbers and letters. A64172XC. There was some writing above it—it looked like Spanish—but it was pencil and so smudged and compromised by the water that got into his shoes and socks, I couldn't read it."

"Any idea what the number means?"

"Nope. Not a clue. And happy to know that you will figure that out. But let's have lunch soon. I miss our chats."

Irv gave Max a hug and headed to the coffee shop on the corner outside of the public health building for a cappuccino. He sipped on it while staring at the numbers in his notepad. A64172XC. What did it mean? He hoped it was something and that he could figure it out. He couldn't think of any other way to go further with this investigation. And he was getting surer and surer that it was important for him to do so.

Chapter Twenty-Six

2020: HealthMost Board Meeting

"Do I have a second for the motion to approve the financial report for last quarter?" queried board chair John Holmstrom as he scanned the faces of his fifteen fellow members of the HealthMost Board of Trustees. They were assembled at the plush corporate headquarters of the corporation in downtown Chicago. The view out the large windows in the penthouse boardroom on the 96th story gave one the sense of looking at the Atlantic Ocean on one side and the Rocky Mountains on the other. In reality, it was Lake Michigan to the east, and the only mountain in sight was Mount Trashmore, a local dump that had ascended to such heights that Chicagoans renamed it a mountain.

"I second the motion," said Meredith Johnson, a longtime board member and former head of a southeastern natural gas company. She was appointed to the board as she was leaving her CEO position, just before the company declared bankruptcy and left creditors, employees, and regulators grabbing at straws to reconcile debts. She was now board treasurer of HealthMost. "Shall we also call the question?"

"Not so fast" came a voice from the far end of the rectangular oak table. It was Frank LeClair, the consumer representative of the board. One year into his three-year term, he had been hesitant to say much at board meetings, and sensed that his fellow board members and management preferred it that way.

Frank had only been appointed on advice from corporation counsel that the organization's status as a not-for-profit corporation under federal, state, and local law would be more secure. Millions of dollars were at stake with that legal designation, so the board's nominating committee accepted the intrusion of Frank's sort into their club. They were less interested in hearing from him during meetings or otherwise.

"I still have not heard an acceptable answer to my question about the revenues and expenses in Footnote Twelve."

"I thought that this was suitably explained by Mr. Goldwin. And we have too much to do rather than reconciling every line item in the corporate financials." Chair Holmstrom was also a retired CEO, of a local telecommunications company created by the breakup of Ma Bell in the 1970s, and he was used to having his way in meetings.

"Mr. Goldwin only said that management was working on a special project to implement the new value purchasing arrangement with ALI Insurance. He didn't explain why there were several million dollars in cash payments required to do this," said Frank.

"Well, I found it to be more than an adequate explanation. We know there are things that need to be done to make that contract work. It involves perhaps a billion dollars of potential revenue, and the footnote you are questioning is budget dust in terms of the scale of that contract and its net earnings impact." To be sure, even a million dollars was a microbe of cost for HealthMost, a national health care system with holdings and contracts in almost every state in the nation. "I also did not recognize you, and we are indeed calling the question. All in favor of accepting the report signify by saying aye."

Fourteen ayes reverberated across the room, and Frank was left to abstain from his assent to the board action. "So noted" was the best he could get from his questioning of Footnote Twelve.

"Next up is a report from our CEO Performance Review and Compensation Committee. Meredith, can you present a summary of the committee's meeting? Materials supporting this item are attached to your agenda under Appendix VIII. I must remind board members that this is confidential and privileged information and is not to be shared with any person outside of the board of directors." Holmstrom glanced toward Frank pointedly.

Meredith was anxious to get to her report. The sooner the board finished their work today, the sooner she could shop on Chicago's Miracle Mile. There wasn't much in the way of high-end shopping when one lived in Selma, Alabama, even if you had the resources to buy expensive things, as she did. She also was looking forward to getting ready for the board's reception at the Chicago Lyric Opera, to be followed by VIP seating for the performance that evening.

"Mr. Chair, our Review and Compensation Committee met with Mr. Thrust and reviewed his goals and performance for the year. We found that he had another excellent year, as evidenced by the profits we just reviewed in the Financial Reports." HealthMost ran an operating margin of 11 percent for the past year, and a total margin of over 18 percent. "A written performance review is included in the materials in the Appendix. We are recommending to the board that you accept our finding of outstanding performance by Mr. Thrust and the payout of his bonus attached to this finding per his employment contract. Additionally, we are recommending that we extend an offer to Mr. Thrust to renew his contract for another five years. The draft terms and agreement are also included in your materials."

"Thank you, Meredith. Board members, do you have any questions for Mrs. Johnson?"

Several questions were asked by various board members. Frank concluded that these softball questions were planted and intended to make the coming action a simple and fast conclusion. After ten minutes of declarations of how fortunate HealthMost was to have Richard Thrust at the helm, Frank raised his hand.

"Yes, Mr. LeClair. Do you have a question?" asked Chair Holmstrom.

"No, more of a statement."

There was no denying the glare from Holmstrom, Mr. Thrust, and almost everyone else in the room. The others did not have much interest in his thoughts on this matter—or really any matter—but Frank knew it was his right to speak up and decided it was necessary in this case.

"I find it hard to conclude that we had such a stellar performance as a company when our board review comes through summary financial statements and special topic management reports. Moments ago I was told that my questions about even one footnote were inappropriate. This has been the pattern I've experienced since my board appointment last year. So, maybe we did have a great last year, but I can't be sure of that, other than to agree that, yes, our profits were very large. However, I am not sure that this is the ultimate test for any health care organization, let alone one registered as a charity in order to maintain its not-for-profit tax status."

Chair Holmstrom interrupted. "We discussed this at our last meeting, and I believe the rest of the board would agree that your point of view is not one held by others. I don't think there is any doubt that HealthMost had a tremendous performance last year and that Mr. Thrust's leadership was essential to that performance. We voted on the former at our last meeting, and today's report is to support the action of ensuring that Mr. Thrust will remain at the helm of HealthMost for the foreseeable future."

Frank knew his questions about valuing corporate performance were shot down by the full board at the last meeting, but he was not going to let go of today's implications without a fight. "Yes, you are correct that we moved forward with this thinking at the last meeting. But today's conclusion is not only that we approve an $8 million bonus to Mr. Thrust, on top of his annual salary of $5 million, but that we extend his contract with a raise of $2.5 annually and bonus provisions that could pay out as much $20 million over the next five years. To me, that just seems excessive for any health care organization and, again, certainly for a charity."

Chair Holmstrom glared down at the end of the table toward Frank. "Meredith, I know that your committee spent much time reviewing the basis for Mr. Thrust's compensation and came to this recommendation through that and meeting with Mr. Thrust. Could you review that for Mr. LeClair and other board members?"

Meredith reviewed materials in the Appendix, emphasizing a compensation survey for the industry and comparable organizations that suggested Mr. Thrust would be in the top 25 percent quartile of compensation among his peers. She noted how fortunate they were to have Mr. Thrust and that it was essential to compensate him at a level that prevented him leaving for greener pastures.

Frank knew these surveys were provided by management, and they might even be accurate. His point was that the compensation for Thrust's peers was also excessive. He knew this was not likely to generate much sympathy within a board filled with current or former chief executives who were paid these salaries at some point in their career, or hoped for the same.

Chair Holmstrom turned to his left to the object of the discussion, president and CEO of HealthMost Corporation, Richard J. Thrust. "Richard, it seems only fair that we get your thoughts on this. I would like to congratulate you on another stellar performance. I believe that the full board is prepared to extend our offer to you with the great hope that you will agree to be our CEO for another five years. Perhaps you can shed some light on today's discussion and help convince anyone who might be hesitant to agree that they are mistaken?" That he was looking intently at Frank as he made the last statement was not lost on anyone in the room, certainly not Frank.

"Thank you, John." Richard J. Thrust stood as he addressed the board. He was a large man, bulky and closer to fat than athletic in physical presence. At sixty-eight, he tried to use his size to intimidate others, though all knew he would never get his hands dirty. He would harm people in his own way though—and everyone knew that.

Employees who disagreed would be escorted from the building with a HealthMost security guard. Volunteers, like disaffected board members, would find a similar, though more intricately constructed fate.

Thrust wasn't a handsome man to look at—pale white, balding, and with a prominent nose and largish ears. His brown eyes were set high on his forehead, much like a crow. Beauty was not how he had made his way through the past forty years of conquest. He did dress up for his part, almost always wearing expensive Italian three-piece suits. He always wore a suit when in the office, once in a while removing the jacket, but not the vest.

Calculating, always contemplating new ways to advance his interests, Thrust considered his brain his greatest asset and thought himself the smartest person in the world. If there was any doubt, all you had to do was ask him.

He was also socially awkward. Colleagues, classmates, and even those he considered to be his friends found him aloof and arrogant. He didn't care about these assessments. All that mattered were results.

He had achieved these results in his long health care career—making money for him and his employers on a grand scale. This only fed his confidence in his abilities and his view that the ends justify the means. Forty years later he found himself at the top of one of the largest health care organizations in the world, and one of the largest in any industry in America. To him, his perch was well deserved.

He thought it only the beginning of his conquests. As the nation's economy shifted from a manufacturing base to services, with health care at the top of the service pyramid, he saw himself a titan of the nation and world, on par with the Fords, Rockefellers, and Carnegies of the early twentieth century. No, better than even them.

It was time to put the matter of his value to rest quickly at this board meeting. "As Mrs. Johnson noted, my compensation level is set by comparison to my peers. I don't think there is any question that HealthMost is the leading health care system in the nation, thanks to my leadership and the changes we have made during my time as CEO. The truth is that I should not be paid on the basis of top quartile salary comparisons, but at the top of the compensation level. It is my gift to you to be willing to do this job at reduced compensation. If that isn't enough of a sacrifice for you, then I will need to make some other choices." Thrust was scanning the room as he stood in place and spoke, his eyes looking at and through each of the board members with a haughty stare.

"Rather than waste time reviewing my compensation, I suggest we use our board time to review the top tier strategies that I am deploying to increase our market share. For example, our joint venture relationship with ALI Insurance will bring significantly more money and control to HealthMost Corporation. This is on today's agenda. I, and only I, can successfully identify and implement strategies like this. So, if you want to waste your time reviewing me, go ahead. I find it tedious to even engage in these conversations with you. You do so at your peril—and I suggest we just move on."

That was that. The board, or fourteen of the fifteen members of it, understood it was time to move on. Frank wasn't convinced at all, but even he found it useless to dissent as the board unanimously accepted the committee's recommendation of a new contract for Richard Thrust.

Chapter Twenty-Seven

1960: The Jones and Medicare

As the 1960s began, Patrick Jones thought it unlikely he would ever see the Recommendations of the Committee of the Costs of Medical Care come to fruition. He was about to turn sixty-five, with at most another five years left in his career. Patrick was already turning over projects that he once would have coveted to younger colleagues. He was willing to make one more run at a big health policy change like that offered by the committee, but it seemed more likely that his lot was now to turn over the health policy reins to the next generation of leaders.

The Age of More had continued to merrily roll along. Americans were generally happy. Postwar posterity had a long tail, and expanding the capacity to provide medical care to the American public was generally welcomed as a good thing. There were more hospitals, more practitioners, and more health insurance. Now 60 percent of the public had some form of coverage.

The Cold War was still a thing, though the vitriol of the McCarthy era was gone. The greatest national health concern was that nuclear war might wipe out much of the nation. Regular civil defense drills didn't fool many into believing that our defenses, or health care system, could save much of anyone if it came to that.

On the positive side, one could at least talk about social solutions to problems like health care without fear of being called a traitor. It just didn't seem that there was much reason to do so since there was such little appetite for overturning the status quo.

Patrick had enjoyed a stellar health policy career, advising and influencing policy makers on American health policy and contributing greatly to the Age of More. He took pride in what he had done, but still regretted the failure to do more about the overall dysfunction of the American health system.

The Committee on the Cost of Medical Care had described it as not even a system in 1932; now, a system had accreted into place over forty years of disparate health policy. But these policies did little to resolve the problems with the overall system; in many ways, they only made the system more dysfunctional as a whole, no matter what their discrete policy benefits.

Patrick had hope for the future, though. It was how he was wired. He could also see a new wave of those who might solve the fundamental problems of the health care system, including his eldest son, Christopher.

This seed had been sown for quite a while. Patrick had learned from his parents how to proselytize at the family dining room table. They emphasized to him in his childhood how family members must repay their debt of gratitude to America. Patrick did the same as a dad in nightly sermons to his children. His message had gotten through to Chris.

Christopher was a keen listener at these dinnertime talks. He was a quiet boy, accepting of the premise of service, and more interested in the details of whatever Patrick was discussing than generalities or political barriers. How would we do that? Why was whatever a certain way? Could the change be put into place practically? Patrick used to joke that Chris was the most talented policy analyst in the family as just a child. The joke had given way to reality.

Patrick nurtured Chris's natural interest and abilities. He encouraged his studies and directed him to the best classes in preparation for becoming a policy leader. Patrick was working at one of the leading policy institutions in the nation in Harvard, and he regularly brought his son to work. From the time he could walk, Chris would sit in on meetings, lectures, and conversations with Patrick's colleagues at Harvard. By the time he was a teenager, faculty members considered Chris to be another member of the Harvard family.

It was no surprise when Chris attended Harvard as an undergraduate, or that he graduated in the top 10 percent of his class. He was sharp as a Bowie knife and had the curiosity and drive to be an extraordinary student. Nor was it all that surprising that he attended law school after college. Legal training seemed like an excellent way to sharpen his already superb analytic skills, as his father had done before him.

It raised eyebrows when he attended Georgetown Law School. Most thought that more of Harvard would be coming. Following in his dad's footsteps at Georgetown made the move seem less bold, and Chris explained the choice by his need to find a school where he could double in advanced health care studies. Through special arrangements with the deans of both schools, he was allowed to also take classes in the Georgetown School of Public Health and attain a graduate degree in public health along with his juris doctorate.

The greater reason was a deal he had made with his dad when he turned eighteen. Patrick would help Chris get into Harvard as a long-term career proposition but only if Chris went to a school outside of Boston first and got experience working in the actual delivery of health care to people.

Going to school at Georgetown had satisfied condition one. For the second, Christopher chose to learn about health care delivery at the nation's Veteran's Administration as he graduated with joint degrees from Georgetown. He was chosen for a two-year administrative residency with the chief executive officer of Walter Reed Hospital in DC.

Shadowing the CEO, Chris saw up close and personal what it took to run a major health care institution. He was regularly brought into the daily intrigues of running this hospital, and worked on a series of special project assignments related to clinical and administrative challenges.

Meanwhile, Chris also got a healthy dose of how American government worked. The VA was always in the midst of a national health policy controversy, and the CEO of Walter Reed was in the middle of the political response within the agency. There were special project assignments galore for Chris in this realm too.

Chris proved to be most capable in fulfilling the assignments in both the institutional and policy arenas—so much so that he was offered a job as Director of Planning for Walter Reed at the close of his internship.

He served in this capacity for three years, and ably so. In 1960, he also got involved in the national presidential election. He wasn't a fan of politics, but knew the Kennedys from his time at Harvard. The thought of an Irish Catholic progressive being president intrigued him, and he became a foot soldier in candidate John F. Kennedy's run to succeed President Eisenhower.

Christopher was noticed during the campaign by key aides to the candidate, mostly through invites to campaign parties. When President Kennedy assumed office, these same folks were now transition advisors to the president, and Patrick was offered a job in the national health agency, the Department of Health Education and Welfare, more simply called HEW. In 1961, he became the Assistant Secretary for Policy and Planning, advising the secretary on how to improve American health care.

Chris quickly took to this job, much like his dad had when opportunity arose. The challenges were interesting and the possibilities endless. Patrick was a regular source of advice to Christopher, though by then Chris was building his own intellectual arsenal on the health care issues of the time.

The murder of President Kennedy was a harsh blow to Chris's confidence and place. It was a stunning event in its own right, shocking the nation. Added to Chris's angst was seeing how intent the incoming administration of Lyndon Baines Johnson was to change things across government, including at the upper levels of HEW. Christopher was technically a civil servant but practically a political appointee, and was asked to step aside because of his perceived loyalties to the Kennedys.

It confused Chris as much as it angered him because President Johnson had declared his intent to pursue major policy change in consonance with what Christopher believed in—something akin to the programs and laws of FDR's New Deal.

President Johnson called the policy change his Great Society, and it included efforts on civil rights, voting, housing, a war on poverty and, yes, national health insurance. Chris was well versed in the CCMC and its Recommendation 3. He and his father were excited to see another major opportunity for its adoption and were plotting how Chris could help move this along in his leadership role at HEW. It was a stunning setback for both of them when he was asked to leave the agency, and for imaginary political reasons.

Chris moved back to Boston, sensing that he had been branded an outcast in DC purely because of his political affiliation with the Kennedys. He accepted an adjunct professor position within the Harvard Medical School, a new position that his dad worked to create for him, teaching health policy, much like his father had done years before. Patrick had honored his deal with Chris, just when his son most needed a helping hand.

Patrick welcomed his son's return to Boston. While Chris was in DC, his father had been able to visit him on a fairly regular basis since trips to the Capitol were an important part of Patrick's role as Director of Policy at the Medical School. But it couldn't beat the regular contact of living in the same city, and especially not working at the same school and department.

For Chris, it was a soft landing after his political disappointment. Even better, he found a new way to engage in his interest in national health care reform. Working together, he and Patrick injected Harvard's voice into the need for the Great Society to include key CCMC ideas in its social reforms. Top on the list was a health coverage program covering all Americans. Chris and his dad were both excited by the prospects for it.

Disappointment on this front soon followed, and again for political reasons. Advisors of the Great Society quickly shifted the aim of national health insurance from protection and health for all to a more targeted and incremental focus on constituencies in need. President Johnson was a congressional deal maker. This was where he had gotten his power in the United States Senate. Already embroiled in a big political fight with Southern democrats over civil and voting rights, he targeted his health care solutions to the elderly.

What followed was the passage of Medicare in 1965: a national program of health coverage for the elderly and the disabled, funded largely by a payroll tax on workers and companies. It was accompanied by targeted efforts to provide the poor some health care too, as a supplement to their welfare benefits. Medical Assistance, or Medicaid, was created to do this through a federal matching grant program to states willing to provide care for the poor within federal standards.

Patrick and Chris agreed that this legislation was important and good in its own right, probably an earth-shattering advance for older Americans, who were more at risk of disease and most likely to not have coverage to help pay for medical diagnosis and treatment. Yet, they could also see it was another lost opportunity in the bigger picture—it did not create something to cover all Americans.

What's more, they feared it would further erode the efficacy of the American health care system. Medicare would overnight become the largest bloc of covered patients in the United States. What the government decided to do in terms of implementation would affect the overall system greatly, and perhaps not for the better.

No one was sure where the Johnson Administration was headed with this implementation—their focus had been on the congressional fight to pass legislation. The new law creating Medicare was not all that detailed; it was a series of amendments to the Social Security Act. HEW had been given broad direction and a lot of discretion to build this new program into the government and the American health system.

Early on, Christopher could see that the approach and scale might make the overall health system even more complex and fragmented, rather than simpler. When Blue Cross and Blue Shield plans became fiscal intermediaries for managing Medicare and paying providers, thereby inexorably altering their original identity as local health community organizers, he was sure of it.

Patrick decided he'd seen enough of the same old health policy act, and chose to retire. He would do what he could to help push American health policy forward, but from a new perch—his home. He would clear the deck at Harvard so his son Christopher could grab the policy leadership stick from him and take the fight forward.

Christopher was as ready as anyone could be for this challenge. Well steeped in policy and bruised by politics, he thought the big problem of system inaction must be attacked in a new way.

There was a way built in to what would come next from the passage of Medicare, he thought—the tremendous cost of the new program. Congress had largely ignored this with lowball financial estimates. Chris saw it would require a massive infusion of federal resources. It wasn't clear that the payroll tax could foot the program's bill when it was fully implemented, and he was sure it couldn't come close in its early years before the tax revenue could even be collected.

He also figured that the cost of this would soon become a political controversy. His dad reminded him that it was the high cost of care, in 1927, that had triggered the CCMC study. Now, there would be several more zeroes added to those early cost projections. Chris needed to be ready when the cost problem hit the fan this time around.

It would mean finding ways to control the costs of Medicare, and perhaps all of American health care. There were ways to do this, he thought, even with the hodge-podge of federal health policy that had accumulated over the previous thirty years. Most important, he believed, was to reframe the context of the debate to a quest for system-wide solutions. Away from the postwar emphasis on More and toward a perspective that managing scarce resources in a rational way was the nation's new health policy imperative.

This would be the next era of American health policy, and Christopher would be ready to be a leading voice in it. His aim was to create a moderation in costs and make health care more affordable for Americans—one of the principal aims of CCMC. But also to use this platform to build a rational and far more effective health care system in America. The CCMC Recommendations would be his guiding light.

Chapter Twenty-Eight

Irv Contemplates Evidence in a Sock

The more Irv stared at the number written on the sock of his mystery corpse, the more mystified he became. Eight digits. A combo of numbers and letters. It was not a social security number—too short and it had more than numbers. And it was too long for a license plate, at least for the states he knew about. He would do a national search to make sure.

Maybe it was a banking number? A personal password? A product ID number? A case number for an investigation by some civil or criminal authority? Coordinates for some mapping approach that he was not aware of?

He did a Google search of the number, but nothing showed up. He then did a random search of numbers and letters. Among the possibilities to appear were special codes for various purposes. Maybe that was what this was. It would certainly fit with something stashed in a special hiding place like a sock. But it seemed a bit odd to find on a corpse. The dead man also looked like an itinerant laborer, and Irv couldn't imagine a use for such a code.

Why was the number in his sock? What did the smudged words above it say? Who was this man? Why was he found dead in a cabin in Kent, Washington, with indications of a contagion that wasn't? Why did he have potato derivatives on him from an antiquated masking agent used decades ago?

None of it made sense. But it was something, to be sure. Otherwise, why would there be an effort to contain this situation by higher-ups in the government? Exactly which one he wasn't sure, but Irv could smell a cover-up like a mouse smells cheese.

Maybe he should just let it go, he thought. There was plenty to keep him busy at work, and personally. Digging into this might cause him to lose his job—maybe worse. Why was he always getting into these difficult choice situations?

He knew the answer to the last query—because he could handle it. What was the old adage—God only gives you the challenges that he knows you are up to? Irv had faced many in his life and career. People telling him that to take one road would be folly. Impossible or a dead end for him or his career. For whatever reason, he liked to think he made his choices based on his manifest destiny to pursue what was truthful and right, not what was easy.

Most times, his choice proved to be the right one. Though sometimes he would have a long wait to see that in any evidentiary way beyond his own confidence. His wait was still on within the Public Health Department over his last rogue operation—his taking up the dirty restaurant problem had uncovered a major public health problem but had left him with a personnel file that seemingly had "troublemaker" stamped on the top.

Quietly bowing out of this search was not in his cards, so he continued to ponder the eight digits. Nothing was coming to him. He checked in with friends who were savvy in the ways and technologies of the world. Without getting into the why of the number set or even the actual numbers, he asked about such a thing. They couldn't think of anything either, though some had new ideas—a passport number for some country, a ticket number, a secret government ID number for the CIA. It was possible that the latter was it—but he really had no way of confirming that!

Unfortunately, Irv had other things to do, including a couple of old assignments at work. He spent most of his time reviewing what he knew about this suspicious death and cover-up. Maybe there was something else he was forgetting? Was this number the only way forward? If it was, its nature or origins would need to get figured out. Maybe it would happen through the magic of an open mind. This was part of his method to impossible choices in the past—a belief that things will work out in the cosmic order.

Tuesday became Wednesday, and Wednesday turned to Thursday. Nothing was hitting, on the numbers or the case. Patience would be necessary, it seemed, and patience was not his strong suit.

Irv awoke on Friday morning and went into the office early. He needed to take a long lunch for his annual physical examination. Mary Beth had been the one to prod him to set personal health goals, and this annual get-together with his primary care provider was part of his method. He spent some time in the office in the morning filling out a "What the Doctor Should Order" form so he could take control of the exam.

He walked to the clinic in the International District of South Seattle around 11 a.m.; it was about ten blocks from his office. He handed the receptionist his form, as she handed him his. They would both need to get ready for the exam. "And I will need a copy of your health coverage card too," she added. Irv got his insurance card out of his leather wallet. There it was, plain as day. The mysterious number was an insurance number!

Chapter Twenty-Nine

Young Johnny Goes to Congress

John Gibson became a United States Congressman in January of 1985. In the same election, President Ronald Reagan easily won reelection to his second term. Johnny was headed to DC. in the middle of the Reagan Revolution.

That revolution didn't matter much to him. Really, little about American political life did. This was not your normal first term congressperson. Johnny Gibson had hit the mother lode, as far as he was concerned. He was now a congressman and on his way to Washington, DC, for his next adventure, courtesy of the United States taxpayer. It amused him that he would be paid for this gig.

Money was not what he was after. Rather, it was adventure, and especially people to meet along the way. That this was the perfect spot for him was confirmed quickly. Most of the role was meeting and talking to people. Every day was filled with appointments, many with constituents who wanted to bend the ear of their new congressional representative. Johnny enjoyed these meetings; they provided a slice of the life experience of others to add to his own. It didn't matter what they might ask him to do—that was a whole other deal than learning of their issues and lives.

Other meetings were with lobbyists from a wide assortment of corporations, associations and other groups—an A to Z cornucopia of special interests looking for favor from him. It was obvious to even him that most were sending their lower rung of advocates rather than their heavy hitters to these meetings.

Johnny was a freshman congressman—an independent, no less—with no seniority. Few in political circles believed he could win reelection, since it seemed a lark he was voted in the first time. Why would any of them invest in him as an asset to their advocacy plans? None of this mattered to him—they were still interesting to meet, and he was learning much about life from them too.

It wasn't all roses though. Most distasteful to Johnny were the rules of Congress—and there were a shitload of them. He had spent his life ignoring or breaking rules, and it seemed strange that he would now bend his knee to a rulebook. At first, he resisted and broke the rules regularly. One day the House Parliamentarian walked into his office unannounced, sat down, and asked him what the hell he was doing.

They had a two-hour talk that afternoon, and it was one of the more important meetings of Johnny's career in Congress. The Parliamentarian told him that he was making a fool of himself, and for no good reason. Johnny fought back, saying that the rules were stupid and made it hard to produce legislation or anything else.

The Parliamentarian got up and threatened to slap him across his forehead. "Of course it makes it harder—the point is to make it hard to get something passed in Congress." He further explained that most of the ideas coming from its members were dumb or impractical, and that the brilliance of our parliamentarian system was that it made it really hard for these to get enacted into real law.

"Huh," said Johnny. "That changes things." The Parliamentarian encouraged Johnny to look at the rules not as a typical set of social boundaries that he had rejected most of his life, but as the rules for a board game like Monopoly. He should learn them, play within them, and above all else, look at them as just part of a game. Someday he would use them to do something he cared about, said the Parliamentarian. Johnny couldn't see that possibility very clearly, but that this was just a game appealed to him greatly. If so, this could be fun—play by the rules, he would.

The real downer was what his freshman classmates were sharing about their lives as new congresspersons. The party staff were orienting them to their new role, something Johnny did not have to suffer through since he was an independent. But they shared what these operatives were telling them—the job was 60 percent fundraising, and they needed to get on track with that right out of the legislative shoot.

His freshmen colleagues were told the first objective of their job, and maybe the only one, was to get reelected. Playing ball within party structures was one important ingredient. But the other, and bigger one, was to raise money for their reelection campaign. It was one thing to win a seat in Congress, and another to retain it. Millions would be needed, and they should devote at least two or three days out of every week to building a war chest of money. This would mean sucking up to rich people and organizations with major political dollars at their disposal, and worse yet, needing to show concern for their particular issues.

If this was a rule, it was one that Johnny was ready to break. If he ended up being a one-term congressman, so be it. He would cross the reelection challenge when it came upon him and, in the meantime, would devote almost all of his time to meeting with constituents and interest groups, whether they had money or not.

It didn't take long for Johnny's lack of power in the House to become clear to him. Others in Congress were ready to point it out to him if he didn't see it himself. Leaders of both parties were courting him to join their party, or at least caucus and vote with their side. They told him that being an independent was a lonely and weak place to be. "Just look at the piece-of-shit office you were assigned," they said.

That it was, agreed Johnny. His committee assignments were even worse. He justified them by declaring that someone had to serve on the Post Office Committee—so why not him? His other committees weren't much better. Johnny figured this gave him more time to forge relationships within DC. While his counterparts were debating important national matters on C-SPAN, he would do what he came to do—meet with people.

He found this interesting and personally rewarding. Sure, there would be the occasional blowhard. Johnny would flip a mental switch in these meetings, imagining that he was writing a novel and that these asses were the villains in his story. Mostly, he met with people with real-life grievances and in need of help from somewhere—maybe from Congress, maybe not. He would always listen to their stories, letting their problems wash over him as a vicarious adventure.

Once in a while, Johnny found a way to be helpful—rarely with legislation, as he had little influence within the House or Congress as a whole, but a telephone call or a letter from a congressman, or even his office staff, did mean something in this town. He was at his most useful when these were issues brought to him by constituents, not interest groups. He began to build a capacity within his congressional office to intervene in their cases. That he could do.

Chapter Thirty

Irv Explores Insurance Numbers

Irv hoped his discovery that the number in the victim's sock was an insurance number would be the breakthrough he needed. But it wasn't like it was a complete answer to the many questions confronting him. If it was an insurance number, why was it hidden in a sock? What was its purpose? How could he find that out in the absence of even knowing who this person was? Nor did he have any way of knowing which of the hundreds of insurance companies the number might belong to. But it was something, and a lot more than he had other than his suspicions.

He thought about who might help him unravel the insurance number mystery and recalled that one of his classmates in the MHA program had gone to work for Group Health Cooperative and spent time working in its insurance arm. The Cooperative had tried to grow their influence and market share by introducing a variation from their staff model HMO product in areas of the state where they did not own facilities or employ physicians and other practitioners. The contracts they used to assure service to enrollees was much like a standard insurance offering. Managing this relationship was Irv's classmate's assignment.

Irv opened his alumni directory and found the entry for Antonio Sanchez. He tried the personal cell phone number listed, as he had a vague recollection of Antonio having left Group Health over the last few months. Something he had read in the alumni newsletter, or a comment from a mutual friend on the Seattle streets?

"Hello, this is Antonio."

Irv was pleased he had found him, and on one call.

"Antonio, Irv Tinsley here. Good to hear your voice. Hoping I can talk with you a bit about an insurance issue I am having and see if you can head me in the right direction." Irv thought it best not to connect his inquiry to a work investigation. "You always were the one in our class who seemed to understand this world best. Is this a good time?"

"Hey, Irv. This is a surprise. It's been a while. Glad to help you out, but right now I need to do a conference call for a client. You might have heard that I left Group Health this past summer. Started up a consulting practice on health insurance matters, and I've got to keep my customers happy. If they want to talk on a late Friday afternoon, that is what we will do! I can call you later this evening, or maybe we can get together tomorrow for coffee or something? Do you still live in north Seattle? I just bought a home there, and we might even be neighbors now."

"Yes, same place as where we had the party many years ago." Irv remembered that Antonio was there; it might have been the last time that they had spent much time together. "I am open tomorrow for whenever works for you. Maybe at the Starbucks off of Forty-fifth? Is that close to where you live now?"

"Only a mile away. Let's get together at ten. I've been telling myself that it is time to look up my old buddies. My new partners tell me that I need to work the Rolodex and get some clients into the firm if I want to carry my weight. You always knew a lot of the right people, or maybe you knew somebody who knew all the right people—wasn't it John Gibson who used to come hang out with us when he was in town?"

"The one and only. Ten it is."

"I'll be there. I got about a minute before I need to get on my call. What's the general topic for your insurance issue?"

"Insurance numbers. I have one and am trying to figure out how to track down some information about the policy and such."

"Sounds pretty dry for a guy like you. Why do I have a feeling that it will get way more interesting when we talk tomorrow."

Antonio was sitting at a table in the corner of the Starbucks, with a large mug of caffeine and a portable computer open on the table in front of him. It was one of the more private tables in the coffee shop, which was good because it was pretty busy on a gray Northwest Saturday morning. Irv waved, ordered up a grande latte and banana bread, and nestled in the chair next to Antonio once his order was filled.

The two classmates exchanged pleasantries and got reacquainted. They were good enough friends during the MHA program. After graduation, they continued to socialize, but these get-togethers faded as did so many others under the influence of distance and life demands.

Antonio was one of the few diverse students in the MHA program. The son of Panamanian parents who had moved to the Seattle area in the 1960s, he had spent all of his life in Seattle, so he mostly saw the world as a Seattleite. He had taken one trip to see his grandparents in Panama City back in the 1980s, and the extent of his diversity was mostly what he learned from his parents and the appearance his name and Latino looks got him.

Despite the school's attempt to add diversity to its student candidates, the MHA program classes were made up of mostly white students. Over 50 percent of these were women, as they were ahead of the curve on balancing the sexist ranks of health care leadership. Seattle, and the applicant pool to the program, was just too white to make a bold statement on racial and ethnic diversity. At least, that was the case with respect to Black and Hispanic applicants; there were a healthy number of entrants in the program from Asian descent.

Almost all of Antonio's classmates were welcoming and friendly, but he felt a stronger bond to Irv from the outset. They both did internships at Group Health their first summer in the program, and sharing a commute deepened their bond.

Irv was impressed when Antonio accepted a position as director of Insurance Marketing at Group Health on graduation. Group Health was very different from most health insurance companies, so diversity as a general matter was not a foreign concept. Their insurance division, needing to develop and sell a more conventional insurance product than their local HMO offering, was by necessity staffed mostly with folks from conventional insurance. There were lots of white men in starched white shirts trying to figure out what a Hispanic was and why he was managing them.

After about ten minutes of catching up, the two friends turned to the task at the heart of their meeting. Antonio kicked it off. "So, tell me more about your insurance issue."

Irv was far more comfortable getting into the details with Antonio now that they were face-to-face, and he had confirmed that Antonio was the man he had known for many years. "The truth of it is, Antonio, it isn't a personal health insurance issue. I just wasn't comfortable saying anything else on the phone. It is a matter related to a case I am investigating in the department. Probably the less you know about that the better, for you. What I can tell you is that I am trying to figure out why a public health victim might be carrying a number with him and holding it somewhat secretly. I think it is a health insurance number, but maybe I am even wrong about that."

"You can't ask your victim about this?" queried Antonio.

"I could, but he is too dead to answer."

"I had a feeling that was the case. Let's take a look at that number." Antonio was all in on helping Irv out. He could tell there was some risk to doing so, but trusted Irv to watch his back as much as he could.

Irv flipped open his small case notebook and thumbed through to the page where he had written "A64172XC" in large block writing. He put it down on the table in front of him and Antonio. The burnt notes of espresso beans wafted through the coffee shop, their odor adding to the air of mystery of the moment.

Antonio picked up the notebook and looked intently at the numbers. He put his right index finger to his chin, thinking hard. After about thirty seconds, he spoke up. "Yes, I think you are probably right that this is an insurance number, and maybe a health insurance number. Let me check a couple of things here before I say too much more though." With that, Antonio began to peck away at the keyboard of his personal computer.

It felt like far more than five minutes to Irv before Antonio said, "Again, this does look like an insurance number. The first problem is that there are almost six thousand insurance companies, and no easy way to confirm that it is a number used by any one of them. It is also possible that it is a company based out of the country. That is a pretty big 'n' for a search without any central landing place for inquiry. Insurance companies have been pretty smart—although you might call it something else—in ceding a regulatory role over their activities to government agencies and then capturing those agencies so that most of their business practices are hidden from the world. They also do this at the state level, so the local politics and variation only make it that much harder to find anything out.

"But the X is a clue that it is an insurance number. More likely a life or property or casualty insurer than a health care company. One of my projects for Group Health about five years ago was doing a review of potential competitors who might enter our market, and I got to know what was out there in the data world. That is how I know about the X—normal folks would not have a clue. The A64172 is likely a client identifier. Possibly a case number, but I would bet it is more likely an identifier of the policy holder. I don't have any idea what the C might mean—never seen that in my travels."

"Why would someone have a number like that on them?" asked Irv.

"It wouldn't normally be a surprise for it to be carried by someone. You carry around a card with your car insurance coverage, right? And a health insurance card? Never know when you might have to show it to someone when you leave home. A little more strange for a life insurance policy—those are normally attached to wills or in safe deposit boxes or otherwise to be found once a person dies."

"I guess it is possible he knew his life was in danger and wanted the policy information to be found if something happened," Irv said.

"That is possible. In fact, during WWII there were some less than patriotic life insurance companies that sold benefit packages to American GIs that would pay out far more than their government death benefits. Once they were killed in the battlefield, there was little evidence to confirm that they had bought the policy, and these companies were able to deny claims because of lack of confirmation of their coverage. It was such a lucrative practice that a couple of the companies started to sell special policies to immigrants into the United States. This time they used language gaps to confuse claims on benefits, but it was effective nonetheless. It wasn't as big a payout for them but a good enough business model. The investigation into all of this mostly got swept under the rug by the government; the whistleblowers who got it out into the open were fired, and little more was ever heard about it. All to say it is possible that your John or Juan Doe was trying to make sure his policy information would be found and paid on his death."

"Possible," countered Irv. "But that doesn't seem all that likely. By all external appearances he was an agricultural laborer. Legal or illegal, it is hard to imagine that he would have made enough to be able to afford a policy like that. Or, if somehow he got involved in an insurance scam, it would seem more likely that it would be some type of personal injury scam around automobile insurance."

"Makes sense, but why would he have a code on him hidden away? I have read about these scams, and the claims are usually asserted by a third party who groups these claims. Law firms, for example. They would be the ones who would want the number; the victims most likely just got some small cash settlement or bribe from the third party in exchange for assigning their rights and turning over their benefits."

Irv and Antonio looked at each other across the table in silence, both deep in thought. It felt good to ground the number in some possibilities, but the reality was that Irv was not much further along in being able to press his investigation. They both knew it.

"Let me try one other thing. It is a bit of a flyer, but who knows." Antonio went back to his personal computer, clacking away on the keys with far more strokes than his earlier search. He looked up at Irv. "We've got about a ten-minute wait to see if this works. Only worth explaining if I get a hit."

Irv nodded, and they resumed their catch-up on lives, wives, and automobiles, oh my, while Antonio occasionally glanced at his screen. About ten minutes later, he dove in for a longer look. A broad smile spread across his face as he looked at Irv. "You, my friend, have gotten lucky. I found your number!"

Antonio explained to Irv what he had done. It turned out that personal insurance information is private and protected, and that has great value. So, every once in a while some hacker or other opportunist figured out how to get access to them. Most of the data was held on private insurance company servers, with fifteen levels of security and almost no chance that it would be compromised. Breaking into Fort Knox and grabbing a few bars of gold would be easier.

There were major weaknesses introduced to this security when health care companies started to get into the insurance side of the world. These companies adopted all the requisite policies and signed all of the right pledges, but were far more sloppy in their execution in protecting client data. Over the course of the past decade, there had been dozens of major data breaches for health insurance, almost all from health care provider organizations who had diversified into insurance. Some were small, local breaches, and some were large and national in scope involving hundreds of thousands of people and millions in transactions. Most were the product of health care executives leaving their laptop on their car seat while running errands to or from work. Car thieves grabbed and go-ed, and then figured out they had something of great value on those computers. Others were a product of ransomware attacks; instead of millions in cash, some providers gave away client data instead to get back control over their systems.

A market developed as a way to translate the value of this stolen data into cash, through accumulators of the data. They made data available to any who were willing to pay for it. The scammers got scammed though, as an insider got control of the data and made it publicly available. In some cases, they were also able to continue to update their databases because of the unwillingness of those who breached data confidentiality to admit to it. The United States Government got involved immediately and protected these websites from any domestic access. But they went global, and there were international websites where one could still get access.

Antonio had done a search of one such international database that he knew about. The query had come back with a series of attached files.

"I don't know what is in these files, and I really don't want to open them while I am using public Wi-Fi. How about we go by your house and I directly transfer them onto your computer? But only if you promise to someday tell me what this is all about."

"I promise. Though if something happens to me, you might have to find my body and look in my sock to try to find out how to learn more." Irv was joking. Sort of. Whatever this was, there was a good chance that there was something on one of those files worth knowing. It was something that very important people, in the government or subject to its directives, didn't want others to know.

Chapter Thirty-One

Early Richard Thrust

Richard Thrust hung up the telephone and rocked back in his leather desk chair. He pivoted his large body and cast his oddly shaped head toward the massive window behind his desk. Chicago's waterfront stretched in a line before him, and beyond the endless waters of Lake Michigan.

He was satisfied. Once more, his plans were succeeding. Why was he so much smarter than everyone else? He didn't dwell on it often. All that mattered was that he was, and that he made sure everyone he met understood it.

Nelson Duncan III was no match for him. Duncan was a dimwit, hardly worthy of concern. ALI would continue to give Thrust what he needed. He already had acquired its national insurance license and the operational architecture to add insurance to his vertically integrated health care system. Now they would provide the cover he needed for the screw-up in Washington State. That error was not to be tolerated, and he made a mental note to dismiss all involved. The head of that division must learn that failure would not be tolerated.

It was Richard's destiny to be in charge, not from some privilege of birth but because he was so smart. Willing to do what was necessary to get big things done. Some of his peers—other CEOs of large integrated health systems—were too concerned with the trappings of the office. They needed people who would regularly tell them how smart, good-looking, and extraordinary they were. Thrust only needed to show all that he was the smartest person in the room and see fealty to his command.

The only person he ever wanted affirmation from was his father. But he had never gotten it, and it wouldn't happen now. His father had passed away decades ago, the year after Richard left New York City to attend the Master of Business Administration program in the University of Michigan. They had quarreled about that. His father was insistent that Richard finish his learning of the family garment business on the lower Eastside of Manhattan, and then take it over as he had from his father.

It was a successful business, but Richard wanted more, much more. The garment store was what Grandpa Thrust started after emigrating from Lithuania in 1901. The family name was Throstowitz, but an agent at Ellis Island found it too long for his liking and shortened it to Thrust on his entry papers. Grandpa was a tailor and used his skills to build a place for his family in the new world, and passed the trade on to his children.

Richard's dad dutifully worked the family business and helped secure a solid financial standing for the entire family. It was all he knew, other than having served in the Army during WWII, avoiding combat by showing an aptitude for logistics management. He became a supply clerk supervisor, and his assignments included organizing the ammunition deliveries to troops after the D-Day invasion. Once the war was over, he returned to New York City to the family business, and started a family with a woman he met on the lower Eastside.

The family company was successful enough to allow the Thrusts to leave the crowded city for a new home on Long Island, right next door to one they also bought for Grandpa. Richard grew up in these suburbs, but still worked weekends and holidays in the old store that remained in the lower east side of the city. This continued through college—Richard got his undergraduate degree at New York University so he could labor in the family business in his spare hours.

Richard resented that he could have attended a more prestigious school but for the family's needs. He had the grades and snuck an application into Yale. He got in, but never told his family. There was no chance that they would agree to him leaving the family nest. As it was, Richard needed to bus tables on weekend nights to make ends meet at NYU—he received only a small allowance for his work at the family business as his father tried to control him through money.

Richard's dad wanted to build the store into a regional business by branching out to New Jersey and southern Connecticut. He dreamed they could make enough money to move the family into the prestigious neighborhoods further east on Long Island. Richard privately scoffed at his dad's vision—he wanted to be on top of something far bigger than a regional clothing company.

As graduation from NYU neared, Richard secretly applied to the top business schools in the nation. His top choice, the University of Michigan, accepted him and even offered a scholarship. He told his dad he was leaving only two weeks before his departure, knowing it would be a major conflict. It was, and he left town with a hug and kiss from his mom and grandparents. Dad had gotten up early and headed to work without a word of farewell or encouragement.

Richard tried not to dwell on the unsaid words between them. He would show his father how rich and successful he would become. That would never happen—but only because of his father's inconvenient death.

Richard was a good student at Michigan. His classmates were bright and as ambitious as he was, but he fought harder. His grades put him at the top 10 percent of his class. Still, it irked him that so many of his classmates had accepted internships between the first and second year at corporate headquarters for major companies, while all he could muster was a post in Detroit with an investment bank.

It was there he learned about the health care industry. One of his projects was to evaluate a hospital company going public with a stock offering. It opened his eyes to the great prospects for health care as a business. He was intrigued by the growing demand, the ability to largely set your own prices, and limited, if any, accountability. It seemed to him the only drawback was that so many of the existing hospitals and health systems across America were the product of communities—local, religious, or otherwise—who seemed to care less about money than doing some foolish social good.

The hospital stock prospectus showed him that there was another way to view the health care world. Instead of a service commitment, he saw enormous profit potential—if one made that the organization's priority. Richard was struck by a recruitment brochure put out by the company to attract business students like him to their company as management trainees. The brochure spoke to the golden handcuffs they offered to candidates—salaries and benefits that were so lucrative, trainees would be dissuaded from ever leaving the company. When he showed this to one of his classmates, his response was that this was the type of bondage he was into. Yes, indeed, thought Richard.

Tempted as he was to accept a position with that company on graduation from Michigan, Richard found another opportunity even more enticing—an offer to be vice president for Finance and Operations in Minneapolis for a regional not-for-profit health care system. While the system had a major teaching hospital in Minneapolis, and several ringing the city, it was also acquiring hospitals in several midsize cities across the American West. The new position was aimed at this aspect of their business. It paid very well and afforded immediate entry into the senior management circles of both the company and Minnesota, a place nationally recognized as a leadership node for health care.

Richard felt a connection to his boss-to-be, Tom Shelby. Like Richard, Tom was an MBA grad, not an MHA grad, a physician, or other clinician drawn to health care as a calling to serve others. It was an opportunity to make money, to gain power and control and ultimately recognition. Richard thought Tom would be a mentor who could help accelerate his career.

Richard thrived in his new environs. There was little control; he would meet with Tom several times a month to get general direction, but it was really up to Richard to grow the company's new line of business. He got tactical advice about how to build the business, along with tips on how to manipulate boards, make payoffs to politicians, and cut side deals with labor unions, but it was his baby.

Tom did also offer up moral advice. He told Richard making promises was easy, but keeping them not something to be worried about, unless the risk and guilt were too much for one to take. Such things didn't bother Richard, and he applied himself to building a regional network of hospitals beholden to him. And he was most successful at doing so. Richard made a lot of money after several years at the company and was becoming recognized as a rising star. But he found he wanted more, much more than just money, and now, not later.

His opening came when the parent company undertook a strategic review because of a whistleblower complaint. Many thousands of dollars were at risk, and it triggered a company-wide evaluation of its business plan. Some thought the company should return to being the leader of health care in Minneapolis and perhaps across the Midwest. Richard's portfolio of business in cities like Denver, Albuquerque, Las Vegas, and Reno was in conflict with that thinking.

Richard saw this opening. Over the course of his travels, he had met a businessman from South America interested in health care. He had silent investors, with substantial capital, looking for opportunities in America, and health care was one of their ventures of interest. That they were more interested in the pharmaceutical aspect of health care led Richard to wonder where their money came from—not that it mattered. Money was money.

Richard convinced these investors to make an offer to his company to buy the regional business. He would help put together the proposal, but as their hidden partner. He would also work within the company to make sure the offer received consideration.

The investor group made a generous enough offer to the Minneapolis health system. Richard got the offer on the board agenda and ran a quiet campaign to convince senior managers and board members that the time was right to focus more locally on the company's future. He did not disclose his conflicts of interest around the proposal.

His boss Tom became the primary obstacle to the board accepting the deal—he pressed key leaders to understand that their best future play was national, not local. Tom argued that long-term profitability was to be found in the lower cost marketplaces outside of Minneapolis. They could pay far lower rates for labor in these mostly non-unionized cities and charge as much or more than they did in Minneapolis.

Richard knew this was an accurate assessment, and that Tom was beginning to win the day on the strategic debate. So, he seeded rumors that Tom was the whistleblower who had brought the charges threatening the future of the company. There was no truth to it, but it stuck to Tom like stink on a skunk. His standing in the company immediately shrank under this cloud of doubt, along with his influence. The deal went through.

Tom was fired. He figured out that Richard was behind his demise and confronted him angrily one day, prattling on about loyalty. His rage and comments blew by Richard as little more than a dusting of pollen in the spring. Richard Thrust was a protege no more.

The final piece of the deal soon was put in place—Thrust would become the CEO of the new company. Only five years out of school, Richard Thrust now found himself as CEO of a multibillion-dollar health care system that spread from the badlands of the Dakotas to California—HealthMost. It was a good start. With so much more to be done. He had . . .

His memories were interrupted by a buzz of the intercom on his desk. "Mr. Thrust," bellowed his executive assistant, "Mr. Bridgewater is here for your meeting."

Mr. Bridgewater was the principal lead to HealthMost's outside lobbying firm. "Send him in, in a couple of minutes." Thrust made it a practice to make all who came to meet him wait for him. There should never be any confusion as to who was in charge.

Chapter Thirty-Two

1966: The Age of Health Care Rationalization Begins

Christopher was right. President Johnson's new Medicare program blew up the federal budget. Its initial cost projection of $5 billion per year was proven a mirage—maybe even a lie. In the first year alone, hospital costs increased by over 20 percent and physician costs 7.8 percent. The original actuarial projections that Medicare costs would slowly grow to about $12 billion annually by 1990 were being revised with the fear that this would be well over $100 billion. Wage contributions and premiums would not be enough to finance the program at that level, requiring the federal government to find a different way to pay for it or to raise these taxes or premiums.

The cost spiral was similar for the new Medicaid program. States were signing up for it, as it was a relatively easy state budget choice since the majority of the costs were paid by the feds, not the state. Its cost was close to doubling each year.

National health expenditures for the nation were shooting up like a rocket. As a percent of the Gross Domestic Product, the 1965 rate of 5.6 percent shot up to 6 percent in 1967, 6.2 percent in 1967, and 6.5 percent in 1968. Something would have to be done.

Part of the explanation for the numbers was the intentional underpricing of the cost by the Johnson Administration and congressional allies. More troubling to Chris was that the numbers also reflected a failure among leaders to recognize that cost control should be a major design issue for the new programs. HEW leaders were still deeply rooted in the paradigm of More, and Christopher's political replacement as Assistant Secretary for Policy and Planning showed no aptitude for the challenge at hand. As the saying goes, when one's only tool is a hammer, that is what gets used. For HEW, their tool was "more" and they applied this to building Medicare.

For example, a major question was how to pay the hospitals for service to Medicare recipients. Hospital costs were the great majority of health care costs then, and paying for these was at the core of the base Medicare program. Medicare Part A was the portion financed by the payroll tax, with physician and other service costs largely covered under Part B of the program, which was funded by additional client payments.

The number, size, and costs of hospitals had grown significantly since the end of World War II, largely because of government incentives. HEW ignored—in great part because of deals made in Congress—the reality that virtually all hospitals would have agreed to participate in the program under any reasonable compensation, and instead encouraged hospitals to be part of Medicare by paying them on the basis of their individual hospital costs. What's more, they added a "plus" factor to reflect the need for a hospital profit on top of reimbursement for their costs.

A cost plus reimbursement system did exactly what one would expect. Hospitals were most happy to be serving Medicare recipients, if that was the point of the payment incentive. And they saw little reason to constrain themselves in what they provided to them, as they would be compensated for almost anything. Medicare would pay for more salaries and wages, more staff, more equipment, and more facilities.

With such an incentive, it was little surprise that hospital and Medicare costs exploded upward. Medicare became the poster child of government excess in short order. Medicaid policy was right behind it in building up financial problems for the federal government.

Solutions to the cost problem were needed and soon—Congressional leaders were especially anxious to hear how to control health care costs. Even officials at HEW now saw the problem and were anxious to find different ways. They took out the "plus" in cost reimbursement, but far more was needed to put the program on sound, long-term financial footing.

This was the moment Chris had been waiting for. He had been working with his colleagues at Harvard and in study groups across the nation on cost control methods for when the time was right.

Christopher thought he must lead with practical ways to stem the tide of the Age of More before he could offer larger systemic improvements. "More" had, in economic terms, dramatically changed America's health care supply curve. There was a time for such thinking, but that time had passed. Solutions were now needed that would stem this supply, or change the demand curve such that better prices would be found.

Members of Congress and their staff didn't really think in these economic terms, and Christopher and his counterparts in the policy community branded a new range of solutions in different language around common-sense solutions. They found an anxious and receptive audience. Chris himself participated in over a dozen legislative and administrative policy efforts to control cost over the next decade.

Some of the key early programs enacted to stem the high cost of health care included:

> *Redefining "Cost": This approach was to restrict the nature of "cost" by limiting it definitionally to certain things or amounts. For example, the operative change for hospitals was that they would be reimbursed only for "allowable costs." Whether by statute or administrative action, disputes grew over what was "allowable."

> *Professional Standard Review Organizations (PSROs): This idea was to reduce use of service by Medicare beneficiaries through national clinical standards developed and enforced by peer review of medical care treatment decisions. Other physicians would review admission and other clinical decisions and, through these PSROs, determine that certain care was not medically necessary and therefore ineligible for payment through Medicare.

> *Capital Controls: To tamp down the urges of the medical care system to build new facilities and buy expensive equipment, payments for "capital" were split out from other costs, and restricted. This proved to have only a partial effect on the major appetite to build and buy more, as the federal government still paid a major portion of the cost of such investment choices. Officials began to

consider ways in which they could have a say in approving or rejecting new capital as a Medicare cost.

*Hospital Rate Setting: Several states adopted programs whereby they would set a payment rate for hospitals. The most innovative of these programs set a rate that would apply to all payors. The calculation would be made for each hospital by developing and negotiating specific annual hospital budgets through a government rate review process.

Some of these were federal solutions; others played out at the state level. Christopher was a prominent voice in proposing and shaping these cost control ideas over the next five years. He had hope for some of the methods, but was generally skeptical that costs would be controlled absent major reform. If the ideas worked, great. If not, he hoped to have made the case and earned the credibility to explore more systemic solutions that would redesign health care—the types of ways embraced by the CCMC.

There was a mixed track record of success from these early efforts. Costs were not going down as a result of a shift of philosophical orientation and the adoption of cost containment tactics, but they were at least not accelerating as quickly as they had before. But they were still going up, rapidly. As expected, Medicare was also proving to be the trendsetter in health system development since older Americans constituted the largest share of hospitalized patients. By 1975, health care had risen to almost 8 percent of GDP.

Chris thought it time to unleash more pervasive systemic solutions. His view was that the nation was still in the early stages of a much-needed Age of Rationalization. Practical solutions to the cost problem would be part of recreating a more sensible American health care system. But, so far, smaller solutions were not having much of an effect. It was time to think bigger, or the age of rationalization would be remembered more for its foolishness than being a golden age of American health policy. Chris shifted his attention to finding and pushing these bigger solutions.

Chapter Thirty-Three

Young Mary Beth Meets Nancy Jones

Mary Beth Collins was liking her new life as an independent woman. She had rejected her family's call to become a wife and mom, and instead was blazing her own trail in north Seattle. Still, she saw the irony that this had somehow devolved into living with her boyfriend and working in a bakery. Not all that different from what life would mean if she had decided to work while raising a family. Sans kids for sure, but drifting toward a very normal life.

She didn't really mind it all that much, though. Irv was an interesting love partner, and he was also intent on unshackling themselves from ordinary life. Just how to do this was the question, collectively and individually. Irv was trying his best to figure it out, and she thought it important to do the same.

Her answer was, in part, to volunteer her time for causes she believed in. Her former roommate Tina had gotten her interested in this through a referral to a shelter for domestic abuse victims. Mary Beth was now on the board, and the organization was organizing and growing. She was also helping the owners of the bakery grow their community footprint with a not-for-profit food bank venture.

Both these organizations needed some professional help to move forward and Mary Beth had volunteered to reach out to a consultant she had met while working for her dad. She called up Nancy Jones and asked if she would be willing to meet with her. Nancy remembered her, which flattered Mary Beth. Nancy suggested they meet for lunch at a restaurant near her office. This was far more than Mary Beth expected, and she jumped at the opportunity.

The Theory of Irv

It proved to be a pivotal moment in Mary Beth's life. She arrived early for their lunch at a small restaurant overlooking Elliott Bay in Seattle's Pike Place Market. She wanted to gather her thoughts, nervous as she was about meeting a woman as successful as Nancy.

She thought about how she would describe herself if Nancy asked: a local girl who had challenged her family's expectations by moving away from home rather than getting married and having kids. A young woman with no security, but surrounded with interesting people. A woman with a passion for organizing and running things. She was happy, enjoying her life's ride and her own growth. Yet there was a wall in front of her that she thought would greatly limit what she might do in the future.

Nancy was running a little late, so Mary Beth had time to ponder this wall. It was not so much about a woman's place in what remained a male dominant society. Yes, there were some limits from that, and she implicitly understood that any choice to go beyond those limits would be difficult. But those limits were not at the top of the list of what would hold her back—it was more her own personal limits that would make it hard to find a more meaningful place.

She knew she had the smarts and the social graces to contribute to social good in a bigger world, a belief fed by her growing role in the bakery's community venture and her volunteer work for social and political causes. It was satisfying to be a part of these things, and she imagined how she could have a growing role in them and be able to more closely observe such efforts. She might even be considered a bit player in the social change movement.

Rarely, though, other than in her dreams, did she realistically think that she could be a leader in these efforts. Leadership roles were reserved for the outgoing and assertive; those who aggressively claimed their place in society. Television shows, her ventures into the business world, and observing her more extroverted brothers told her this must be true. She was too reserved, too introverted, and too quiet in nature to be in the lead.

She wasn't frustrated by this; it was just the way it was. She understood who she was and had no inclination to fight that destiny. She would contribute how she could, and perhaps someone like Nancy would help outline new possibilities in this regard for her.

Nancy did, but far beyond what Mary Beth ever imagined. The surprise began soon after Nancy arrived for lunch and sat down at the table with Mary Beth. They looked at each other. Time seemed to stop as seconds ticked away in silence. Mary Beth was the one who finally broke the awkward quiet. "Ms. Jones, thanks so much for agreeing to meet with me. I don't know if you remember meeting me at my dad's company a couple of years ago?"

"Of course I do. I was so happy that you followed up from our introduction. Let's have this young man get our order in. This restaurant gets pretty busy, and I would hate to tie up their table all afternoon."

They quickly scanned the menu, with Nancy ordering the meatless bean burger and sweet potato fries, with an herbal tea. Mary Beth was so nervous about the meeting, her introvert pleading for escape, that she found it easiest to just say, "Make it two."

With that, the waiter left, leaving the two women to be with each other and the view. Mary Beth smiled at Nancy. Nancy smiled at Mary Beth. One fidgeted with the fork in front of them, the other a spoon. It mattered little who did which, nor who cast their glances across the restaurant or the view of the water and mountains out the window. Among the voices and clanging of dishes, and the sweet smells of cooking food, the winning voice was the silence between the two women.

Seconds passed, maybe even a minute or two. To Mary Beth, it seemed like hours. Here she was with one of the most successful women in Seattle, and she couldn't muster up anything to say. Several times, words started to form in her head, but the gulf of quiet swallowed up her ability to roll the vowels and consonants needed for language. She had never felt less confident of herself and her abilities. Maybe marriage and family was the ticket for her to punch.

Then it hit her, like a mallet on a gong. Yes, she was struggling to find some words to say; that was very clear. And she would have to figure out how to manage her introversion if she was to do more of these visits with other leaders. But what was even clearer was that Nancy was even more uncomfortable than she was!

How could that be? Leaders were extroverts, comfortable with people and the spotlight—certainly not scared of interacting with pipsqueaks like her, that's for sure. She knew Nancy was one of those leaders in the community. She had checked her sources, and they had said that Nancy Jones was one of the top women leaders in the Seattle area, certainly for social causes.

Wait. I am introverted; I know it. And have been trying to cope with it. But I can see that Nancy is too, painfully so. I know the signs. She's even more introverted than I am.

A lifetime of assumptions and limits deconstructed before her, like grains of salt and pepper pouring from the shakers on the table. It would take some time for the full ramifications to fully form in her brain, but her understanding of the natural order of limits and expectations had just been shattered. And it had all happened in less than three minutes.

It would be up to Mary Beth to carry the conversation to its next place. That much was clear.

"You weren't able to convince my father to run for office that day I met you, and I was wondering why." Mary Beth awkwardly tossed something on the table that they had in common.

Nancy perked up immediately. "Oh no, he was interested. I was the one who wasn't sure that he had what it would take for the chamber of commerce to get behind."

"Oh," replied Mary Beth. "I am surprised by that. Not exactly how he told the story over our dinner table that night. What was the problem?"

"Nothing sinister, my dear. It was just that . . . how can I say this delicately . . . it was just that he was such a *man*. And we've got more than enough of those types running around our power structures in this town. I was looking for something more. Something like, well, you."

Mary Beth blushed. First her world order had been blown up in a couple of minutes, and now she was being flattered. "That is so nice of you to say, Nancy, but I have no idea what you mean."

By now, Nancy was more comfortable and began to beam like a summer dawn. She was an introvert but had learned how to roll back the curtains quickly as she found herself in business settings. She was intrigued by how quickly she had relaxed with Mary Beth. It boded well. "Oh, Mary Beth. We have so much to talk about. You just don't see how special you are, do you?"

With that, the two were off, getting to know each other, and themselves, a lot better. Ramifications were to follow for years and decades to come. They talked through their veggie burgers, tea, and dessert cookies, and then adjourned to a park bench just outside of the restaurant, overlooking the water. Two hours later, they hugged and went on their way.

Until they saw each other again the next week—Mary Beth's first day as a part-time employee at Nancy's fledgling political action firm. Nancy could only afford, and Mary Beth could only fulfill, a few hours in the late afternoon each day after the end of her bakery gig. Nancy was experimenting with new techniques of group process and thought that Mary Beth could help develop them. It was a start, though, a beautiful start.

Chapter Thirty-Four

Irv Finds Some Useful Clues

Irv stared at the computer screen in his home office. Antonio had downloaded the files linked to the insurance number found in the sock of the corpse. Irv had caught a major break with the number being in the pool of data breaches made publicly available through international sources. What were the odds? It reinforced his sense of destiny and purpose.

He could see that analyzing what he had would be a major brainteaser. There were three files attached to the number that were now on the hard drive of his personal computer. One was an insurance application and enrollment form, filled out for a "Rodrigo Lopez" applying for inclusion in a health insurance program called "BestCare." Antonio's place of residence on the form was Phoenix, Arizona, and BestCare was apparently a product line of an entity called HealthMost. Irv recalled a major health care system by that name, though he was fuzzy on any details about them.

A second file was an emergency room report of service. Rodrigo had apparently gone to an emergency room in Phoenix, complaining of chest pains. An evaluation of his condition had been made, and he had been discharged the same night.

Irv understood the nature of the first two files, and there was nothing extraordinary to be found in his fast review of what was on the actual forms. It was notable that Rodrigo resided, or had at least applied, in Phoenix—far from Kent and the Pacific Northwest. Phoenix was not exactly spud-growing territory either. But perhaps Rodrigo was an itinerant worker who moved with the crops and their seasons.

If so, Irv could see from the recorded date of service, his mystery corpse had been back in Phoenix only a couple of weeks ago—quite alive—before his demise. Irv thought it possible that Rodrigo had left town after his discharge and that whatever happened to him occurred subsequent to the ER visit. On the other hand, he didn't see any mention of flu-like symptoms in the ER record.

This was his first cursory review of the files, and Irv didn't want to dwell too long on any of the specifics yet. It was helpful to now know who the victim was, where he was from, and have a record of a recent health care experience. He would dig deeper once he saw the universe of possibilities held in the last file.

It was this third file that had him scratching his head. It was labeled an "Assignment of Benefit and Security Integrity" form. It referenced the number that was found in the sock and was the data origin for the files he was looking at now. There was a signature on the bottom, but not Rodrigo's. The document was only a page and consisted of a couple of brief paragraphs that referenced a series of other numbers and a data host name of ALI. He had no idea what this form was about.

Irv went back and reviewed all three of the files again, in greater depth. He didn't get much further than his first impressions from any of them. A health insurance program application for a Rodrigo Lopez. An emergency room visit two weeks ago by the same. Most likely this was the person whose corpse was found in Kent, though he was recently in Phoenix. Irv would do some additional searches into Rodrigo Lopez using his government access codes available at work. His instinct was that he wouldn't find too much more about him—the absence of other record linkages suggested that Rodrigo was flying low on the electronic information highway. But it was still worth exploring.

Irv remained baffled by the third form. Looking at the clock, he observed that it would be another few hours before Antonio returned. He was off to a Seattle Sounders soccer match and then would need to commute back to their neighborhood. Irv watched the end of the match on his television and waited for Antonio.

He didn't have to wait long—the match was one-sided for the home team, and Antonio left at halftime because of his great curiosity over Irv's project. Irv told him what he had found so far.

They homed in on questions about the third file. Antonio's guess was that it was a data transfer form used by insurance companies when they relocated client files to third parties. The data protections in law for health information were strict and severe in consequences. Confidentiality breaches related to mental health records even carried criminal penalties. It was one of the reasons he found the sloppiness of health care providers in handling records so shocking—the insurance world understood the seriousness of security and was thorough in setting up protections.

Most likely this form was the legal ass-covering allowing the placement of files for A64172XC into another company's server and information system. He guessed ALI was an insurer in some other line of business who had gotten involved with health care in some way.

This matched up with what else Irv found while waiting for Antonio to return. He had done an online search of HealthMost and had read up on the formation of this national health care system. Its corporate office was located in Chicago, and it owned hospitals and other health care facilities in many states, including most western cities. Phoenix was one of them, including the hospital that operated the emergency room from whence the second form derived. More relevant to their quest was that a life insurance company named ALI had entered into a joint venture with HealthMost last year, some type of capitated payment arrangement.

Maybe it was as simple as ALI holding the insurance files for this joint venture. So far, nothing about this case was simple or to be accepted as normal. Irv would follow up on all three forms. He had some vacation time coming and thought he might take a few days and head to Phoenix. A little digging in person at the site of Rodrigo's care might bear fruit—and he wouldn't mind a little warmer weather.

Chapter Thirty-Five

Young Irv Ponders His Life

Johnny had gone off to a new life of politics. Irv knew that this meant his own life would need to evolve in significant ways, but he took his time in making changes. Johnny had been his partner in all forms of adventure and, along with Mary Beth, was the anchor to his life. Irv's first response was to try to hold on to the tightness of their relationship, and he bought a used car so he could travel out to see Johnny on the east side of the county on a regular basis.

It soon became difficult for the two to maintain any regular adventure schedule. While they had regular get-togethers over Johnny's first year off to the east, Johnny's marriage to Reena made these less frequent. Then Johnny began to find his footing as a politician, and time became even more precious.

Johnny found that life as a King County councilman required attending meetings, many meetings, most back in Seattle. Irv could sit in on the public meetings and maybe find some private time with Johnny around them, but it was not the same as before. The challenge became great when Johnny was elected to Congress and moved to Washington, DC—the forces of separation were now infused with several thousand miles of physical distance rather than forty.

It wasn't just Johnny's life shift that was at issue. Irv found himself at his own crossroads of an undefined sort, feeling something was missing in his life. For a while, the void was filled with more Mary Beth. The two moved in together, leaving their group home basement for a small cottage in North Seattle in a community called Wallingford. It was closer to the bakery where Mary Beth worked, and a stone's throw from Gasworks Park, a strange collection of rusting gas refinery and storage parts on a scenic plot of land jutting into Seattle's Union Bay.

There was much to do around their neighborhood and the greater Pacific Northwest. They were in love, and soulmates who enjoyed each other when they were together. This certainly took the sting out of Johnny's leaving, but it couldn't fill the total gap.

Irv was working his way up the ladder at the coffee company, adding some purchasing duties to his shipping role. It was good enough money, and he found the stability of a regular job oddly comforting at times. It got him out of the house doing something during the day, and limited the time available to ruminate over his circumstances.

Irv welcomed the opportunity to go to work on most days, though not all. There were days when hangovers, cosmic misalignments, or Mondays left him with little enthusiasm for the task. This was to be expected. What troubled him was that he regularly found he had an ever-present itch underneath these specific down days that he just couldn't quite scratch.

He was out "doing" as his mom had told him to, but there was a monotony beginning to gnaw at him. His on-the-job learning had slowed to a crawl. The routine of getting up, going to work, and coming home was beginning to be very repetitive. It was also hypnotic; he felt like he was in a trance on some days. He pondered how to spice things up and wondered if he would wake up in forty years and realize that this was all there was to his life.

He tried to make changes. He began to read again and adopted his mom's alphabet parade at the local library. He exercised, playing basketball every Wednesday evening with friends. He and Mary Beth would make sure to go out at least one night every weekend. All of these things helped to make life more enjoyable, for a while. But it didn't soothe the rising beast within Irv.

There needed to be something more—if not for now, for some time in the future when he might really need more "doing" to be happy. He needed to find this, but didn't want to lose the part that included Mary Beth.

What to do? He struggled mightily with this question. No answers were to be found, and his existential gap grew into a perceived crisis. As close as he got to a solution was figuring out a way to process an answer—a road trip. He wondered if he could recruit Johnny to take a trip with him.

But where? He recalled they had planned a hiking trip to Southern Utah as part of Johnny's bachelor party for his wedding, but had to postpone it when the King County Council gig came up. Then, soon after, Johnny was off to DC. Maybe Irv could now convince Johnny to finally take that trip. It was worth a shot.

Chapter Thirty-Six

Young Johnny Ponders His First Year in Congress

The first year of his time in Congress—1985—passed quickly for Johnny. There was so much to learn and so many people to meet. Early in the second year, he started to realize that he would soon have to consider whether he wanted to bother with running for reelection. His freshmen colleagues were well underway on that decision, while he had only barely thought about it.

Nor did he really want to think much about it even then. He made a mental note to check in with Nancy Jones during spring break to figure out what he should be doing, if anything. Johnny was more interested in spending time with Reena and his new family than planning his future, but he knew that decisions had to be made soon.

A couple of weeks later, Johnny went to his Capitol Hill office early in the morning and found an elderly Black woman sitting in the small lobby. She didn't have an appointment, but was hoping to meet with someone to talk about what happened to her husband late last year. She lived just outside of Johnny's district and had been turned away by the staff of her own congressman's office, and both Senate offices for Washington State. Someone had said to try to see him, since he was always open to taking a meeting.

Johnny was, and he brought Mrs. Ruth Benjamin into his office. Her tale was a sad one. Neither she nor her husband were eligible for Medicare, or any other public or private insurance program. He was an agricultural worker and she a housewife, so they slipped through the cracks of the public program rules. It wasn't a problem until her husband got sick one night, and they went to a hospital emergency room in the suburbs of Seattle. When it became clear to the hospital staff that he was uninsured, and without other resources to pay for care, they refused to see him and told them to leave the emergency room.

The Benjamins did. They first went back to their house, not knowing what to do. Some friends told them to go to the public hospital in Seattle—they would take anyone. As they were starting to do so, her husband had a heart attack and died in their driveway. His symptoms when they went to the suburban hospital were the warning signs of this heart attack.

It was hard enough on Ruth that her husband had died suddenly, and maybe needlessly. But what was worse was that she couldn't find anyone who seemed to care about it. The hospital was sympathetic to her loss but not apologetic; they said it was not possible for them to provide care to people who couldn't pay for it. She had even consulted an attorney. He told her that their case was a weak one—there was no duty for a hospital to treat the sick, and he didn't think that her case was worth trying to change this common law fact. Take it to Congress, he told her.

Ruth knew the lawyer was just trying to get her out of his office. But she had a sister who lived in DC and had taken a Greyhound bus trip across the country. She would stay with her sister and find someone in the government who just might care.

She was not having any luck with that, she told Johnny. He took Ruth's hand and told her that he cared, and would do whatever he could to help. He brought in a legislative aide to document details. "Give us a couple of days to do some research, and let's meet again on Friday," he said, "if you could come back then."

Ruth did. Johnny did not have much good news for her. The attorney had gotten the existing law right—there was no duty of the hospital to treat her husband. This was the case even though the hospital was a not-for-profit, exempt from federal income taxes; even though it was built with Hill Burton funds back in the 1950s; even though the hospital would use underpayments as part of the prices to inflate what they would charge private payors. This was the "cost shift" of health care.

The hospital was more diplomatic with Johnny's staff than with Ruth; the inquiry of a congressional office mattered. They were courteous and apologetic, but underneath, this tone didn't take any responsibility for the death of Ruth's husband. Johnny got a follow-up call from a lobbyist from the state hospital association, offering up their explanation of the tragedy.

Ruth began to cry as Johnny shared the product of his office's research, which upset him. He was usually able to find some way to bring some comfort to constituents who came to his office with complaints, enough that they would feel better even if there was no real solution to their problem.

"What else can I do for you?" asked Johnny.

"Oh nothing," said Ruth. It wasn't really about her any longer. Her loving husband was dead and there was nothing to be done about that. She went to a lawyer not to get some money because of his death, but to make sure it didn't happen to anyone else. Could Johnny do something to make sure it didn't happen to anyone else?

Johnny sat back in his chair. *Of course I could, in theory,* he thought. *That is what we do in Congress—pass laws.* It was the first time that he really understood the potential for his new role in life to be of great use to others. *It will take some new thinking about how I approach this job,* he thought. To Ruth, he promised to figure out how they might change the law to make sure this never happened to anyone else.

Johnny's meeting with Ruth Benjamin over her husband's death had a great effect on him. How could something like that happen? What could he do to make sure it didn't happen again? What did it say about this whole adventure and experience?

He talked to some of the friends he had made in Congress over his first year and a half. Few had dealt with this specific problem, but they had their own set of personal tragedies that had been put before them by constituents. We can, in theory, legislate and fix these problems for the future, some said. But it will take a while to solve any of these big issues. Most said that it was important to steel up to the reality that they can't help everyone. Pick your issues, they said. And don't forget to get reelected or you won't have any power to solve these problems.

Some on Johnny's staff also suggested that he pick his battles and try to put Ruth's behind him. Instead, he began to meet with her every week. Johnny wanted to keep her problem alive and fresh as he assessed what else could be done for her.

His staff reported back to him that this was a growing problem across the nation. There had been a change in policy orientation within the Reagan Administration implying that health care was now a business. Entrepreneurs were moving into the field, some through for-profit organizations but others who went to work for nonprofits. They were realizing that great profits could be made by limiting their care to the best paying patients, and that it was especially lucrative to avoid uninsured patients. They justified this by asserting that public hospitals were the ones obligated to care for these patients.

There were objections to this in Congress and elsewhere. All hospitals were reaping the benefits of the federal and state government investment in care for different populations, and not-for-profit hospitals also had distinct benefits arising from their tax exempt status. Not having to pay federal taxes was an enormous financial boon to them, and it was even bigger practically since this translated to exemption from state and local taxes too.

Some had thought this would be a problem resolved by the Internal Revenue Service through its interpretation of the law of charitable organizations and their tax status. Surprisingly, the IRS avoided saying that not-for-profit hospitals wishing to qualify for exemption from taxes under Section 501c3 of the tax code had to take care of all who needed care.

Johnny became part of a rump group within Congress, from both parties, who wanted to do something about this. It was his first real legislative effort to pass a law to solve something he considered to be a major problem. The group began to settle on some policy solutions that would make sure Ruth's experience would not happen to anyone else—a duty to treat for any hospital that offered up its availability to provide emergency care by having an emergency room.

Johnny was encouraged by this—and began to learn what it took to make an idea a law in the nation's capital. He was faced with one harsh reality—it was not going to happen overnight. The idea had been planted, but with it being an election year, he was only relevant to the battle over the issue if he committed to run for reelection. Otherwise, he had no power base to leverage his influence. The rump group needed all of its members to succeed, since industry groups were questioning the need for legislation.

THE THEORY OF IRV

It was this moment that forced Johnny to publicly declare that he would run for reelection—it would give him leverage to help pass legislation that would make sure that what happened to Ruth's husband didn't happen again. The legislation passed—the Emergency Medical Treatment and Active Labor Act, enacted as part of the Consolidated Omnibus Budget Reconciliation Act of 1986.

Johnny felt great pride in having helped change the law. He brought Ruth out for a public ceremony celebrating the legislation, and her hugs and tears moved him. There was much more to this politics thing than just the experience, he realized. It could lead to some real good.

Still, Johnny was not completely convinced that being a congressman was for him. Running for election was one thing; working to get reelected was another. He had gotten into this as an adventure where he could meet people. And he had. Now he could see that there was more to it, potentially much more. But was that for him?

He needed time to step back and figure things out, but the pressure of starting up a reelection campaign was pressing upon him. He had just gotten a call from Irv, something about that trip to Utah they had never taken. His first reaction was to say no to his friend, but maybe he should reconsider. Time away with his buddy might be exactly what he needed to clear his head—and his future.

Chapter Thirty-Seven

Irv Takes the Investigation to Phoenix

Irv steered his rental car through the gate at the Holiday Inn near Sky Harbor Airport in Phoenix, and took a left out of the parking lot. He needed to find his way to his final destination here: the west side of Phoenix and HealthMost's Westside Medical Center, and the emergency room where Rodrigo Lopez had gone to get medical care because of chest pains.

First things first. It was an easy enough transition from the Northwest to Phoenix. Irv had found a room and a rental car in short order through Expedia, at decent enough early summer rates in the 110-degree weather. It was hot, but manageable if you could avoid being outdoors in the afternoon and evening.

The bigger challenge was to find a way to get inside of the Medical Center's emergency room and dig for evidence that would help his investigation. It wouldn't be easy, but Irv was an expert on the processes of the health care system, and he would take advantage of its weaknesses to find what he needed.

He drove to a public library just outside the downtown core of Phoenix and brought his computer with him. He found documents outlining the local medical scene in the library and used these to focus his online sleuthing.

HealthMost had three hospitals in the region, one more in Tucson, and an assortment of urgent care centers, diagnostic centers, and nursing homes across greater Phoenix. Westside Medical Center was not their flagship hospital in the area; that was the 450-bed tertiary hospital located near downtown. Westside was a flailing community hospital

HealthMost had bought in the midst of the retirement communities on the west side of town. Its primary service base was retired Medicare beneficiaries who had relocated to Phoenix, or who spent winters there as snowbirds.

Irv found an electronic version of a hospital directory from the state hospital association on their website and outlined the hospital's leadership on a piece of paper in his notepad. He Googled the names and took notes that profiled key elements of the career and personal histories for the executive staff and management within the emergency center.

He also found government documents in the library that helped him construct a rudimentary picture of how health care was regulated by the government in greater Phoenix. He didn't need much more than that, enough to build credibility as he made his next play.

From there it was on to the local public health department. Irv had set an appointment for that afternoon with the person in charge of the local trauma system. He had learned much about EMS systems from his time in Seattle. The local public health department would undoubtedly, in connection with a state agency, manage local emergency transport patterns and systems. His cover was that he was on special assignment looking to better manage these patterns in the Seattle area. It was unlikely that anyone would even check on this beyond seeing his valid identification card from the local health department. If they asked for official clearance, his plan was to give them Rose's name and number. She would cover for him.

His goal: to find the local expert who would provide him a way into the emergency room of Western Medical Center. Sally Jenkins was the local EMS director, and she was more than happy to meet with him and tell him everything she could about how things worked in Phoenix. Things generally slowed down during these hot summer months, and she was glad to have the distraction of an out-of-town visitor. Sally spent a couple of hours putting on a dog and pony show for Irv.

Like many cities, Phoenix had far more of a laissez-faire attitude toward emergency referral patterns than Seattle. Harborview was the Level I trauma center in Seattle, and a step-down hierarchy of eligible hospitals flowed from that. Ambulance companies were required to get centralized approval regarding where they brought patients, mostly based on the condition of the patient but in part built by daily surveillance of capacity in local emergency rooms and inpatient units.

Phoenix had most of the elements of the system in place as in Seattle, but was plagued by a policy decision to designate multiple hospitals as Level I trauma centers. There were nine in all, probably eight more than a rational emergency care system should have, even in a large and spread-out city like the greater Phoenix area. It was the product of competing hospitals trying to get the best and most patients, or at least those who had insurance.

Irv thought it a stupid system. In this instance, though, he cared less about the local problem and far more about how to build a credible storyline that would get him the access he needed inside of Westside Medical Center. As Sally went on about the local EMS system, the story was written for him.

He asked Sally to get him an official referral to the director of Emergency Medicine at Westside. He asked her to mention that he was from Seattle and doing an investigation with the local public health department. All that was true enough.

At Westside, he would use his charm and experience to work his way into the emergency room information system. His cover would be that he was reviewing case files for a Seattle area person who had contracted and died from a rare and severe case of the flu, and that reports had suggested that this victim had been treated in the Phoenix area just before, possibly at Westside Medical Center. Again, all was factual enough to satisfy Irv's need to be truthful.

Sally got on the phone and secured him an appointment to meet with the Westside Medical Center emergency room director the next afternoon. He was ready to go, and returned to his hotel to get a little rest for his big day tomorrow. He thought momentarily about exploring the Phoenix area, but it was just too danged hot to do so.

Chapter Thirty-Eight

Trapped in Canyonlands

Irv had been looking forward to this trip with Johnny, as it had been almost three years since their last major adventure. Over that time, Johnny had become a successful politician, first winning a seat on the King County Council and then shocking the world by winning a seat in the House of Representatives in 1984, representing the eighth district of Washington State as an independent.

Johnny was now commuting to DC just about every week, and busy with constituent events. Johnny and Irv would get together on the weekends as much as they could, but it had gotten harder and harder to do so. A big chunk of whatever time was left for Johnny was spent with Reena and his new family.

Irv missed his friend greatly, but was generally happy with his own new life. Mary Beth was a big part of his joy, and really the biggest reason for his happiness. They had built a life together in the Northwest, and Irv was tickled pink that he had found such a wonderful woman to spend his life with. He also had a job and hobbies, but it was Mary Beth who made the Pacific Northwest feel like this was indeed his home.

Still, there was something missing, he reluctantly admitted to himself. Maybe it was that life just wasn't as magical as it had been when he first found Seattle and Mary Beth and Johnny. The place and people were revelations, but there was also something to how he discovered himself during these first years in his new home.

Irv's mom had given him his marching orders on her deathbed. She told him he must experience life and satisfy his curiosity, not through books or secondhand accounts of the world, but directly. *Go out and do* was what she said. Going to college at UCLA and experiencing new things from that base had been a start to that calling, and a good one.

But it was only when he landed on a whim in the Pacific Northwest that he really understood what she had been saying. It was then that his life had leapt to a new level. Every day he was learning something new and exciting, trying new things in his new home. Irv liked the experiences themselves, and was enthralled with what he was learning about himself. He was an able adventurer and friend, fulfilling his promise to live by a theory of doing things, not just watching.

To be sure, he was still doing a lot now. He was learning a lot from these activities, and still liking himself and his lot in life—just not as much as before. The cosmic spark to it all was no longer so evident. Grand adventures and discovery were slowly giving way to routines of life: the schedule of a job, the need for regular sleep, and the rhythm of being a good boyfriend. Was this what growing up was all about?

He was sure there was another level to life to be discovered, but he wasn't confident he was on the path to find it. *Maybe it will become apparent further down the road*, he thought. Johnny had figured out how to do it and was now off on a new path to his own life story. Mary Beth was trying to figure out this same thing, in part with him but also around her own career quest. Perhaps he just needed patience.

But Irv found patience hard. The more patient he tried to be, the more discontent he sowed. The more he thought about the next thing, the more elusive it became. Looking around, it seemed others had figured out their paths. Classmates of his had settled into careers, families, and new patterns of life. Once in a while he would see them, and they seemed happy enough. He felt like a bit player in their new stories, which frustrated him for no apparent good reason. His only solution was to put more space between him and them.

He tried doing entirely new things, with new people, but sometimes these experiences just saddened him more. Most troubling was when these attempts brought him to much older people who shared their frustrations of life lost. Far too often, they told tales too similar to where he now found himself, but with a sad conclusion. Sometimes they had plans for still pursuing their dreams but rarely seemed to have done so. Irv worried that this would be his fate and feared that he would be them in another twenty or thirty years.

There was something else he needed to figure out. He had tried to work some of it out with Mary Beth, and they had good conversations about the future and his need to find something new, but it was hard—

she was not a part of the problem and was instead what he cherished most. It was hard to explain his underlying unhappiness to her when she was the center of his life. How could he manage this without screwing up the thing he cared most about?

Who better than Johnny Gibson to help him navigate this dilemma, he thought. Irv had given him a call and asked if he could find time to take a trip out in the American West. It would be hard, said Johnny at first ask; his reelection campaign would be ramping up then. But Johnny called him back the next day and suggested they take a ten-day trip to the Southwest over the congressional break around Labor Day.

They left on a Thursday evening, packing camping gear and other supplies into Irv's Isuzu Trooper. It was one of Irv's big investments over the last couple of years—a new car that could four-wheel him to normally inaccessible points on the globe. That this was the first such trip he had taken only highlighted his current quandary.

It was two days' drive to southeast Utah and the remote Canyonlands from Seattle. Irv and Johnny could have driven straight through but decided instead to stay a night at a motel in southern Oregon, splitting the drive in half. This got them to the national park at about three in the afternoon. They registered at the trailhead and then four-wheeled out into the massive and desolate park, randomly scrambling their way across ravines, ridges, and dried-up rivers. With hundreds of miles to wander in any direction, they would let fate dictate where they landed. It was difficult to keep some sense of basic direction, as there were few roads and no one to be seen in any direction.

Irv felt some stirring in his soul as they wandered, but no answers. He knew these deep matters were not to be rushed and wasn't sure it was fair to expect that he could find his way by the end of the ten-day trip. But with Johnny, he was encouraged. Johnny hadn't changed very much. Sure, he had a whole bunch of new stories from his time as a politician. These tales, though, were just Johnny being Johnny and doing what he said he wanted to do—experience his life journey with people. Irv was lucky to have such a person as his close friend, and happier still that he had him now when he needed him most.

Then the axle broke on the Trooper as they were traversing a high ridge and some sharp boulders. They were able to leverage it off the rocks and then roll it slowly down a hundred yards to a canyon. They set up camp there and settled in to figure out their predicament. They had an early version of a cell phone with them, but service in this remote area was out of the question. With enough water and food to last another week or more, they decided to wait for a few days to see if they might run into someone who could take them back to civilization. If not, they would pack enough supplies and walk out of the wilderness.

They had great fun for the first couple of days waiting for help—confident that someone would show. There was no reason to worry for a couple of days anyway. They took short hikes around the area, finding high ridges to sit and gaze through their binoculars. Natural wonder was all around them, and they enhanced its beauty with occasional puffs from some weed Irv had bought for the trip. He also had a couple of buttons of peyote he had bought from a friend in preparation for this trip; they thought it best to wait on that should they miss out on being rescued while tripping across the desert.

It was hot, well over ninety degrees, and the sun blazed down viciously on them during the daylight hours. When it was high in the sky at midday, they would sit under a tarp that they had set up in their base camp for shade. It was just like the old days—they would sit and ponder the questions of life and their role in it. Irv was feeling his answer draw closer, but he couldn't make it out yet.

What surprised him was that Johnny was going through his own midlife crisis. Like Irv, Johnny was largely pleased with how his life was advancing. The political thing had been a hoot, a fun experience in its own right and, as he had hoped, a perfect perch for meeting people and learning from their experiences. It had surprised him that he was as successful at it as he was. He was confident enough to believe in himself, but had gotten into this thinking that he would be at best a second-tier politician. He wasn't even sure why he thought that then—maybe because he was told the best and brightest were trying to do this, and that these people were typically Type A individuals who would work extra hard at succeeding. Johnny just wanted some fun and experiences.

But succeeding as a politician began with one's ability to relate to people, and Johnny was a superstar in that respect; his aloofness and independence only added to his interpersonal mystique for many. He looked for opportunities to bring people together to make things work better—

The Theory of Irv

not on grand policy questions, but the practical problems of living life brought to him by his constituents—and found doing so made him even more likable. It turned out this political thing wasn't that complicated.

Johnny had been a success as a King County councilman because of these traits, and they served him even more when he won his seat in Congress. Because of this, he could have years ahead of him as a United States Representative, should he so choose.

So, what was causing Johnny's angst? In part, it was watching the dysfunction of American government in action. There was an old saying that one wouldn't want to watch sausage or American laws being made. He hadn't visited a sausage plant, but he was in agreement on the lawmaking dimension. It was messy, and sometimes downright stupid.

Thankfully, it was also sometimes amusing in its incoherence and happenstance. When Johnny started out, he found this entertaining. It was an experience, and he had a front row seat. Even now, there were many occasions where this was still his reaction to the nonsense at play. Sometimes, in more philosophical moments, he also thought it a positive aspect of the system—bad ideas were rooted out not by their idiotic features but by an idiotic process around them. The genius of the founding fathers? Perhaps, thought Johnny.

But Johnny also spent much of his time meeting people and learning of their troubles. It was not hard for him to discount the woes of those who were greedy or seeking political power; he didn't begrudge them these ambitions, but their pleas didn't invoke much empathy from him. He had plenty, and it was reserved for those who were really suffering from a bad situation or just trying to survive. Many suffered from illness, business failures, and bad luck—a myriad of woes, sometimes their fault and sometimes just random acts of God or Nature. These people were looking for solutions to their lot in life and asking Johnny and the system he was a part of to help.

Surely the system, and he, could do more for these people. Sometimes he could help, but usually in some smaller and incomplete way, which frustrated him. How could he be so successful in being a politician in all normal appearances, and still fail to achieve what the job should really be about? Johnny was struggling with this question when Irv had inquired about the trip. When he reconsidered Irv's request, he realized that his friend was asking for help, and that he also needed some. And who better than Irv to help him figure this out?

Like Irv, Johnny felt some stirring in his being on his question while they were waiting out their rescue in the hot canyonlands. He sort of hoped that help would not be found for a few more days. He was having too much fun. Odds were that the Crockpot of this experience would give him an answer—but it could wait a few more days.

So he felt a little disappointed when Irv and he spotted the dust trail approaching from the west. It was a jeep with three men in it, scooting through a dry wash toward their campground. Oh well, they thought. They could get the help they needed and then finish off their vacation after getting to safety.

The three men parked about twenty feet from their camp and spread out as they walked toward Irv and Johnny. They looked like they had been out in the wilderness for a while themselves. Their clothes, dungarees and work shirts, were filthy, and their hair slick with grime. All three had major stubble on their faces, not beards but many days of missed shaving.

The leader of the group stepped forward to meet Irv and Johnny, with his friends spread out on his flanks. He introduced himself as Bob, which made one of his friends giggle. He scooted down and looked under the Trooper, which they had propped up with a rock as they tried to fix the axle. "Looks like you got some trouble here," he said.

Johnny stepped forward and introduced himself, leaving out the part of being a congressman. He explained how the axle had broken and how they would appreciate a ride out or if they might at least notify the authorities to send help their way. Johnny offered a couple of hundred dollars for the help.

It was then that "Bob" reached into his waistband to the rear and pulled out a handgun. As he did, so did his two companions. "We'll take that two hundred dollars, and everything else you got, boys. Drop all your belongings on the ground in front of you."

Irv and Johnny did. It didn't help that they had smoked a bowl half an hour ago.

"Now lay down on the ground, with your hands over your head." They did as instructed. Bob's companions then approached them and took the belongings they had tossed to the ground, frisking them to make sure they had everything. Irv had a watch that Mary Beth had given him; they took that too.

Then they moved to the Trooper, opening all the doors and riffling through the contents. After getting a mental inventory, they took everything of value to them—the food, the water, the liquor and pot, the cell phone, backpacks, and even the sleeping bags. They packed it all into the back of their jeep, now stuffed with Irv and Johnny's supplies, and Bob began to back up toward it.

"Sorry, boys," he said. "It was nice of you to come along when you did. We were running low on supplies. Not much traffic out here. And it can get mighty hot. Some interesting critters too. You might even survive for a few days. Wish you luck though." He took a long swig from a canteen, swirling it around so he could hear how much water might still be in it. At best, it was half full. "Don't say I didn't do nothing for you though." He tossed the canteen halfway between him and them.

With that, he ran to the jeep, jumped in the driver seat, and they drove off with their loot, leaving Irv and Johnny to figure out what to do. The pair forgot all about their questions about life choices now—this was now a red alert. It was time to figure out how they might survive.

Chapter Thirty-Nine

Hiking Out of Canyonlands

At about three in the afternoon, Johnny and Irv found themselves in the sweltering heat of Utah, in the desolate locale of Canyonlands. Robbers had stolen virtually all of their supplies and left them to fend for themselves. Irv's four-wheel drive vehicle was of no use because of a broken axle, and they had a half canteen of water. They could either wait for help to magically appear, or they could try to walk out of Canyonlands. It would be many miles of travel over rough terrain to do that—perhaps well over a hundred.

They searched the Isuzu Trooper to find what was left of use to them. There was little: a couple of candy bars in the glove box, a blanket, and some clothing. After discussing their situation, they concluded the best option was to walk out—and soon. The odds of running into others in the park were low, and *really* low if they just waited in this spot.

They would have to choose a direction. Using a National Park Service map they were handed on entry, Irv and Johnny did their best to retrace their route, plotting what they thought was the shortest line to what they hoped would be help. Southeast would be the general direction of choice.

They would leave in the evening as the sun was setting, allowing them to travel at night out of the sun. They took down the tarp and the ropes and poles. Shade would be important when they rested during the hot afternoon. They put all the useful possessions in the tarp and folded it over so it functioned as a container, then tied a piece of rope to either end of the tarp. Each held one end so they could carry their supplies like a stretcher.

As the sun set they began their journey. They agreed on the location of the North Star from their several nights of observing the Utah sky and plotted a course to the southeast. There were a couple of campgrounds in that direction and, as best as they could figure from the map, no marked obstacles in the way of their escape.

Of course, they knew this may or may not be true. Looking a hundred yards in any direction revealed dozens of formidable obstacles, and none of these were on the map. There were boulders and ridges that they would have to walk slowly over or around. Nor did they have any certainty about how many miles they would need to travel. They guessed it was at least fifty miles, but with a miscalculation of any type, it could well be a hundred or more.

The odds were low, no matter how they cut it. They would see how far they could get with a half canteen of water and two candy bars. Off they went.

They walked all night, taking three short breaks. As expected, there were many detours around the twisting rock landscape. The North Star provided a good target, and they moved what they thought was due southeast throughout the night. When the sun rose and the North Star faded away, they fixed a mountain peak in the distance as their aim point, and kept moving. At about 11 a.m.—they were guessing since they had no watch—the sun started to really cook them, and they stopped. They set up the tarp so it shielded them from the sun; each ate half a candy bar and took a gulp of water. They slept as much as they could. They were tired, hungry, and thirsty, and their feet hurt.

They guessed that they had gone about twenty-five miles. Maybe fifteen hours of walking, a half an hour to a mile? They had taken plenty of detours though, and there was no way that their pace was the same as when they hiked on flat trails or city streets and sidewalks.

At about seven the next evening, they did it all over again. Their tanks were much emptier though. They had only taken two more swigs of water over the course of the day, and craved water even before they started the night's trip. They also decided to hold off on the remaining candy bar until the next day. When they stopped the next morning in a small ravine, they knew that they had traveled far less than they had the night before. They were slowing down, and hurting. No one was to be seen or heard, and they saw nothing on the horizon, when they could even see a horizon, that suggested they were getting close to help.

Irv and Johnny looked for water around their daytime campsite for a few minutes, or anything that might serve as food. They knew that cactus sometimes would have pockets of moisture that could be sucked for sustenance, but there weren't any of those around. Rather than burn more energy in what they thought a useless search, they set up the tarp and rested as best they could.

As the sun began to set, they ate the last of the candy bar and took another drink from the canteen. It was almost empty. They began another night of walking, and their pace continued to slow. They stopped for a break in the middle of the night.

The odds were getting lower on their survival—of that they were sure. They both took a drink from the canteen, which was now empty, and leaned back against a boulder and looked at the sky. At least it was cool this time of night. A shooting star flashed across the sky.

"I say we follow that trail," said Johnny.

"Affirmative," said Irv.

"We got anything at all left to eat?"

"Nope," said Irv. "Wait, I do have one thing left." He pulled the peyote buttons from his shirt pocket. The bandits had not thought to look there when they frisked him. "Hungry?"

They smiled, and then laughed. If this was it for them, what better way to go? And what better way to increase the odds that they might survive too.

They each nibbled at their button, savoring their only meal for the day, and prayed that the trip would be kind to them, however it turned out. They got up and began to walk some more, following the general trail of the shooting star. It was roughly east, but really, who cared anymore?

Chapter Forty

The Theory of Irv

Somewhere in the canyonlands of southeast Utah, two tired adventurers were stumbling across the harsh landscape by foot, while juice from peyote buttons flowed through them. A half hour later they were more floating than walking. A bass note trebled in their ears, and they felt a coolness on their skin. It masked much of the hunger, thirst, and pain of their current circumstances.

Their pace slowed, and they were no longer on a mostly straight line to the east. They were meandering, toward the shooting star, around more obstacles and toward whatever moved them at the moment. They weren't focused on any real destination, or even a plan for survival. They were now good friends out for a walk, which they hoped would end happily enough for them, somehow.

"So, Johnny, how does Congress get your replacement when they find your body out here in the desert?"

"Beats me. They probably first have to find it and identify it. Might be a few months before they even get to your question."

"Huh. I'm not sure they will even bother to look for me."

"What do you mean? Mary Beth will, for sure."

Irv was saddened to think of her. "Yup, good old Mary Beth." They walked another twenty steps or so, still hanging on to the tarp with the ropes between them. "Johnny, I would give anything to see her one last time. She is the best thing to ever happen to me. Now, you are a strong second, brother, but . . . you know what I'm saying . . ."

"No offense taken, Irv. I know exactly what you are saying. Truth be told, I've always been jealous of what you two have. Would give my right nut to have a woman like that."

"Well, you know you probably could have. She's always had a thing for you. I knew that the first night I stayed in that house and your name came up."

"Oh, we had a thing for sure. But it wasn't like your thing. More like brother and sister. You and she—you are the real cosmic deal."

They trudged along another twenty yards.

"I got a confession to make, Johnny."

"What's that?"

"Remember when I moved into your congressional district when you first ran for election to Congress?"

"Sure. You did some campaigning for me too."

"Well, I voted for someone else. Got in the voting booth intending to vote for you, but when I got there, well, I just couldn't do it. Kind of screwed up, huh? Don't know what I was thinking. Probably that you were going to go away, and leave us far behind."

Johnny laughed. "I take that as a compliment, Mr. Tinsley. And good judgment on your part. What the hell am I doing in Congress anyway?"

"Oh, you are a fine congressman. Probably the best one I know."

"Do you know another?"

It was Irv's turn to laugh. "No. But if I did, you would still be number one. But tell me, was it what you thought it would be?"

Johnny thought about Irv's question, his thinking mixed with wavy visions in the shadows around him. "Not sure what I thought it would be. I thought it would be a great way to meet people and expand my adventures through them. That it has. Been some frustrations for me too."

He shared with Irv, for the first time, his struggles with the lot of being a legislator. It had been top of mind throughout the trip, and he had occasionally fished for Irv's thoughts about career and ambitions. He figured it would come up before the trip was over, but it looked to be now or never. Not that it seemed like a very relevant question anymore, as he anticipated their end to this trip.

Irv was surprised to hear of Johnny's angst. He had always believed that it was the journey that mattered to Johnny, not the outcomes along the way. And yet, it seemed to him that this was what was ailing him. It tugged at Irv like tight underwear.

"John, I don't think you are alone in your thinking." Irv shared with Johnny his own struggle about where he was with life. The happiness mixed with the frustration of thinking that there was something more, or next that needed to be put in play.

"How frigging bizarre that we are trying to figure this out when we are about to become coyote snacks. After we pass out from dehydration, hunger, and heat stroke!" exclaimed Johnny.

Irv laughed, and listened to his voice roll across the canyonlands. "Go figure! But what if we somehow made it out of this? What would we do? What's our thing?"

"Yeah, we need a plan. A backup plan?"

"No, I don't think it's a plan. That's a little too linear. For us, and certainly in our current state." The stars were jumping around in the sky, playing a video game beyond his understanding.

"So, what is it?" asked Johnny.

Irv pondered the question as they stumbled forward. "I got it," he shouted. He jumped up and down, dropping his rope and the tarp on the ground. "We need a theory!"

Johnny dropped his rope to the ground too, realizing that he wasn't going to be very successful dragging the tarp ahead by himself. He looked around—they were on a small plateau overlooking a little canyon to the north. To the east was a large rock formation that they would have to walk around. It would be a lot of work. This would be a good place to watch the sun rise, he thought. *And to die with my friend.* He sat down on a boulder and patted the space next to him. "Come on over here, my friend. Let's just wait here for a while."

Irv came over and sat down next to Johnny, who wrapped his longish right arm around him. "As good a place as we can find, Johnny. It's all about the company, anyway."

They sat and looked out over the canyon and the open range to the north for a couple of minutes, processing their thoughts and what remained of the peyote juice. It had been several hours since they had eaten the buttons, and the effects were wearing off. The extra surge of energy from the buttons was starting to wane, and behind it they both knew were some serious problems.

Johnny decided to fill his last times with a meaningful conversation with his friend, just like so many times they had before. "So, you were saying we need a theory. If I remember right, a theory is, loosely speaking, an idea that sets a course of action. It could be a principle or a moral or something else, but it mostly serves as a guide for what one might do over time. Much like how we have been following that comet."

"Correct again, Johnny. Yes, a theory. But not a theory—*our* theory." Irv stretched; he was beginning to feel some sharp pains in his back that were now merging with the burning hole in his stomach and the dryness in his throat. They didn't have long. "Our theory. How about something like this: That it is not enough to just experience the world. That one must try to do good in the world. Not lose oneself in the trappings of the experience or the power that might accompany the pursuit, but just to try and do good, for others and the society we are within."

"I am liking it, Irv. So, as a politician, I would try to do more than get more powerful. I would commit to trying to make a difference, and even a bigger difference if I have the opportunity to do so. I like that."

"And I, Mr. Gibson, would find a way toward some career that might put me also in a place to do good. I could keep living my life with Mary Beth but start to plan for something more too." A sadness came over his revelation as Irv realized the irony of the moment.

Johnny sensed his friend's sadness. He must keep his attention from what was likely to come soon. "If you could solve one thing for the betterment of others, what would it be?"

Irv looked at him. "Seriously? Like that matters now."

"It does to me."

Irv realized that he also must make his friend feel better about what was soon to come. If it was talking and theorizing about the future, so be it. He focused what was left of his reserves on the question and thought.

A couple of minutes passed. They were both beginning to lose consciousness. Their vision was wavy, and the air was still around them. "Okay." Irv revived enough to answer Johnny's question. "Health care. I would do something about health care." He figured that was not enough for Johnny and filled in some of the gaps behind it, starting with the death of his mom. "It was screwed up, how it worked, and I've been doing some reading about it. It doesn't have to be that way."

"You are just the man to do something about it," said Johnny, his words trailing away as he passed out. He fell toward Irv, who did the same in the other direction. They would take a short nap together, maybe for eternity. But at least they had a theory—the Theory of Irv.

Chapter Forty-One

Rescue

A light was approaching. Irv could see it. Just like those stories he had read about death experiences. It was true. *There is my light. I should follow it.*

Then he realized that the light was coming at him. The closer it got, the brighter it was. It was familiar. It was . . . a flashlight?

The man holding it shined it fully in his face. "Hey, he's awake. Come on over here." Another man and woman came closer to him. The man turned the flashlight off. Irv could now make out that he was lying on a bed in a cramped room. Maybe a camper?

"You gave us quite a scare there, fella. If my son hadn't woken up in the middle of the night to take a pee, we may never have heard you. I don't think you and your friend would have lasted more than another hour or two at the most."

Irv had a splitting headache, making it hard for him to process the words and images before him. He tried to sit up a bit and found it hard to move. Picking up just his head, he looked around some more. Yup, a camper.

"Where the hell am I?" he asked.

"We are in a campground in Canyonlands National Park, about a half mile from where we found you and your friend. You were both unconscious, and we rallied some other campers to help us carry you back to our rigs. That was about four hours ago. You two camped around here somewhere?"

Irv shook his head. "No. We were car camping, and our axle broke. Some bandits took all of our supplies, and we have been walking across the parklands for the past few days."

"No shit? You guys are lucky to be alive."

"Where's my friend?" Irv was worried about Johnny not being in the camper with him. Was he okay?

"Oh, he's next door in another camper. He just came to a few minutes ago too, though hasn't said anything yet. Seems pretty dazed. But alive and coming around."

Irv smiled. "Not like Johnny to be so quiet. Just be warned—once you get him talking again, he might not stop."

"Lay back down, fella. I think it is a little too soon for you to be telling jokes. Let's get some more food and water in you. So far all we've been able to do for the two of you is wash you down with wet towels. One of the other campers is a paramedic, and he's been helping us to revive you both. He is with your friend Johnny now."

Irv had no energy to argue. "Okay. I could use an aspirin or something for this headache I got too."

"We are going to hold off on that just a little bit till we can move the two of you. Our paramedic friend says that both of you need to get to the hospital. We have been waiting for daylight to make the drive over this rough terrain. It's probably two hours to the hospital. We'll take you as soon as you think you are ready."

"Let's do it soon," Irv said as he put his head back down on the pillow. Sleep was calling him. Though a meal and some water would be nice too. "I need to make a phone call too. Got to talk to Mary Beth."

"Is that your wife or girlfriend?" asked the man with the flashlight.

"Yup. Got to tell her I love her. And that I have a theory . . . " *I will see her soon*, he thought before passing out again.

Chapter Forty-Two

Westside Medical Center in Phoenix

Irv drove to Westside Medical Center in Phoenix early in the morning, beginning this phase of his investigation by meeting with the director of Emergency Services. He had spent part of the last evening in his hotel room, researching the director online in order to find a way to relate to him personally. Irv began their meeting with small talk, maneuvering this to the director's guitar hobby, which he had found on his Facebook account, while also name-dropping a couple of the upper management people at Westside Medical Center, suggesting he knew them personally.

The approach worked—the director let down whatever defenses might be making him reluctant to cooperate and soon was opening up. It was also clear that he had other things going on that day and had limited time to talk. After twenty minutes, he excused himself, gave Irv a business card should he have additional questions, and assigned a unit clerk to help him with any of his specific needs. Perfect. Irv was now in.

His first stop with the clerk assigned to him was the Medical Center's electronic medical record system for patients. She logged in with her password and was ready to run any search he needed. He directed her to patient care files for Rodrigo Lopez. As expected, the file Irv already had found in his investigation popped up. But no others. It looked like this was a one-time stop for Rodrigo.

The clerk checked other portals in the system for records, such as insurance and billing information. All were empty, save for an asterisk and a code number. He wrote the number down in his notebook. The clerk asked him if he wanted a paper copy of the record, but Irv declined;

he already had the necessary information and didn't want to trigger any notice to higher-ups that someone was going through this record.

What he was really after were paper records that might tell him more about Rodrigo's visit to the hospital. He knew from his time working at hospitals that while health care leaders liked to brag about their expensive electronic medical systems, these were far from effective. In order to fill information gaps and do their jobs, clinical and other staff regularly created ad hoc paper systems.

He presumed that Westside Medical Center's emergency room would have its own unique paper systems, and he wanted to see what he could find. He reviewed standard care and record protocols within the ER with the unit clerk, searching for the record link.

One protocol seemed promising—every outstanding emergency room patient case was identified and reviewed during the change of shift. Physicians and nurses on days would summarize where things were for the evening shift, and the same happened for the night shift, and so on. It was particularly important they transfer information about patients still in their care as shift change happened. Just in case memories failed, a paper record of the handoffs were made by the unit clerk. These notes from shift transfer were stored in a file cabinet, along with any paper records that came up during the case reviews.

The unit clerk brought Irv to where they stored these shift change records. He thanked her for her help and encouraged her to go back to her regular duties. He needed to review the records, and there was little she could do to help with this part of the research. She was ready for a break and left him alone in the small office with the multi-drawer file cabinet.

Irv found the records pertaining to Rodrigo's visit to the ER in about fifteen minutes. Rodrigo had been in the emergency room over a shift change, and there was indeed a case review for him. The conclusions discussed at shift change were brief, noting that a thirty-year-old Hispanic male had presented with chest pains, was undergoing the usual standard tests, and was expected to be discharged soon.

More helpful were several paper reports for Rodrigo attached to the case review. One was a series of standard lab tests. Irv knew enough about medical tests to know what to look for. All indications were that Rodrigo had chest pains that might suggest some underlying cardiac issues. Some seemed particularly troubling to Irv, but he was not well versed in cardiac health issues. Most importantly, the tests showed there was no chance that Rodrigo's symptoms had anything to do with the flu; that was Irv's wheelhouse, and all the lab values pertaining to that were normal to the extreme.

The other record stapled to the review was more puzzling. It was a general notation to the medical record that was attached to his ER admittance form, inserted by the unit clerk when they formally processed him as a patient within the Medical Center. There was little to it: his name and the same number found on the electronic record.

Irv waited for the unit clerk to return. He told her how helpful all this was, trying to put her at ease and make sure she didn't sense any danger in what he was doing. He casually moved the conversation to the documents he had found for Rodrigo related to the change of shift, and homed in on the document related to his patient processing.

The unit clerk shared with him that when a patient presented at the ER, the center would input their insurance information so that billing information would be forwarded immediately to the finance division. It was usually a pretty simple process—finance clerks would check insurance for the patient using an electronic system, and confirm coverage was live and sufficient for the services to be rendered. If the patient was uninsured, or if their insurance coverage was insufficient for their presenting diagnosis and likely treatment, the hospital was to refer the case immediately to a finance caseworker whose job, as much as the clerk understood it, was to make other payment arrangements by the patient or to transfer them to another health care facility.

She added that every once in a while, the system would flag a patient as a special case. Rather than referring them to the finance division, they were to immediately send a message via the hospital's landline phone to a special number. No one really understood where this message actually went or what it meant, but there was some concern among the staff of the emergency room that there was an audit underway that might affect their job. So, they had begun to put a paper flag on these cases to make sure all staff knew which cases they were. It was an underground warning to other emergency room staff. The document he found in the shift change record just meant that there was a paper flag for the patient in question—in this case, Rodrigo.

Irv was intrigued. "You don't happen to have copies of the actual documents that triggered the flagging, do you?"

"Sure. If they are not attached to the shift reports like for the case you found, we put them in a file in the second drawer." She pointed to the second file from the bottom.

Irv opened the drawer and got out the file. There were easily a hundred of these files, maybe more like 125. He quickly flipped through them. They were just like the one for Rodrigo, each with a name and the same type of number. He asked the unit clerk if he could make a record of these other names just in case they needed to reconcile some documents. He also asked if she would be able to go through the names on the electronic medical system to see if there was information about those patients available within the computer database.

Alarm bells were beginning to ring for the unit clerk as to why his research was getting so broad, but Irv had convinced her that he meant her and her colleagues no harm. She intuited that his digging might mean that somebody in HealthMost management could get into trouble, but she cared little about that. They treated her poorly, while they took home big salaries. She compiled a summary report of patients like Rodrigo over the rest of the afternoon.

She also introduced Irv to members of the unit staff; he talked to them while she was putting the report together. A couple of nurses were willing to talk about the record flags, in part because they found the approach to these cases unsettling. They were to complete their evaluation and then transport them out of the ER, once stabilized, by calling the special telephone number. They would prepare them for discharge and escort them out to the portico of the ER, where a hospital van would pick them up and take them to wherever they were going next. They did not know the destination, nor did they have any records that would indicate it. One staffer noticed that the van, while a normal hospital vehicle, was manned by a transport aide who he never saw come for any other patients.

Irv returned to his hotel room and contemplated what he had learned at the hospital. Rodrigo had gone to Westside Medical Center and been diagnosed for a heart problem, not the flu. His presence in the ER was flagged by reference to a central database for the health system, but otherwise was largely missing in any formal record keeping.

The shadow paper systems showed that someone had taken him away. Where he went was unknown, at least until he was discovered dead in a house in Kent, Washington. In between, he had presumably been flown from wherever he went after the hospital, maybe to Moses Lake, and transported somehow to Kent? There were another 117 case records at Westside Medical Center of patients who were similarly flagged in the ER. Did they all meet the same fate, or some version of it?

What he did know was that the names on those 117 cases were almost all Latino. Irv thought it possible that this was HealthMost flagging patients who might need more care and support because of their diverse background; it was well-documented that non-white patients fared worse in terms of health care risks and outcomes. No, he quickly concluded this was not the case here. It might happen at some other mission-driven hospitals, but Westside had the feel of a hospital focused on making money, not spending extra amounts out of their own pocket for those in greater need.

He thought about calling the telephone number provided to the ER staff. But it might only work through the hospital internal system, and he didn't know enough about phone systems to be sure. More importantly, he decided not to let whoever was on the other end know that someone was digging around these records. One of the few things he had going for him was that no one knew that he was on the trail of whatever it was. If they knew, the trail would likely get much harder to find.

There had to be another way forward. What he needed was to relate what he had found at Westgate Medical Center to the bigger set of records in the database at ALI in Hartford, Connecticut. It seemed to him that HealthMost's system defense around Rodrigo and other patients like him was to limit patient records within clinical care files that were available across the system, and instead to get most of the data pertaining to such patients into another location. It sure seemed likely that was behind the firewall of their new partner life insurance company, ALI.

Irv would not be able to bluff his way inside of a company like that as he had at the emergency room. Insurers were different cats. They cared little to nothing about public health needs, certainly when lined up next to the security of their information and financial systems. A health insurer might offer a little sympathy for a fake public health investigation, but for a life insurer, it would take an act of Congress to get even an ounce of interest.

Of course. He knew someone in Congress! That could be his ticket. He still had several vacation days left, and it would be good to see Johnny. A quick text confirmed that he was in town and would find time for him. Irv researched flights to Washington, DC, found a red-eye leaving at 11 p.m., and made his way to the Phoenix airport.

Chapter Forty-Three

1980: Chris Jones Looks for Bigger Policy Answers

As the calendar turned to the decade of the 1980s, Professor Christopher Jones thought the time had arrived to test bigger and more comprehensive solutions to the problems of the American health care system. His certainty came from personally spending much of the past decade helping federal policymakers test smaller and more incremental solutions. The end result, he concluded, was an even more confused and inefficient health care system.

It wasn't for lack of trying. One of the earliest attempts to shift toward bigger solutions came, oddly enough, in the 1970s during the Nixon Administration. Leaders within the administration were seeing the financial impact of the health system's failings upon the federal government and began to look for more efficient models for delivering health care across America, especially within the Medicare program.

Some observed the existence of several Health Maintenance Organizations across the nation. These HMOs used the concept of prepaid health care organizations, which were the underlying principle of state Blue Cross plans that had grown across the country in the 1920s and 1930s, and applied it to an even more integrated model. These organizations would not only finance care by accepting enrollees, but actually deliver health care services to these enrollees through their own hospitals and staff.

There were a number of HMOs then, and studies suggested that their cost savings might be as much as 40 percent from the traditional fee-for-service-care business model. Some of these entities were formed by necessity in the New Deal era. The public works projects of FDR brought multitudes of workers to isolated areas of the country where care was not available, such as in the building of dams. Companies like Kaiser Permanente created their own capacity to provide health care to these high-risk workers. It was an industrial model of health care delivery and showed promise to be a major reform vehicle if it could be made available to many more Americans.

There would need to be a lot more of them though. While the ones that existed were doing a good job, a much greater supply would be needed to transform the American health care production cycle for health care and make a meaningful cost reduction impact nationally.

Christopher was influential in convincing the Nixon Administration to provide incentives for the formation of more HMO supply; these incentives would be somewhat like the construction grants for hospitals of the 1950s. With many more of these HMOs in place, Christopher thought it would then be possible to direct Medicare, and all of American health care, toward a different solution. The notion of HMOs also contained many of the features of a great health care system recommended by the CCMC. It would be coordinated care, and the incentive would be to make and keep people healthy, rather than just provide more and more expensive treatments and other services.

As the HMO grant program rolled out, Chris momentarily thought that the needed revolution for bigger system change was at hand. But it quickly lost its allure, as the forces of the status quo exerted itself upon the political arms of the agencies and Congress, and soon changed the notion of what it meant to be an HMO.

Almost all of the models being used to demonstrate the value of the concept were what became known as Staff Model HMOs. They owned and controlled most of the inputs of medical care, such as their own hospitals, clinics, and clinical staff, allowing them to organize and coordinate care more aggressively—and to apply cost savings strategies as a major factor in their economic decisions, including substituting labor inputs, the greatest cost element of hospital care.

Medical professionals and others fought against this notion, in particular the AMA, as it was the actualization of their fear that corporations, not physicians, would be put in control of American medicine. Also, there were those who saw an opportunity to make a buck, and they pressed policymakers to add an option that would allow them to start up HMOs without major entry barriers and get in on the financial action. The Nixon Administration proved sensitive to these overtures, as were many in Congress.

The Nixon Administration decided to allow non-staff model HMOs to qualify for the program. These new types typically contracted with provider groups and others to provide the care they were paid for by a client, but did not have the same level of control as the staff HMOs. Many of these hybrid HMO models were formed by physician groups, who were intent on maintaining fee-for-service payment methodologies and practicing pattern autonomy like those of the existing system. Because of this, studies suggested and experience proved that such entities would only marginally cut costs, if at all; nevertheless, they were added to the program.

The HMO program became largely another failed cost containment program. There were some success stories through additional staff model HMOs, but not enough in place to trigger a comprehensive re-sorting of the system of American health care, and its cost.

In subsequent years, the grants for the creation of these entities faded away as a policy option. But there was a residue of the concept inserted into Medicare policy—the notion that the federal government could outsource its Medicare obligation to private health plans. While short-term marginal cost savings were built into the effort, the bigger strategy game was to transfer government obligations to the private sector so that, ultimately, it would no longer be a government obligation to care for the elderly. Advocates of this were happy to get Medicare beneficiaries to sign up with private health insurers who largely operated outside of Medicare protections for those clients who stayed in the base program—whether they provided necessary care or access to physicians and hospitals in reasonable ways or not.

The bloom came off the rose of this innovation for Christopher early on, and when he saw the way the option was being used to whittle away at the federal role for health coverage by Americans, he further distanced himself from the effort. HMOs—*real* HMOs—might have a place in the ultimate system answer, he said. But it was not the big answer needed to solve the fundamental problems of the American health care system.

Chris's favorite innovation was the notion of comprehensive health planning, and he spent the second half of the 1970s trying to make this work. Comprehensive health planning was, by definition, intended to be thoughtful, comprehensive, and rational. After all, a failed system reflected exactly that there had been no conscious planning in place to design and manage the American health care system. Chris thought it still possible to do so; that is, we could put the horses back in the barn for America's health care policy, through a comprehensive new federal requirement for local health planning. Doing so would be real rationality in the Age of Rationalization.

By the time Chris presented this option in 1972, the growing cost of health care had risen to a national crisis. Chris worked with other health policy advisors to devise a national framework of local health planning agencies that would convene citizens, health care leaders, and politicians toward creating rational decisions for allocating health care resources in their communities and states. The local planning recommendations would be given force by their incorporation into decisions to be made through a "state health planning and development agency" within each state.

One set of teeth the law provided was that these SHPDAs would have the authority to approve or disapprove capital investments within the state and their eligibility for federal reimbursement. Built upon this notion were state laws that required "certificates of need" for providers to add major new services, such as a new hospital, major pieces of medical equipment, and in some cases, even a service line.

Public Law 93-641 was passed in 1972, and soon dollars were flowing to states and localities to develop their local plans. Hundreds of people got involved in these efforts, and it was a regular occurrence for American communities to convene on weekday evenings to discuss how to improve their local health care. It was CCMC Recommendation 4 in essence: community based and coordinated care planning.

Chris's belief was that these entities would devise pragmatic resource allocations in a way that would yield massive savings to the system, all while reshaping health care into a real and more effective system. It would be driven more by what users of the system wanted and needed, rather than what those who profited from it would like. The Age of More had created far more health care than we needed, and there had to be a way to tamp it down to a more reasonable level. Since we the people were paying for the excess, it would also solve the cost problem.

Health planning had a good run, and it showed potential to achieve Chris's lofty reform dreams. Resistance was expected, and the status quo didn't lie down easily. One problem for the planning mode of redesign was that it would take some time to yield results. First the plans must be developed, then implemented, and then one would have to wait and experience the actual benefits of rational redesign.

Opponents pointed to the lack of clear benefits in the early years of planning, and many in Congress wanted a quick fix. Also damaging was the inclusion of the capital approval process in the model. Providers who had their proposals rejected by local or state agencies began to use the courts to challenge these decisions, sometimes on constitutional grounds of "taking" without due process. These lawsuits slowed down the process dramatically, and some states and agencies began to settle the disputes rather than fight on. Providers soon learned that lawyers could get them what they wanted if the agencies disapproved.

Politics was the real enemy, and the election of President Ronald Reagan in 1981 was the real end to health planning. The Reagan Revolution promised an end to government overreach, and the network of health planning agencies was one of its symbolic targets. It was time to get the government out of American life, just when it was finally rationally inserting itself into American health care.

What was even more painful to Chris was that the Reagan team did away with health planning through budget techniques, not some clear policy debate by the American people on how best to manage American health care or Medicare or Medicaid. Budget bills at the federal level, some of the first "reconciliation" bills used to fund the federal government in the face of partisan conflict, included provisions removing federal support for comprehensive health planning, and this budget cut was effectively its end.

The federal Certificate of Need requirement was also soon repealed, though many states kept their own CON requirements on the books, many times due to lobbying by existing hospitals and other providers who were intent on using such laws to prevent new competition. In some states, the status quo was even able to get the government out of the business of reviewing their own expansion plans, while using CON as a tool to keep out new competition.

Chris was frustrated over the demise of health planning, and the nonsense around capital approvals only made him see more policy red. He thought comprehensive health planning was the best chance to rationalize the American health care system, short of taking control over it at the federal level. He thought that the innovation was working fairly well, despite its slow pace of change, and could have worked as a solution.

By the early 1980s, reforms like health planning had been repealed and replaced by hype about how marketplaces and private competition would come to the rescue. This was the philosophical branding for a series of policy solutions over the next twenty years, asserted first by the Reagan Administration, and then through subsequent Republican administrations or Congress. The policies were more talking points than real and serious proposals, but the rhetoric was translated to legislation that became part of American health policy. Some of the laws might even have made some discrete policy differences, but almost all ultimately just made the whole of American health care even more fragmented and dysfunctional.

An early example of the fallacy at work was the adoption of a new methodology for paying hospitals adopted by Medicare in 1981. It was the notion of doing this through payment based on Diagnostic Related Groups, or DRGs. These were the codes used to denote the discharge diagnosis for patients. Researchers at Yale had been working to organize costs associated with these different diagnoses and assigning them different relative values in terms of cost. Christopher thought it to be a scientifically sound effort that offered a lot of promise to rationalizing the prices paid by the government and others for hospital care.

The Reagan Administration captured the idea and targeted it for adoption into the Medicare program beginning in 1981. Their DRG Payment System for Medicare would eliminate the old system of paying for hospital care and largely end the past fights over what was "allowable" as a cost, since a relative price for diagnosis would become the basis for payment. It would also allow for a slower rate of increase in these costs, since the update would now be an inflation factor within the payment formula, with the level set by Congress.

Chris had no quarrel with doing any or all of this. What he found objectionable, and even dangerous, was how this was labeled as the introduction of competition into America's health care. It was anything but—it was just sophisticated rate setting by the government. But the rhetoric opened the door to more "marketplace health policy."

A favorite stalking horse for those pushing market solutions was that Americans needed more skin in the game. That is, if their care was financed by first dollar coverage, there would be no limits to the use of care. Chris understood that this was the economic concept of moral hazard, an artificial incentive that would increase demand for a good or service.

He thought it was true that this was real. But it was far less of a factor than pushed by its proponents. Chris knew well that many Americans wanted no part of more health care service, regardless of the financial incentives. Among men, it was hard to find many who had even seen a physician for years. If they did, it was usually because their wives had browbeaten them to do it, not because it was covered by insurance.

Nor was the solution all that useful to addressing moral hazard, to the extent it even was a major factor. Usually, the answer was to make Americans pay more for service, through copayments, either of their insurance premiums or their receipt of health care. The reality was that these decisions were usually made by their health care providers, not them—and the incentive for most of these providers was to order and do more.

Chris observed that the thoughtful application of such a concept might have some useful policy value, but was used instead to displace financial obligations of employers and other payors by pushing rising costs on to consumers. Use of service didn't slow because such decisions were made elsewhere since health care was not a traditional consumer good. The approach became part of the problem more than a solution.

Nor did other more traditional additions to American health policy stop during these times. "More" continued to be added, as new opportunities and needs arose politically in the 1970s to 1990s. Medicaid was one of the leading areas of addition. Congressman Henry Waxman figured out how to politically leverage the principle of categorical eligibility within Medicaid for sub-populations at risk. The needs of these patient cohorts were sold politically, such as the priority of health care for pregnant women and children. Some of these were optional programs for states, but state politicians soon discovered, again, that they could provide major benefits to their citizens and address major state health care problems using mostly federal money.

Some additions were necessary and worthy, Chris thought, and at times, he was an ally for these new efforts. For example, AIDS/HIV had been a shock to the country when it became a major health issue in the mid-1980s. A significant national effort was needed to fight this deadly disease, and the Reagan Administration had at first ignored the problem.

Chris thought it fundamental to national health policy that the federal government lead the effort to address new maladies facing Americans, especially those that arose through mutating viruses, bacteria, or other invisible contagions. AIDS/HIV was eventually tackled and contained, though not eliminated. Chris greatly hoped that politicians had learned their lesson, but privately thought that this would remain one of the greatest weaknesses of the American health care system going forward.

There were also much older maladies and needs that were finally getting addressed. Some were byproducts of the fragmentation of American health care; these were also isolated by the nature of their source. A notable issue was mental health. Many Americans suffered from some form of psychiatric disorder, and some were in extreme danger because of it. Yet, mental health was a condition that the nation wasn't even comfortable identifying and talking about, let alone treating. As its broader devastation became more apparent, and cultural norms shifted a little bit, doing something about mental health care became a monstrous American health care issue.

Oral health was another. The mouth had never really been fully considered to be part of the body, and the practice of dentistry was largely isolated from the advances of medical care and new health care system design. Part of this was from dentists wanting to assert professional autonomy, part of it from ignorance. Research was beginning to show that diseases of the teeth and gums had much to do with overall health conditions and risks, including heart disease. American health care policy was starting to recognize the need to connect the dots, but very slowly.

Individual diseases were also making their own strides in being understood and acted on by American health policy. Much of this was funded and organized through the National Institutes of Health and its different institutes for diseases—Cancer, Heart, Lung, and more. The medical specialists working within these fields emphasized their uniqueness, and not-for-profit organizations who raised money to fight these diseases also reinforced a separateness in thinking about them. Soon, almost all major diseases had sprouted a unique and significant lobbying base competing with others for attention and resources.

Meanwhile, more objective health policy was recognizing that diseases were far more integrated in how they played out for people. Diabetes became a leading example. Not only was it accelerating rapidly because of the bad behaviors and health system problems of society, but its consequences were typically things that related to other subsystems—heart disease, circulatory problems, amputations, and more. Even more pressing was the growing understanding that some of America's most important health research breakthroughs were general research that was not aimed at any one particular disease or condition—though lobbying by the different disease constituencies limited these investments so that there was more for them. Wiser American health policy-makers slowly began to understand that we needed to address the holistic reality of disease and how it applied to people.

All of these new efforts and thinking were being added to the already weak superstructure of American health policy. It became clear that adding on new things to an inefficient and unworkable health system, even if they were the right things, might not work all that well. Somebody must tend to the overall garden, thought Chris, or very little will grow into the future.

Watching the slow and perverted advance of American health policy also reminded Chris of how politics could and would prevent sound and sane American health policy from moving forward. He saw that one of the enemies of the good was money—health care had become a lucrative endeavor, and defenders of the status quo were now spending millions to make sure that change was resisted. These groups and individuals learned how to use lobbyists, and major campaign contributions, to protect their turf and fortunes.

Health care was also becoming a source of political power—that is, Americans were increasingly starting to vote for candidates based on their frustrations and views over health care. Some observers began to describe health care as the new "third rail" of American politics—touch it and you will get destroyed. Better not to touch it all was a common refrain from candidates. The status quo, of course, was the winner in such thinking.

Christopher thought this to be idiotic. The voter concern over health care was born out of frustration with how health care was working, or more to the point, not. In particular, voters disliked how costly it had become, but also the problems they experienced when they used it. Shallow solutions were usually easily dismissed or vilified by one political party or the other. Republicans generally flailed away at any solution that had a government role, while Democrats chomped away at the imaginary marketplace of Republican solutions.

Americans, on the other hand, Chris thought, just wanted solutions. They were less ideologic in their relation to them, and more accepting that whatever these solutions would be should draw from both political camps in some compromise. The ability to use health care as a political tool in campaigns made it, ironically, less likely that anything to fix it would be seriously proposed.

Maybe, just maybe, thought Christopher, this irony could be flipped in a way that would open the door to fixing the system. It was time to put aside the Age of Rationalization in American health care and shift to an Age of Reform, he thought. Rationality should be incorporated into the reforms, for sure, but health care should now be approached as a political matter that needed votes to enable major and comprehensive reform, rather than incremental strategies. The public just might support this, and politicians would have to follow if there were enough of them.

Figuring out how to do this, and what the next iteration of American health policy might look like, became his next career obsession.

Chapter Forty-Four

2020: Patient Dumping Hearing in the Senate

"The committee will come to order," Senator John Gibson barked into the microphone on the raised dais, while spraying a look across the hearing room. It was a sizable room, more ornate than big because of the high ceilings, massive chandeliers, paintings, and arty light sconces on the wall. It was DC at its best, democracy "of the people, by the people, and for the people" in a setting more suitable to French royalty than the mobs outside of the castle.

The "committee" was the Subcommittee on Public Works and Resources, which was part of the United States Senate Post Office and Government Operations Committee. It was not exactly a plum political assignment in Congress; more like where one was put if one was a newly elected independent senator who had to run for reelection next year. That would be Johnny.

Johnny took what he could get and figured that he would find some opportunity within it. The ranking senator from New Hampshire declined the opportunity to chair the committee, wanting something more visible. No one else wanted the job, so Johnny took it. He would at least be in charge of nothing, if that was all he would get to do.

It was a creative turn of events that made his assignment now relevant. Patient dumping was a violation of federal law, and cases were growing around the country. Congressman John Gibson was part of the group that had helped pass federal legislation to stop this back in the 1980s, when he was a freshman legislator in the House. These laws had helped then, but reports of problems were now commonplace again in 2020. There was a little loose talk about trying to tighten up the relevant statutes because of what was going on, but no real energy was building to do anything about it.

Then a patient dump happened in Johnny's home state of Washington. An elderly woman named Helen Neederdam had died as a result of an alleged dump, and a complaint had been filed with the federal Department of Health and Human Services Office of the Inspector General.

It seemed destined to become another forgotten dumping incident and statistic. With knowledge of the federal law, and local constituents asking him to help them out, Johnny put his chief of staff, Lance Givens, on the case. Lance was a creative sort and had a law degree that provided useful insights to the task at hand. He figured out that the hospital in question had received government funding through local property taxes. This, per ancient Senate protocols, technically placed their behavior under the investigative power of Johnny's Subcommittee on Public Works, and gave him the leverage to use the committee to press an investigation.

Worse for those who wished the issue would go away, Johnny had also worked with legislative allies, including old friends in the House, to insert an instruction on the issue in the budget reconciliation process. Well before Johnny's time in Congress, the Appropriations Committees of the Senate and House had found tremendous power by making the monetary allocations to programs across the federal government. They not only set broad policy by asserting what pots of money could be spent on, but they spent considerable time in hearings and markup sessions drafting legislation and conference reports that detailed particular funding decisions.

The Reagan Revolution of the 1980s took away much of this money power by creating a budget process that included something called "reconciliation instructions," which called for Congress to adopt a budget map for each year. Attendant to it would be instructions to various congressional committees to set out their sub-agendas in dollar terms. This was just when then Congressman John Gibson began his time in Congress, and he learned this new system well.

As partisan divides and modern election campaigning began to drive a wedge through bipartisanship on the Hill, "reconciliation" soon became the primary legislative vehicle for making policy change—by allocating money. The necessity to act on the federal budget was about the only thing that could push through the friction and inertia of the modern legislative process on Capitol Hill. Johnny figured out how to work this process, and was doing so this time, now decades later, by threatening HHS's funding unless they dealt with the patient dumping issue.

He also wanted to use media attention to exert even more pressure. So, Senator Gibson's committee scheduled a hearing to review patient dumping allegations, and invited the Secretary of HHS to testify on the issue. Johnny had won his Senate seat through the power of digital advocacy, and asked his staff to raise a social network stink about what was going on. A story had gone viral, making the hearing a topic worthy of the nightly news. No way that the White House was going to pass on the chance to defend their record.

The hearing began innocently enough. The audience was filled with the usual suspects—lobbyists, hill staffers, and a row of news reporters. Most were barely more than teenagers—interns or employees representing principals who had little time to actually sit and listen to a public hearing in person. If they cared enough, they might listen in on television. More likely, they would wait for the report from their staff on what happened, and then compare it with the *Washington Post* story or reports provided by trade associations, party organizations, or other interest groups.

Only two of the five senators on the committee, including Johnny, were even in the room. The junior senator from South Carolina was there, though still off on the wings behind the stage, talking with his legislative staff. Johnny figured he would be around to ask a question or two, and then leave. *That's okay,* Johnny thought. If no other senators were there to stop him, he alone would own the agenda for the hearing and the issue. Showing up was part of the job, he knew, and those who weren't there would learn this again.

"The committee will come to order," Johnny barked into the buzz of the large hearing room. As people began to quiet and settle, he continued. "We are meeting today to review the administration's recommendations from Health and Human Services regarding the issue of patient dumping. We will begin with a presentation by staff."

Lance walked up to the table in front of the dais where the senators sat. He moved the microphone closer, identified himself, and then provided a thorough report. He described the current state of the law and the history of patient dumping. He emphasized the recent rise in the number of alleged dumps, and then spent ten minutes describing the catastrophic case of Helen Neederdam.

When Lance was done, Johnny made a few critical comments and then turned to the Secretary of HHS. "I would ask Secretary Ben Olsen to present the administration's recommendations to the committee on this. After his presentation, we will open the floor to questions from committee members."

Secretary Olsen strode to the hearing room table, trying his best to look confident and in control. But there was no mistaking who was in charge in this room at this moment. The problem for Johnny, and other senators, was that there was little influence beyond these moments by Congress on issues like these. There was so much complexity that Congress mostly accepted what administrations did. The challenge was to show some conviction at moments like this, and then try to pass laws or budgets that would mold executive action in some small way. Even that was getting hard to do.

Secretary Olsen was a political pro and read through a statement prepared by his staff. "Thank you, Mr. Chairman." Secretary Olsen proceeded with his performance, as much for the television cameras as the senators and others in the room. The only ones hanging on his every word were the teenagers in the audience, taking note of everything he said and every twitch he made, hoping to turn their report into something that would get them noticed by their supervisors. Olsen outlined HHS's recommendations detailed in his written testimony, using flowery rhetoric that would play well in TV clips that night.

When he was done, Chair Gibson opened the floor for questions. The Republican senator from South Carolina went first. As expected, he asked two softball questions and then picked up his papers and left the hearing room. It was Johnny's turn.

"I do have one more question for you, Secretary Olsen. I've got a copy of the president's proposed budget, and there is a footnote that says the agency is proposing to reduce the money spent on the enforcement of federal hospital antidumping statutes. You might recall that I was one of the original House sponsors of that legislation when it passed back in 1986, and that it passed with bipartisan support. My view is that these statutes have done much to constrain the improper behavior we found back then around hospitals turning away patients needing care in their emergency rooms and clinics. Why would you see a need to cut back the funding, especially with incidents like we have heard here today?"

Secretary Olsen looked up from the desk and made eye contact with Senator Gibson. He knew that committee staff had asked this question of staff a month ago when they shared the evolving administration budget proposal for HHS. They seemed satisfied with the answer then, and they had not anticipated it would come up at today's hearing. It would make for a bad headline if Olsen said the wrong thing, and saying the wrong thing, not lousy performance on real health issues, was what could get someone fired in this White House.

"Mr. Chairman, as you know, things have changed dramatically since the 1980s, when the underlying legislation was passed. Back then, millions of Americans, about 15 percent of the population, were without health care coverage. Since then, we have expanded Medicaid and provided coverage through the Affordable Care Act and the health exchanges. The uninsured rate is now down to less than 10 percent, and the reality is that most Americans are receiving and paying for health care through private health plans. It has become the case that how hospitals provide care to patients in their facilities, including emergency rooms, should be now managed more by the private health plans than by the federal government. The budget recommendation is consistent with this shift in how health coverage now works—we no longer need as thorough a federal oversight of hospital duties in this regard."

"Secretary Olsen, I would agree with you that there have been some significant shifts in how and to whom health coverage is now offered. I would remind you that the president, and you, opposed most of these changes. And your position was that the market and private companies operating on a voluntary basis without government interference would be a better way to move forward. Are you saying that you agree with the policy recommendations we made to pass the Affordable Care Act now?"

The political trap had now been fully set. Secretary Olsen was once governor of Oklahoma, and he was no novice to politics or health care coverage wars. He had led the charge against Medicaid expansion under the ACA in his state, promising to veto any bill that came to his desk, despite strong polling for the notion from Democrats and Republicans in his state. He knew the contradictions, hypocrisy, and talking points that would smooth through the inconsistencies, or at least, confuse the matter at the heart of the debate. He also knew that he was now in trouble.

"No, Mr. Chairman, we continue to believe that this was an ill-advised approach to providing health care to Americans. It has led to increased costs for everyone and a crisis in medical care across the nation." Secretary Olsen knew well that health costs had actually seen their lowest rise in decades since the passage of the ACA, but these were facts inconvenient for the truth as he, and the president, saw things.

"What we are saying is that privatization is the policy that should be advanced to improve health care for the American people. Letting health plans take the lead in managing how the hospitals that they pay take care of their enrollees is a better way to manage health care than having federal workers enforce how they operate. Our intent is to reduce the federal bureaucracy enforcing this legislation in lieu of asking health plans to manage this issue. The statutes remain on the books but are an antiquated solution to a problem that barely exists anymore."

Johnny was not surprised at the answer. He knew that Secretary Olsen was a talented political adversary on this issue, and a host of other social issues on which he disagreed. He expected that the secretary would sidestep the trap and prattle on about the private marketplace. But Senator Gibson was not about to let go of his grip on this tiger's tail.

"Mr. Secretary, I think your confidence in the private marketplace is ill-placed. Some health plans have stepped up and done an excellent job in the new national marketplace for health coverage, and others have not. I believe we need to set a floor for their behavior on matters such as this and other priorities for the American people rather than just hope it all works out for the better. And we know, absolutely know, that millions of Americans continue to go without health coverage because of the opposition of people like you and the president to actually making health coverage for Americans a universal right rather than a benefit that everyone hopes they qualify for. We also know that many health insurance companies are finding new ways to restrict their enrollees' access to actually receiving health care, and this is leading to many Americans showing up in emergency rooms for their needed care because of the protections of these statutes. It hardly seems time to loosen our grip on this issue or these reports of health plan denials."

"Mr. Chair, you and I will continue to disagree on this point. It is a major policy issue that will undoubtedly be a big topic in the next election. And perhaps in Congress's policy committees." There was little doubt of this, nor many prospects that the dialogue and results of either would lead to a clear resolution of the matter. "Meanwhile, we are willing to work with you and your staff to find a budget number that you are comfortable with in terms of enforcement of the antidumping statutes. We are not yet proposing to repeal these laws, and it is currently more a matter of emphasis." Secretary Olsen intended to put this matter to rest as easily and quickly as he could, knowing that there could be no resolution and that public airing of the underlying issues remained a losing proposition for him and his boss.

"I appreciate that, Secretary Olsen, and I will direct committee staff to work with you and your staff on a more suitable budget allocation. I also think that you have opened up this topic for further conversation by policymakers and the American people. I think we need to examine these statutes again, along with the philosophy that says they are unnecessary now. Toward that end, I am announcing that our subcommittee will be holding field hearings on this topic over the balance of the year. I would ask committee members to advise whether you would like to have any of these in your states, and I would also extend this offer to my fellow senators in the full body. I can tell you that we will be having one of those in my home state, and I hope that you will be able to attend and hear from the people of Washington State on this important issue, Secretary Olsen."

"I would be honored to attend," the secretary stated. He hated events in Washington State—it was so far away, and it was a blue state, so blue that it seemed like it was part of Canada. He did find pleasure in reaching out to the conservative multimillionaires in the greater Seattle area, so maybe there was a good reason to attend.

"Thank you again, Mr. Secretary. The recommendations and our specific actions with respect to these will be calendared for action at our meeting next week. With that we will be adjourned." Senator Gibson banged down the gavel.

The secretary, his staff, and the audience members drifted out of the hearing room through the main doors. All who remained in the room in short order were capitol cleanup staff and media members rolling up their cords and microphones. Johnny stayed behind the dais with his chief of staff to debrief before he headed off to a leadership luncheon.

"I thought that went pretty well," said Lance.

"I agree. No big surprises, though I do believe our public hearings on the antidumping statutes did catch the Secretary with his guard down. Always a good day when we can make that son of a bitch uncomfortable." Johnny really did not like the secretary, disagreeing with his politics, religion, and essential philosophy about life and obligations to others.

"Any further thinking on where you want to do the hearing?" asked Lance.

"Yes. I would like to do it on the Olympic Peninsula. After all, that is where the dump happened. I would like some locals to tell the story to the committee—that would really personalize the issue. I also know some folks in the area who can help us make sure this is a success."

"Great. Let me know their names and I would be happy to reach out to them."

"I'll give you a list after lunch. Tops on the list is a woman by the name of Mary Beth Collins. She is an old friend and now runs a public hospital district on the peninsula. I will get in touch with her—we go way back."

Johnny smiled as he left the room. Yes, way back. So far back that if the full story was told, he might have to resign his seat in Congress. Much had happened since those days. They had a great deal to catch up on, and that would be a nice addition to doing the people's business in a beautiful part of the world. This political gig was indeed a good one. Now, if only he could make it mean something much more for the people he represented.

Chapter Forty-Five

Secretary of HHS Ben Olsen

Secretary of Health Ben Olsen stepped to the tee box with his driver on the third hole of Congressional Country Club in Bethesda, Maryland. He was happy to be out of the public eye for a few minutes, and felt comfortable with his cart mate, ex-Congressman Sam Bridgewater. In the other cart were two pharmaceutical company vice presidents who were footing the bill for this round of golf. That cost was nothing compared to the campaign contributions he would be directing them to send to the president's reelection committee.

He took a big swing and hit a slicing shot to the right side of the fairway. Sam looked at him as he stepped back into the cart. "Consistently right, Mr. Secretary. Good to know we can count on you!"

He laughed. Sam and he had met at a fundraiser for him in Oklahoma ten years ago, back when Ben Olsen was somewhat of a political newcomer. He was selling used cars after graduating from high school and proved to be a jovial and successful salesman. He liked to get off the lot and volunteered for the used car association within the local chamber of commerce, which got him noticed by political operatives looking for candidates. They convinced him to run for a seat in the state house as a way to bring him deeper into their fold; few thought he had a chance to win. As luck would have it, the election was the blowback against the Clintons for trying to push health care reform. This swept away Democrats in Congress and remote state house seats in Oklahoma. Olsen eked out a surprise win.

State Representative Olsen still didn't know much about politics, or much of anything for that matter. He was an extrovert and a fairly quick learner. Mostly, he became dependent on whatever the Liberty

Foundation advised him to do on issues—this was a conservative think-tank in Oklahoma with ties to ultra-conservative groups nationally.

Ben liked that the part-time legislative role gave him a break from his dull life as a car salesman. It didn't pay much, but he learned that there were ways to generate other revenues through corporate supporters or political action committees. He saw that wallets opened even more to legislators with power, and he watched for opportunities to grab it. After pulling some strings, he was appointed to chair the state house appropriations committee in his second term as a legislator. The money was getting to be pretty good from his new gig, and he quit the car sales job so he could focus on a career in conservative politics.

It was a good time to do so in Oklahoma. The conservative movement had raised a lot of money from wealthy donors and was playing a long game on taking control of American politics. It was essential in this strategy to secure state and local politics in conservative areas like Oklahoma. Ben became known as a capable follower of the new party creed, someone who was a safe investment because of his willingness to play ball in promoting the national conservative movement.

By his fourth term, Olsen had become Majority Leader of the House and was leading efforts to pass a host of conservative model pieces of legislation brought to him by national groups. He was in an excellent position when the Republican governor of Oklahoma resigned for health reasons—if one can call the pregnancy of his secretary a health reason—and Ben became the favored choice to replace him. Supported by copious amounts of campaign cash, including over $100,000 from a campaign event organized by Sam Bridgewater, he won the special election.

It was a satisfying enough job to be governor. It didn't take a lot of effort, given the politics of the state and the party's disinclination toward government. He rode the job for a number of years, though the economic calamity of the Great Recession made it a far more challenging gig in 2008. He was distressed when things got worse with the election of Obama to the presidency. Ben was convinced that it was now essential to be a strong voice in the Republican resistance movement, and became one of the regular talking heads on national television criticizing the president and his proposals.

It was a natural step to become a leader of the opposition to the Affordable Care Act, and especially the notion of expanding Medicaid coverage in Oklahoma once the US Supreme Court made this a state option. Ben didn't really understand the health care issues all that much, but was quick enough to mimic the talking points directed by national handlers.

When a Republican surprisingly won back the White House after Obama's terms, Ben found himself on the short list to become part of the new cabinet. His willingness to be outspoken in opposition to Obamacare led to his selection as the Secretary of Health and Human Services.

Like being governor, the job of secretary was something that he figured out how to do, with help from the right quarters—associates like Sam, for one. Ben liked the job, though he realized that he was a small Oklahoma fish now in a very large and dangerous sea. He needed friends and guidance even more than before.

"I heard how Gibson sucker punched you at the hearing last month," said Sam Bridgewater. "My staff said you did a great job of putting him in his place. I don't know what is up with him—there is no chance that the federal role in health care is going to get bigger. All we have to do is call it socialism to get 40 percent of the electorate to say no, and then scare the shit out of seniors that this is going to mess up their Medicare, and that is that."

"Yep, I couldn't agree more. Just like him to try a sucker punch like that in committee. He is up to something though. I just haven't put my finger totally on what it is. He backed me into a corner and got me to agree to attend a field hearing in Washington State on dumping issues. He would get reelected if he peed off the Space Needle, so he doesn't need it for any campaigning. We've had some harsh words, but nothing that out of the ordinary. So, I don't think it is personal. Got any idea what he is up to?" Secretary Olsen wondered whether he was out ahead of his skis on this one.

"No, but I am digging," responded Sam. They paused to hit their second shots, with Sam hitting a low seven iron onto the front of the green, and Ben pushing a fairway wood into the trap, on the right of course. "And just so you know, he is not all that safe politically—if we have anything to say about it.

"I can tell you that some of the nation's health care leaders are none too happy about his positioning on this, and you can expect their support to stop whatever he is up to. I know that their past support for Obamacare has sometimes made it difficult to work with them, but this might be the time when we can put hospitals and health insurers firmly back in your corner, Ben. We know we don't have to worry about them." Sam pointed with his chin toward the cart of pharmaceutical reps.

"I know you want me to try to stop that hearing, but my people tell me I can't. And the president's chief of staff is insistent that I attend. They are working on Gibson's support for some international matter and don't want me to piss him off by standing him up. We are going to have to find another way to deal with this."

"Is the money the holdup?" asked Sam.

"No. My budget folks have already cut a deal with his committee staff, and we have agreement on an appropriation amount for antidumping efforts within HHS for the next year. We always knew that it wasn't going away immediately and the budget ask was just a political statement trying to start bleeding it dry over time. Frankly, we didn't think it would get that much play. What do you think we should do?"

Sam leaned back in his cart and pondered the question. He had been noodling over this since the issue first popped up in his meeting with Thrust.

"It's not exactly what my client wants, but my thought is to jujitsu Gibson and make this a talking point for the national election on why Obamacare is a failure. Get it some press attention and sucker punch him with some clear examples of what is wrong when you put the government in charge of your health care. Maybe bring some folks down from Canada—we have used that drill before, and that socialist mess is just a few miles up the road from wherever the hearing will be. My folks will be happy to plot some strategy with you. Just give me the word."

"I'll run it up the White House flagpoles. I know they want to make health care a feature of future elections. It would be fun to stick it to Gibson too."

They stepped from the cart and moved toward the green and their next shots. Olsen skulled his sand shot out of bounds over the green. Bridgewater three putted for bogey. They should have paid greater attention to what the tea leaves were telling them.

Chapter Forty-Six

Mary Beth and Johnny Discuss a Local Hearing

Mary Beth Collins looked down at the cell phone on the conference table. It was ringing, and while the mute function stopped any bells from chiming aloud, the vibration of the phone was hard to ignore. She would normally just take note who was looking for her, and unless it was the office with what might be an emergency, let it roll to voicemail.

Seeing the name "Johnny" on the screen got her attention. She stood and strode out of the meeting room, nodding to the chair of the committee in the front of the room and pointing her finger up, suggesting she needed a minute. The chair nodded back, and Mary Beth hit the answer button, though not saying anything into the phone until the door shut behind her.

"Johnny, what a nice surprise," she finally said into the phone.

"Great to hear your voice, Mary Beth. Did I interrupt something? Is this an okay time to talk?"

"Just a work meeting—I do those all the time. Talking to my favorite senator, not so much."

"Oh, you shameless flatterer. Did you even vote for me?" asked Senator John "Johnny" Gibson.

"Once or twice, I think," joked Mary Beth. "But now that I think about it, it might have been some other hippie turned politician."

"Well, if you remember who that might be, let me know. I'll take 'em to lunch and we can reminisce."

"So, to what do I owe the pleasure of your call?" She knew it had been months since last they spoke. It was always great when they did, but time was in short supply, to him and her, and they just didn't find the time to visit as they once did.

"Now that I hear your voice, I wish it was just to catch up." Johnny felt the same way—sometimes he was such a good politician, he forgot about staying in touch with his friends and family in lieu of networking out to people and prospects who would further his political adventuring. "I've only got a few minutes as I've got a Senate floor vote on the defense budget. You might guess that I've got a few things to say about that." It irked him that the defense budget just kept going up regardless of any clear need.

"No doubt. I hope you have some good news to share with me."

"The good news is that we will get a chance to see each other in person, soon. That is, if you will allow us to hold a subcommittee hearing in your backyard. I am making some trouble for the president and his health henchmen and want to get some stories about lack of access to health care out in the open. Got Secretary Olsen to commit to testifying. He thinks I am going to do it in Seattle and that he will be able to make the millionaire rounds around Bellevue. I want to force him to pay attention on my home field and screw up his fundraising plans. One of the constituent complaints that I got is from your neck of the woods. That poor woman who drove off the road after leaving the hospital emergency room. It seems to me that would be just the place to hold a hearing—I make it easy for a constituent to petition their government, screw up the secretary's fundraising plans, and get to see you—a trifecta of good things. What do you think?"

"Johnny, I never could say no to you—and you know that!" So true, so true. "Get me some dates and I'll find a place. I am assuming you will want some good media coverage, so that will limit our options a bit. What's the specific topic?"

"The federal hospital statutes on duty to treat. The administration is trying to press even more of their privatization of health care notion by offloading enforcement of those laws to health plans. Just an early step to their bigger dream of ending Medicare, Medicaid, and anything that has the government in the mix in the health care sector. I assume you are still trying to change the world for the better and this would be something you and yours would care about?"

"Absolutely." Anything that gave private health plans more of a role in health care was of interest, and concern, to her. It spoke to much of what she felt was wrong with the health care system—turning people away when they were most in need of care. "We've had those complaints here, and a lot of them. And I am all in on making sure we don't just turn the system over to greedy insurance executives."

"All right then. I will have my people call your people and we will get something on the books. And I really am looking forward to spending some time with you. It looks like the vote is about to start, so I've got to get on the floor. If you want to chat before I get out there, you know this number is my hotline."

"Go do what you have to do, Johnny. It will be really nice to see you. It seems like yesterday when we were hanging out, and like so long ago."

"Hear from Irv lately? I am a little behind on connecting with him too."

"Yes, a little bit anyway. We still talk every couple of weeks or so, and once in a while get together out here or in Seattle. He's just like you—trying to change the world from his own unique spot. I'll see if he can be here when you are out."

"Awesome." Mary Beth heard some muffled voices in the phone speaker. "Okay," said Johnny to someone else on the other end. "Sorry. Gotta go. More soon. Love you."

"Love you too, Senator."

Mary Beth hit the disconnect button on her phone and put it in her purse. She looked out into the day from her perch on a porch outside of the conference room, noticing for the first time that the fog of the morning had given way to a clear spring day. The Olympic Mountains rose in the distance, filling the sky like stairs to heaven.

She sat down on a chair on the porch, deciding to take a few more minutes before heading back into the meeting. Her mind rolled back to a long time ago, when she and Johnny and Irv were inseparable. They had little then and everything too. So much had happened since, and it was more and more a special occasion when she got to see Irv. Johnny's political life made regular contact with him, other than seeing him on the TV news, far less frequent.

They were all following their life pathways. Once upon a time these paths were the same, but now they only intersected occasionally. She missed them both, terribly. *Why does doing what you think is right carry such a cost?* She knew there was no answer to her question, but allowed herself a moment to wallow in her sorrow. She had earned at least that much, she thought.

But not much more. Minutes later, she took a deep breath and gathered herself. Three minutes was about as long a pity party as she could allow. She looked through the window of the door of the patio and saw committee members still talking. She missed her boys; that feeling wasn't going away anytime soon. Maybe someday it would be different. Maybe not. Either way, she had things to do. She wondered whether Johnny and Irv really understood that she was busy changing the world too.

Chapter Forty-Seven

Post Utah Irv

Irv found himself in a better place when he returned from his death-defying trip to Canyonlands with Johnny. He now found solace in what were only recently boring routines. They were safe, even if still a bit dull, and way better than dying in the wilderness. Being with Mary Beth again was something he really appreciated—he had come so close to losing her forever.

He also found great satisfaction that through this trip he had found his cosmic answer. Neither he nor Johnny could have imagined how they might find what they were looking for. But find it they did—a revelation about their future, just when it looked like they did not have one. Johnny continued to call it the Theory of Irv. Irv thought it more their co-owned theory, but felt pride when Johnny would ascribe it to him.

Whatever it was to be called, Irv understood that he needed to put this theory into motion now that he was back to life as he knew it. Not that how to do this was clear to him. At first, he focused on the basic proposition—that he was built for some greater purpose to his life, for others. Where once living a life of adventure was enough for him and Johnny, these adventures must now include ways to contribute to the good of society.

It seemed a simple leap when he said it out loud, especially since they found it through such a complex plot of sweltering hikes, peyote buttons, and death desert confessions. Why did it take them so long and so much effort to get to this understanding? He almost felt guilty over the delay.

He talked with Mary Beth about it. She finally slapped him on top of the head. "You idiot," she said. "Everybody talks like that. But not so many really live their lives like that. They compromise, settle, and retranslate—maybe without any bad intentions. It is just that doing good, in a purposeful way, is not so easy to achieve."

She didn't stop there. "And you know what, neither is this notion of living your life as a grand adventure. Lots of people do it in their youth, and most talk about it. Just like you two. But both of you are unique in that you have, so far, been able to live that way for quite a while. Not just as kids, but adults.

"What I hear you saying now is that you are doubling down on that personal commitment—and adding to it this feature of doing good for others while you do it. If you do half as well in that as you have done so far with your adventurous spirit, I have no doubt that the world will be a better place for your having done so."

"Huh," he replied.

"You just have to figure out how to incorporate this idea into your adventures and whatever it is that you think is your life plan. That is why it is a theory, and not just some principle or idle thought, right?"

Irv guessed it wasn't as complicated as he thought, or so simple that he needed someone as smart as Mary Beth to help translate it. Whatever, her point was that it was time to stop trying to understand how he had got to the theory and instead figure out how to implement it.

Irv thought that Johnny had an easier task in doing this. He had already set out his course of adventure—politics. Doing good was something that could easily be attached in principle to that. Thousands of politicians seemed to do so every year, or at least pretended that was what they were doing. Johnny could too—and be more remarkable in actually believing it and seeking real good.

Irv, on the other hand, still had to find a nexus to doing good beyond his current circumstances. Sure, coffee was a good thing for people; maybe even cosmically good. But it was hard to see him as an indispensable part of the supply chain; lots of others could grind it and ship it. And really what was the greater good at play?

Closer to a link to a life with purpose was his relationship with Mary Beth. Some part of him must be helping her stretch herself out toward doing good. She was starting to do this, in many ways, with her women's groups and other volunteer work. But that would be like taking credit for a Ken Griffey home run; just because Irv cheered him on didn't mean he could really take any credit for it.

No, he had to find his own unique way to contribute to the social good—his own footprint—all while maintaining his adventurous spirit. The adventure part was probably best found by continuing to do things, whatever things. The connection to good, he thought, might best be found by digging back into a favorite pastime—reading.

He had begun to read more over the last year, and had gotten a Seattle Public Library card. He had been going to the library one night a week; he now doubled it to twice a week, and sped up his alphabetical journey through their collections.

Irv was just starting to move into the "Cs." One of the random "C" books he discovered was the "Committee on the Cost of Medical Care Final Report on Medical Care for the American People." Adopted in 1932, the report was an analysis of what was wrong with the American health care system and what to do about it. He recalled rambling on about health care with Johnny before passing out in Utah.

Maybe this was it, he thought. He was remembering more. Johnny had asked the one thing he might do to create social good. Irv had said health care and thought about his mom.

He dove into the report and found it to be inspirational in terms of what could be done to help people in their time of need . . . and damning in terms of how society had failed to solve it back then. A deep dive into more contemporary health care treatises found that little, if any, progress had been truly made on the systemic failures found by the committee. Yes, much had happened, but in fits and starts and chunks that made little sense as a whole to the issues raised by the committee.

Irv found interest building within him to better understand how things worked in health care, or didn't. It was so important to people. And to him. Maybe there was a way he could contribute to fixing what was wrong. It would be a greater purpose worthy of the Theory of Irv. But how?

Using his library talents to their fullest, Irv researched careers in health care. He swiftly realized its clinical opportunities were not his ticket. He was not bothered by blood and guts and biology, but it didn't excite him in the least to pursue it as a "career." He also saw that his college track had little of the advanced science and math necessary to set him on this path. Liberal arts studies were great for his pass-fail approach to college, but not so much for becoming a physician, nurse, or other clinician.

Soon he was exploring a different trail, as he stumbled upon a publication of the American College of Healthcare Executives. This was a professional society of health care administrators looking to further their careers in health care, mostly around hospital management. Many of its members, he discovered, held high positions within the health care world, as heads of hospitals or large medical practices.

Digging further, Irv realized that the field of hospital and health care management and administration was there for the taking. There were no set requirements. You could work your way up through the ranks as a health care practitioner or other hospital worker, from the medical records department, dietary, or even the storeroom. Or you could jump in by getting an advanced degree that made you marketable. This could be any sort of degree program but was best served by getting a master's in health care administration or hospital management—something that took only a couple of years of school and had no prerequisites other than a college degree in order to apply.

There were only about a dozen programs across the nation offering up this type of degree. Some were linked to business schools, others to more scientifically oriented branches of America's universities. Irv discovered that one of these programs was less than a mile away, part of the University of Washington's School of Public Health.

The plan came together quickly, with Mary Beth's assent. Irv would apply to the UW program and build a career in health care. Mary Beth would accept a promotion at the bakery to help foot the bills, and Irv would keep working part time at the coffee company to help out.

Irv's grades at UCLA were good enough, and he noted that the local master's program preferred their student candidates have life experiences rather than going straight into the program from college. He figured his experiential plate was more than full enough to fit this bill—and communicating this to them was more a matter of making sure that he left out the parts that an admission committee would find too scary or even objectionable.

It was drafting the essay for the entrance application when health care truly became Irv's passion for applying the Theory of Irv. In addition to reviewing his academic and general life experiences, he shared thoughts about his own health care experiences. This brought him quickly to his mother's death, and the words started flying from him. He recounted the pain that he experienced then. The gaps in diagnosis and treatment that put her at death's door, and the systemic failures to treat and care that made a terrible situation far worse. He sprinkled the essay with links to the Committee on the Cost of Medical Care's report and its conclusions.

Putting his mom's story on paper tugged at Irv's soul. He had subconsciously pushed so much of that time behind a wall of protection in order to move on. Once he opened the door, the thoughts and feelings poured out. Tears flowed, memories rose up like smoke from a cedar fire, and he unearthed a yearning to really do something about what was wrong in health care. Purpose was oozing out of him like sap from a maple tree.

What if he could really do something to solve the problems in the health care system? He wasn't going to heal anyone, nor was he going to find a cure for cancer in a laboratory. Still, he could find a way to fix, really fix, what was wrong with the American health care system. He would get into the UW program and find a career in health care management—not because he wanted a job, or more money, but because this was a thing worth doing, with passion and purpose, with his life. Yes, this was his calling. His Theory of Irv.

Chapter Forty-Eight

Irv's Investigation Goes to DC

Irv's flight from Phoenix landed at about 6 a.m. DC time. He had called Johnny from Sky Harbor the night before while waiting for his plane, and gave him a brief explanation of the reason for the trip. He was leery of saying too much on the phone, so he used code words that would tell Johnny that it was best that they not discuss this matter on the telephone. Johnny was in town, but had hearings and a couple of public appearances until 5:00 that afternoon. They would get together for dinner at six at a restaurant chosen by Johnny near the McPherson Square Metro stop.

Irv found a hotel room in Crystal City, near the airport and easily accessible by the local subway, Metro. He spent much of the day catching up on his sleep. Irv found it hard to sleep on planes and had spent most of the night flight thinking about the investigation—what he had learned so far and what else he needed to know.

Try as he might, he could not think of how to get the needed information out of ALI. Maybe Johnny would have some ideas.

They met at Cafe Mist for dinner. It was always good to see each other in person. They had a natural affinity for one another that brought immediate sparks to their encounters, and now so much history that any get-together might spontaneously combust. For this visit, Irv was coming with a can of gasoline in his pocket.

They settled in with drinks and appetizers and got caught up on life since they had last seen each other six months ago. Both knew they would get to the special topic in due time and there was no need to rush toward it right out of the box.

Johnny shared he had spoken with Mary Beth about coming out for a public hearing on the Olympic Peninsula. He gave Irv a little background on the hearing and the issue of patient dumping. It wasn't the first time they had discussed this topic. The date had not been set yet, but he told Irv that as soon as it was, he was hoping they could find some time to hang, with Mary Beth, back home.

It was a natural transition from that to Irv's investigation of the corpse in Kent, concluding with what he found in Phoenix sleuthing through an emergency room. He left out none of the details; if he couldn't fully trust Johnny, there was no longer any point to life. Johnny hung on every word and asked questions as Irv ran through the chronology.

"That patient list has bad mojo all over it," said Johnny after Irv ended his tale by declaring that this was when he knew that they needed to meet. "The Republicans in this town found that they could weaponize hatred for brown people in other countries for their political ambitions, and have been doing so on every occasion. What is really crazy is that some of them actually believe it is a righteous cause. Those are the ones we really need to be afraid of."

Johnny took a long sip from his drink and continued. "I don't completely understand why a hospital might have a special process for identifying Hispanic patients. You are the expert on that front. Is there some good reason why they might want to know this?"

"Yes, there is. If you look at health outcomes, almost all studies show that patients that don't look like you or me do far worse. In the public health world, we spend a lot of time showing how this is related to the health risks they live with in their environments, as racial and ethnic differences frequently come with associated risks such as greater poverty, less social cohesion, poor nutrition, and the list goes on and on."

Irv took a bite of his dinner and swallowed it quickly so he could continue his point. "The research is also quite clear in showing that health care gets delivered quite differently too, including in ERs. Blacks, Latinos, and immigrants encounter major barriers. It would be a natural and sane response on the part of health systems to target these gaps and do something about them."

"But you don't think that is the case, do you?" said Johnny.

"No. Most health systems and hospitals largely still ignore this data. They might have a program or two that targets improving outcomes for diverse populations, but these usually have some special payments or incentives attached. They might even have some broad statements about the importance of the issue or the appearance of a corporate-wide initiative, but these are usually done for appearance's sake, not because of some deep conviction."

Irv reached for a dinner roll from the basket in the center of the table, clearing his throat as he continued his health policy lesson. "There are a few exceptions. I doubt very much that HealthMost is one of those. You can usually feel the difference in the culture of the organization and the staff. I felt none of that at Westside Medical Center; the staff might have personally felt an urge to do more, but probably without any support from management. I spent some time researching HealthMost online and could not even find even a mention of concern over what is generally referred to as 'health disparities.'"

"Last year I met with their CEO; I think his name was Thrust," added Johnny. "There is nothing in that man that oozes public good. He was arrogant, for sure, but many of the so-called leaders I meet with are. Most find a way to try to frame what they are asking me to do with some reference to the public good. Not a whiff of that in this case. And now that I bring it up, it was one of the things that brought this whole dumping thing up for me. That and some constituent complaints."

Irv nodded his agreement. "I guess it is possible that this is the tip of the iceberg of some dumping scheme. It doesn't make sense on the face of it though—my corpse and most of the names on the list had health insurance coverage. Dumps are almost always of patients without insurance. Sometimes for under-insurance, meaning the actual coverage sucks so much that they are practically uninsured. But the HealthMost website said their plan is a joint venture with ALI that is paid through the federal government in a demonstration program, and that must include minimal standards for these things."

"Yup. I remember demonstration programs being in the Affordable Care Act legislation," Johnny said, "and we insisted that these minimum standards be a part of them. The administration had been approving waivers for states to go around them, but it's not possible if it is a federal program without Congress's blessing. Puzzling."

"I know. Meanwhile, every instinct I have is telling me that I've got the tail of something pretty big and need to keep pulling it. But I also feel that I can't let anyone on the inside know I have it—at least before I find enough evidence to prove my instinct correct."

"I'm with you on that, Irv. In more normal times, I would be able to have my staff do some digging with the agency and maybe get some answers. Now, any request is dealt with as a political fight. We have even issued subpoenas and seen them ignored. All while I can almost hear the paper shredders running full time down the street from my office. I can't even trust committee staff to keep a request like this under wraps politically—it is all too volatile in this town."

"Any ideas on what we could do? I know I have to find out what is behind the firewall at ALI, but that is far easier said than done."

"It makes total sense as the right move—maybe the only one." Johnny picked up his glass of bourbon and swirled its ice cubes as he thought about what they might do. "Here's an idea. This patient dumping thing is already out there as an issue of mine. I even got the Secretary of Health to commit to attending a hearing on this in Washington State. That is the gig I mentioned to Mary Beth when we wanted to find some time to hang. What I said was that there would be a series of hearings. It was to encourage my colleagues to step up and volunteer. Most of them are far too beholden to the health care industry for campaign contributions to want to do so, though.

"Senator Burke, from Connecticut, did tell me that he might be interested. He's not running for reelection and is willing to take some risks. So, what if I schedule a hearing in Hartford on this? And find an alleged dump that is somehow, some way affiliated with HealthMost and ALI? With a little bit of luck, we might find a case that could be a profile of our hearing. Funny how a little light of day turns the godless to believers. We can see what crawls out from under their corporate rocks."

"I like it, Johnny. The hearing is nothing that wasn't going on before my corpse made its appearance, so it shouldn't raise any big flags. I know HealthMost has a few hospitals in the Northeast, and it would be a surprise if somewhere along the line they weren't at least accused of dumping. And, if the list I found in Phoenix comes from a corporate strategy, it might even be that there is a system for dealing with patients like Rodrigo across the nation."

"Gives me a shiver to hear it suggested that this might be the case," said Johnny. "Speaking of which, why don't we get out of here and finish catching up on the steps of the Lincoln Memorial? One of the best spots in this city to feel the good we can do here. Beautiful too. Better than a shower to get the stink off from some things that I deal with on Capitol Hill."

"You're on." Irv smiled as he immediately began to recall the dozens of beautiful places where he and Johnny, and sometimes Mary Beth, had camped and considered the possibilities of the universe late at night. "Didn't they legalize recreational pot in this place?" he added.

"Yes, indeed," noted Johnny as he winked. "And while they drug test staff on Capitol Hill, they wouldn't think of doing it for senators."

Chapter Forty-Nine

Post Utah Johnny

Johnny was thankful to have survived his travails with Irv in Utah, and pleased that it had also given him an answer on whether to put in any real effort to get reelected to Congress. This question had forced him to be more introspective than he liked, but that was now behind him. He couldn't figure out how to tell his staff or mates in Congress about the peyote trip when he got his answers, so he took some liberties in recounting the tale of how he found purpose in the Utah desert.

He did share the full story with his political consultant, Nancy Jones. She was captivated with the tale, and thrilled with the conclusion. He said he wanted to run for reelection, but even more, find ways to pursue good as part of being a more active member of Congress.

Nancy was tickled pink that Johnny now had a passion to actually engage as an elected official. She saw him as a natural politician, and if coupled with real legislative aims, he had great potential to make a difference.

She also thought he had a good chance to win again and didn't think it would require oodles of money. She pointed out that incumbency had its advantages. One was name recognition and the fact that he alone could identify himself as Congressman Gibson. People in his district would now be used to this moniker, and for many, that should be enough to get their vote.

She cautioned him that both parties would want to take him out. "Should I pick one or the other?" he asked. "Would that give me more prospects to pass legislation too?" Her suggestion was to meet with people from both parties and make his own decision. Any way he chose would have a cost, and a benefit.

Johnny knew that Democratic and Republican Party staff were eager to recruit him, as it would be a prize for either to pull him into their ranks, so he decided to meet with party leaders to get a read on both options.

The party leaders provided him policy papers and statements that identified their thoughts about a wide array of issues. These were to be his guideposts if he chose them. They would advise him how to vote on any important issues that came before the Congress; it would make things easier for him, they said. If he played ball, if he became an effective fundraiser for his election campaign and the party, and if he followed the traditional rules of power, he had a promising career in front of him.

Johnny didn't like what he heard. The staff were smart and likable—he found most people likable—but what came out of their mouths about power and politics and governing seemed to be 90 percent horseshit and 10 percent air.

Still, Johnny considered their advice. At the end of the day, he decided to remain an independent, a natural conclusion for someone like him—not some ideological matter but practically keeping his life options open. He invoked Woody Allen when pressed on the matter, and he would question any club that would have him as a member. If it turned out he really had to make a choice down the road, he would. That choice might also be to get out of politics and resume his life wanderings in another realm. If so, so be it.

His last big checkpoint was his wife, Reena. The decision would have implications on her and the kids too. Was she okay with him continuing his life on the road, commuting across the country most weeks of the year, and being home briefly on weekends?

A little to his surprise, she was. She missed him and sometimes wished that he was home more, as he was always fun to be around. The kids felt much the same way. He was their new dad and way more available than their real one. But for all of them, it was a worthy sacrifice to have him off doing good works for others. They took great pride in it too. Johnny's father-in-law reinforced the views of his daughter and offered to help his campaign with more cash and connections.

Nancy Jones took on his campaign again and told him that he had chosen wisely. They ran a campaign that creatively told voters they should vote for him for the very fact that he was an independent. Using campaign donations from Reena's side of the family, they ran a series of ads disparaging the two parties, and not his actual opponents. These ads were clever and funny, building off of the comedy used by Rainier Beer to sell their product in the 1980s. They were a hit and so was Johnny.

He won reelection by a sizable margin, far more than his first election. Both parties began to accept that he was a unique force that they needed to accept with only minor resistance. At least he wasn't with the other party, they calculated. It was better for them to focus on other races. By the time the dust had settled on election night in 1986, John Gibson was in a secure seat of Congress, probably for as long as he wanted it.

Chapter Fifty

Irv's Investigation Goes to Hartford

Senator Gibson's staff took on the assignment of organizing a hearing on patient dumping in Hartford, Connecticut, the morning after Irv and Johnny's dinner in DC. Johnny had confirmed Senator Burke's willingness to host a field hearing in his state.

Johnny's staff reviewed the hospital dumping complaint file at HHS and found, as expected, a number of complaints within Connecticut. HealthMost did not have any hospitals or other facilities in Connecticut. They did have a hospital in Springfield, Massachusetts, which was less than an hour's drive from Hartford, and a couple of hospitals in western New York State, only a few hours away.

His staff didn't know exactly why the senator wanted to make sure that HealthMost was on the witness list, nor why he was wondering if there was any link to ALI as part of this. It was enough that he asked them to find a link. They did find a case from the Buffalo area that referenced a patient who was part of the HealthMost-ALI joint venture, and they bootstrapped that to a series of reported dumps in Springfield. HealthMost was not going to be the centerpiece of the hearing, but it would be a topic of some attention. Johnny's chief of staff let the corporate representatives for HealthMost know this.

Irv returned to Seattle and work while the Hartford hearing was being planned. He still had several weeks of vacation time accrued, and a boss who was happy to get him out of sight and mind. The hearing was scheduled for mid-June.

He didn't attend the hearing at the Connecticut State Capitol, but followed it online on his computer in a hotel room less than a mile away in downtown Hartford. Johnny and Irv thought it best that he not be physically present. His cover was that he was in town for a concert—a local band called NRBQ that had a cult following across the country. They were having a reunion show and it was a good enough story and something Irv was excited to attend. Johnny was also a fan, and they met at the show to do some pre-hearing planning.

The hearing went well enough. There was press coverage, print media, and a couple of cameras from the local public television station. Committee staff presented a report that found over fifty patient dumping complaints in the Northeast over the last year. Several patients testified; committee staff asked some of the victims involved in the more egregious instances to tell their stories. After that, several hospitals and health systems were asked to comment on their policies and procedures. HealthMost was one of those, and a vice president for Medical Affairs testified and spoke to HealthMost's great compassion and concern for patients and promised to do whatever needed to resolve any mistakes. People would lose their jobs if they didn't honor the company's commitments in this regard; not him, mind you, but somebody.

Johnny let the committee process run through its natural course of events. It was important that Senator Burke get top political billing, and he deferred to his colleague for much of the hearing. The HealthMost testimony was toward the end of the hearing, when the interest of the media and those in the audience was fading.

Johnny focused his questions to HealthMost on its joint venture relationship with ALI—and whether this had anything to do with the dumping allegations. He conflated the case in Buffalo with the many more complaints filed in the Springfield area, enough to make any uninformed listener concerned there was something really wrong in River City. The vice president for Medical Affairs was not prepared for an aggressive attack from Senator Gibson. He stumbled as he responded to questions about the ALI relationship, as he knew little about it.

But Johnny had him on his hook and wasn't about to let him off. Of course, HealthMost would cooperate with a review of these complaints to make sure that problems had been resolved. Of course, they would get cooperation from ALI with respect to any allegations that related to the joint venture. Anything that could be said in front of the rolling cameras that made HealthMost look cooperative, contrite, and helpful.

At the conclusion of the hearing, Johnny closed by thanking all of the participants, and especially Senator Burke. He noted how this was the first of a series of field hearings on this topic and that the committee would consider any necessary legislation to fix the problems later in the year. He looked at the HealthMost vice president and asked him to follow up immediately on adjournment in order to get some further information on his testimony.

As most of the attendees filed out of the room, the vice president approached Johnny, who was talking with his lead committee staff, Jubilee Lee. He was accompanied by a tall man dressed in a smart suit—Johnny had met him somewhere before, but couldn't place him immediately.

"Sam Bridgewater, Senator Gibson. I used to be Congressman Bridgewater and we crossed over for about a year or so when you were in the House."

"Of course. Life is good for you, Sam, I don't remember your suits being this nice back then."

"Well, we have built a pretty good government relations program since, and among our clients is HealthMost."

Johnny knew of Bridgewater's successful practice; he just had not placed the face with the name and practice. He also knew that Sam's firm's clients were almost exclusively well-heeled Republicans and that he was embedded financially, if not ideologically, with the current administration. Niceties would be as deep as their relationship would ever get.

"So I assume you will be helping them respond to the questions that didn't get answered today?"

"Yes, I would be happy to get some written answers to you next week."

"That won't do. I've got some more field hearings this fall, and we need to prepare for those. If I can't get what I need in time, I might have to ask HealthMost to appear at our other field hearings too."

Sam understood the threat—bad press in every media market where a hearing occurred and the cumulative stain in DC of being the poster child of hospital dumping. Thrust would be unhappy about this—Sam had been asked to get rid of these stupid laws and instead it was becoming a topic where the corporation might become the lead story. There would be hell to pay with Thrust. "I understand, Senator. Just tell me what you need and I will do everything I can to comply." His voice expressed his irritation with the senator; the time for pleasantries was over.

Jubilee outlined a list of questions. Johnny added a few comments to the list. Then he asked Sam, "And I am curious about this relationship with ALI. They are located here, aren't they?"

"Yes, Senator, ALI is a life insurance company with a principal place of business in Hartford, Connecticut. In fact, those towers you can see through the windows is their headquarters."

"I won't be leaving town until tomorrow morning. I am headed up to Boston for some meetings at Harvard, and I would very much like to visit with the CEO of ALI so he can tell me more about the business relationship. If he can't do it, then I want the CEO of HealthMost to provide it, as soon as possible."

Sam recalled how poorly the last meeting between Gibson and Thrust had gone. Nothing good would come from another, and the path of least resistance was the ALI CEO. The CEO didn't really know anything about this topic, or other actual health care things, so what could he possibly say that would create a problem? "Let me see if he is in town. If so, we will arrange for him to meet with you."

"Great," said Johnny. "Coordinate this with my staff. I'd like to do this at my hotel. I have a suite at the Hilton, and we can meet there. I really hope he is available. And I would prefer to meet with just him. I won't even bring committee staff with me if you are concerned with that. It will be an off-the-record conversation—for now, I just want to understand more about this joint venture with HealthMost."

Sam nodded his intent to make this impromptu meeting happen. He moved away from the senator and his staff and placed a couple of phone calls. Ten minutes later, he returned. "Six p.m. at your hotel. Nelson Duncan is his name. Let me know if you have any other questions after you meet with him." Johnny grinned back, thinking of how much he looked forward to the next set of questions he might pose to Bridgewater and Thrust.

Chapter Fifty-One

Early Sam Bridgewater

To know Sam Bridgewater as a young man was to know a clam. There was a tangible thing before you, but it was impervious to understanding more without cracking the shell and taking a much closer look. Even then, one couldn't figure out much.

Nor was it a shell that could easily be cracked. It had formed some very thick layers over time. Sam's father was a military man, a veteran of the Korean War who made the United States Army his career at the end of this armed conflict. He moved from combat to training, and his posts shifted across the entirety of the United States.

About every eighteen months he was reassigned, meaning that it was time to pack up his wife, two kids, and their furniture and move to a new location. It wasn't that big a deal for the Captain, as his kids called him. He was used to moving around, and the real work of making the family transition fell to wife and mom Alice. The Captain would move to the new base and then wait for Alice to show up with the kids and belongings. They would put down shallow roots of a family life while he went off to work every day. Then they would move and repeat the story.

Over the first couple of moves, Sam adapted fairly well—making friends, finding experiences that made him happy, and enjoying life. He soon found the process of getting yanked from friends and connections painful, and then deeply unsettling, and he learned through repetition to avoid forming any meaningful connections to others. Better to keep his distance, he thought, lest he feel the hurt of separation too much again.

It might have been easier if he could have found comfort at home. Early on, things were better. He and his brother Wally played well together despite their two-year age difference, and counted on each other to be their base of personal support.

Since the Captain was frequently on assignment or at the base, it fell to Mom to make sure that her sons had a good home. It was a lonely life for Alice, and she found her support in a bottle of gin. She would take a few shots each night to start, then a gin martini earlier in the evening as she prepped dinner, and soon several from late afternoon until she passed out about nine at night. Her own soldiers, she used to call them—at your command, sir.

The marriage between Alice and the Captain was founded on a wild weekend leave and then the convenience of finding a mate between tours of duty. The moves, the drinking, and the attention of the Captain on his own troops and his career put great distance between the two, move by move, year by year.

Sam's shell hardened during the many fights between his parents. At least he had Wally. The brothers got closer as the world around them got more difficult. They would talk of how it was them against the world, and planned how they would move to Hollywood and become television stars. Everyone around them would be friendly and want to be with them.

One night, after dinner and another fight, Alice came into the boys' room and asked Wally to come with her to the store. They were posted in Georgia, Fort Benning. She needed groceries, and as the older and stronger brother, Wally was needed to help carry them to and from the car. The Captain usually helped with these duties, but this had been a particularly nasty fight, and neither of the combatants wanted to be with the other. Off Alice and Wally went. Only one returned.

The official police report stated that Alice had lost control of the car and hit a telephone pole. That was only because the Captain had convinced the local authorities to doctor up the report and hide the truth: she was shit-faced drunk and had driven off the road while trying to pick up a cigarette that had fallen out of her mouth to the floor of the car. She had gone off road and hit a telephone pole about fifty yards behind a roadside ditch. Wally had been flung through the windshield. He had a seat belt, unused, and died instantly when he broke his neck as he hit the telephone pole.

For Alice and the Captain, it was the beginning of a resurrection. Alice had a concussion and several broken ribs from the crash. The steering wheel had caved in her chest but kept her in the vehicle. The accident shocked her into a new reality—she found God and an Alcoholics Anonymous program recommended by her pastor. The Captain stepped up too; after all, it was his duty. He resigned his commission and used his contacts to get a supervisor's job at the Studebaker plant in South Bend, Indiana. The family moved there and settled into suburban life in 1970 America.

Sam took his brother's death surprisingly well to most observers. He was sad, but coolly so. He made the move with the family and set on with what appeared to be a regular teenage life in South Bend. He had the same school, the same house, the same friends, and was seemingly no worse for the wear than any other teenager facing calamity at the time.

This was the thickest layer of all his shells, the calcification of his isolation from human contact slowly forming every day in South Bend. Never again would he get close to anyone or anything. He would cope and be and do everything he could to avoid feeling again.

On graduation from high school, he turned down an offer to join the service academies in favor of attending Indiana University. The Army would never again run his life, and he would put as much distance as he could between him and the Captain and Alice. State school tuition limited his leap to the three hours between Bloomington and South Bend in Indiana.

He turned this three hours into a continental divide. School wasn't anything that excited him; it was just a means to his escape. He had no need to take hard classes—that would only bring a risk of flunking out and having to go home. He settled into a liberal arts degree and a major in political science.

Sam wanted some sense of belonging, just nothing too meaningful and close. He tested a couple of fraternities, but their overtures of brotherhood fell flat upon his shell. So did several school clubs; they were trying to build on some great interest within him, when he had none except surviving and not being hurt.

Being a political science major, he had offers to join up with the Young Democrats or the Young Republicans. He attended a YD orientation and was put off by the fervor of the group—there was a passion that stirred within them to do things for the social order. He had none of this within him.

The Young Republican club was different in a couple of ways. For one, their mantra was more about keeping things the way they were. There were also fewer of them, so it was easier for him to imagine "belonging" in a more limited way. He joined.

Sam never really came around to the belief systems of the Young Republicans. Freedom, marketplace economics, and wars just didn't whet his appetite. But order did, so it felt comfortable. Even better was that it provided contacts for him, contacts that would allow him to set more distance between him and the Captain and Alice.

The summer between Sam's third and fourth year at IU provided an internship in the Capitol Hill office of Congressman Sumner Jones, courtesy of one of his Young Republican contacts. Jones was a third-term congressman from the Bloomington area. He was Republican, conservative, and looking for hometown kids for his staff. The internship led to a job offer to be a legislative aide for the congressman upon graduation. It didn't pay much, but required a move to DC. Sam's schedule would be built around Congress, and it would make it hard to schedule time back home. The work itself involved long hours, superficial relationships, and was not all that mentally challenging. All in all, it was the perfect job for young Sam.

He took it, and thrived. Sam was a capable enough young man—smart enough to impress, and polite enough to people to not put them off. He was able to form relations with others to get his work done, but without the threat of getting so close personally that it might interfere with the job that needed to get done. More than anything, he was adaptable—able to fit and form himself around the assignment, without having his personal feelings intrude on the task at hand.

Sam stayed on with the congressman for six years, eventually becoming Jones's lead aide. Congressman Jones was building seniority and influence, and was active in fundraising for Republican candidates around the nation. Sam became his right-hand man and met many influential Republican donors and power brokers. Congressman Jones was building his own network, and this turned into an offer for a cabinet position in the new Reagan Administration, in the Department of Interior.

Rather than join him in the agency, Sam parlayed his position into an appointment as the new congressman for the district. People owed him favors, and he called on them. He did so again when he ran and won reelection to the seat.

It was good enough work, but Sam became tired of constituent relations and only served a couple of terms. It was wearing to meet so many people, year after year, when he didn't really care.

He figured he could suffer through this with far fewer people for far more money. So he gave up his seat and accepted an offer to join a lobbying firm. Sam was a good legislative aide and a mediocre congressman. But he was a natural lobbyist. Deals and rewards and power were what mattered to him. There was nothing he wouldn't say or do for a price. Others had their ideologies and passions, but not him. He considered these to be weaknesses and would exploit them when he saw them, whether by friend or foe. He felt nothing for having done so, as long as he was paid.

Ten years later, he found himself a partner in the firm. And then a named partner. They needed more clients and decided to move into health care. Nowhere else was the trough growing so big every year. Even if defense or natural resources or other interests were less complicated, Sam could see that they would soon be overtaken in federal attention by the double digit cost increases of governmental paid health care each year. Certainly there were some big hogs at the trough that needed his services.

Perhaps the biggest hog of all was HealthMost and Richard Thrust. He would figure out how to get them in his corral.

Chapter Fifty-Two

Thrust Plots a Cover-Up

Sam Bridgewater strode confidently into Richard Thrust's corporate lair. The truth was, he was working hard to look so confident. HealthMost was now the principal client of his federal lobbying and political affairs consulting organization, and it took most of his time. Any time he was called in to see Mr. Thrust personally was a moment to be prepared for the worst.

The contract paid him a lot—a base retainer of two million dollars per year plus additional project billing opportunities. His preparation and trepidation were far more about Thrust himself than the organization. Thrust was smart, ruthless, and impatient, and it was imperative to stay in his best graces. He knew these graces would never be positive toward him, just okay enough to not be fired.

Sam sat down in the one guest chair available in Thrust's office. He remembered how this chair was permanently fixed to a height lower than Thrust's, forcing the visitor to look up at him during meetings. Sam knew this was no accident; people like Thrust were forever working to add to their already significant advantages. It was why they hired people like Sam. He didn't judge it, but he would use it if he could for his own purposes.

There were no pleasantries exchanged between the two men before they jumped to the business topics at hand; Thrust didn't really care anything about other people's lives, and Bridgewater was happy to get to business and get this meeting over as soon as possible.

He let Thrust kick off the meeting. "I just talked to Duncan at ALI. We are going to re-secure the files behind their firewall and their platform."

"That's good," replied Bridgewater. "It seems unlikely that anyone will even see that enrollee information, let alone do anything with it. But we should make sure it is secure and beyond the view of anyone. Even people in HealthMost." Thrust nodded his agreement. "Did we ever find out how this one got out of our control?"

Thrust frowned. "It looks like one of our subcontractors took a shortcut. The body was supposed to go to our Olympic Mountain disposal facility. It was a shipment of only one, and some fool gave a driver his cut upfront. He thought he would save the cost of transport and deposit the body at a concrete plant near a small town in western Washington, hours away from our facility. When it didn't arrive on schedule, we used the chip to track it down. Our team found it in a small, unused cabin, where our sub was going to plant it in the cement mixer down the street the next morning. Our people weren't able to acquire or transport it though. Just as they arrived to take it away, some dogs in the neighborhood raised a ruckus, and it was called in to local authorities. We had to take care of it through our backup channels, but we were able to reacquire the body and lock down the information around it." Thrust outlined in cold terms what had happened three nights before.

"I know the end of this story. I was there in Seattle to claim the body and close out the public health investigation." Apparently, Richard Thrust didn't know everything, Sam thought. "It looked like it was over and done in their minds, though I didn't feel good about the public health investigator who had the case. We may just want to make sure he is out of the way. Your folks pick up anything suspicious?"

"No, the reagents we applied to the body worked as they should. The avian flu agent got it focused into the public health system for follow-up and triggered a call to our federal contacts. We were able to get quick access to the body, and it seems that our potato reagent led them to believe it was a migrant farmworker from the east side of the state. Then we got involved and took jurisdiction because of a pandemic threat, the locals didn't want anything more to do with it." Thrust was proud of this part of the disposal process, as it was his insistence that they come up with a backup plan within the disposal system. That was what extraordinary leaders and thinkers like him did.

"Anything else we need to do?" asked Bridgewater.

"Through you, no. I will make sure that the subcontractor will never make that mistake again. Our contractor will also learn that it is a mistake to cheat us." Their failings reinforced Thrust's dismal view of people—they must be punished to learn how to follow orders. "I have also ordered that all of the files from the project be completely transferred to the ALI server and system. Better that we make sure all of the data related to this is secured elsewhere. One step further from any government auditors, and our own staff. You never know who might take a crack at us."

Moving all the files seemed like an overreach to Sam. There were thousands of files, and it only made it more likely that moving such a large amount of data would lead to leakage in confidentiality. That was a clear lesson from his time in Washington, DC—nothing is really secret, and the more you try to hide, the more likely it will be found. He also knew that it was folly to suggest this to Thrust. Working with him was never a matter of teamwork—it was about implementing his orders without discussion.

"I do have a couple of other assignments for you though."

Sam shifted in his seat and crossed his legs in anticipation of his orders, also wanting to show Thrust how attentive he was to his demands through body language.

"I want you to dig up some dirt on LeClair. That asshole has been to his last HealthMost board meeting." Richard seemed to reflect momentarily and rage about the insubordination LeClair had displayed around his compensation package. "I want him off. Get an IRS audit on him. If there is nothing in it, make sure that something goes in. It has to be something embarrassing and very personal—something that allows us to justifiably discharge him from our board for cause."

"Will do," noted Sam. It was not the first time Thrust had asked him to dig up dirt to discredit an opponent—and his third board member. It was standard fare for a DC lobbyist and very doable. "Anything else?"

"Yes. I saw your report on the patient dumping hearing in the Senate."

Sam nodded to acknowledge his report, though it was an intern who had prepared it and put Sam's name on it. Sam didn't even read it, so he was ready to soft-shoe his way around his ignorance of whatever was coming next.

"I don't like it that Gibson is digging around the antidumping laws. He sticks his nose into other people's business and I want you to stop it," Thrust said.

Sam knew they were getting into touchy territory, but he was comforted that he didn't need to know anything about the substantive topic to reply. "I've told you before that I can do many things—and have—but getting a congressman or senator to stop a public inquiry is not one of them, especially if they are the chair of the committee. We can make sure it doesn't go anywhere, and in some cases help it fade away with a press release or an appearance on a news show that will satisfy their constituents. But not when it is Senator Gibson."

Thrust was having none of this. "I pay you a lot of money and expect results, Bridgewater. Get on it and give me a report by this Friday."

Sam nodded his assent. Who was this ass to order him around like that? It only made him angrier that he knew the source of much of this was how dismissive Senator Gibson was of Thrust in their meeting arranged last election cycle. Thrust had insisted on delivering a check to Senator Gibson's campaign in person so that he could instruct Gibson on his views on health care and what he needed from him. Thrust was stunned to find someone who dared disagree with what he said and was even dismissive of his policy demands. It only made it worse when the senator pushed the hefty check back to Thrust and told him that he wanted no part of his money, or his demands on health care policy.

Sam guessed that Senator Gibson's concerns could be managed away with a little finesse, though Gibson was a very hard politician to predict. He had an independent streak in him that party politicians like Bridgewater found unfamiliar and uncomfortable. Irritating Gibson by directly going after him or his ideas was a sure way to make things worse. Again, there was no upside in telling Thrust that; he knew that Richard would only interpret it as Sam's failing and continue to insist on a direct attack.

He would have to do something about this. For now, all he could do was make sure that his client was satisfied. "I will take care of it." He did have one question though. "Is there anything in your ask related to the fact our body problem occurred in Washington State?"

Thrust scoffed at the notion. "No. How in the world would someone like Gibson or anyone in Congress make a link to this one incident?

I told you earlier—we have taken care of that problem, and it should no longer be of any concern."

"As you wish," said Sam as he stood, understanding that this meeting was over and his role now was to quickly exit. Thrust was always so sure he was right about everything, and Sam could never tell him how ignorant he was in the way of politics and DC. Thrust fancied himself an expert on this topic, along with seemingly everything else. Sam knew that odd linkages had a way of coming up all the time in the nation's capital—things that would surprisingly bite you in the ass. *I really hope this is not one of those times*, he thought.

Chapter Fifty-Three

Nelson Duncan III

Nelson Duncan III hung up the telephone, slamming the headset onto the base sitting on his desk. No one should talk to him that way. It mattered little to him that this was generally how he talked to people. Such was the privilege granted to people like him. He knew that Richard Thrust did not come from the same class of family as he did, and it irked him that Thrust thought himself his better, even equal. He also knew that Thrust could make problems for him, so he would have to let this transgression slide. Again.

Nelson Duncan III was born to Nelson Duncan II and his wife, Sally, in Greenwich, Connecticut. The senior Nelson was a Wall Street investment banker, like his father before him, and his before him. The line of Duncans had amassed great wealth, save for the unfortunate losses in the stock market crash of 1927. The original Nelson Duncan had played the market in a big way back then, and had almost lost the entire family fortune. He solved this problem as a gentleman would, masking his suicide as a homicide so that a large life insurance policy payment went to the family upon his death.

Nelson Duncan II held such family secrets closely as he took over the family's portfolio in his twenties. He got a military deferral during WWII and instead made heavy investments into America's defense industries, ensuring that the Duncan fortune rose massively again, even as most of the rest of the world was destroyed. From the moment of Nelson III's birth, his father was insistent that his son would rise to the status worthy of his heritage. Since the other four children were girls, Nelson II thought it essential that his son be the heir to his fortune and destiny.

As a teenager, Nelson III was admitted to one of the best prep schools in the nation. Like Dad, he found himself the beneficiary of a wartime deferral; Vietnam would not be his place of service when he left high school. Rather, it would be entrance to Yale University, to which Dad was a major donor. Then he would go on to receive an MBA from Yale and an internship on Wall Street. Nelson III didn't have the grades, or inherent smarts, to do any of these things based on merit. Doors just had a way of opening for him.

Life got harder after Nelson II passed from a heart attack at his work desk, though there were rumors it was in a hotel room with a prostitute where he really met his demise. Nelson III was then working as a vice president in Prudential Bank in Manhattan, a position his dad had secured for him on his graduation from Yale. The plan was for Nelson to spend a few years building his résumé at the bank and then to make a move into politics. Nelson II thought this was the next step for the Duncans—to rule over others, and not just be above them. He fancied himself another Joe Kennedy, and Nelson the favored child.

Nelson III needed Dad in order to rise in the political world—he didn't have book or street smarts, nor the airs that would allow him to lead men. He couldn't see this himself, but others did. Even his father's plan for a career in politics was based on this evaluation—he thought Nelson would succeed by ordering others, not convincing them to follow him.

Without Dad, Nelson's steps up the career ladder became harder and harder, and a future in politics was out of the question. Nelson found it easiest to just stay put at the bank. A decade later, he was still there, earning an extraordinary salary for little work and almost no risk. The truth was, this was the happiest time in Nelson's life. It provided him many opportunities to enjoy the nightlife of New York City and his secret indulgences.

When Nelson turned fifty, the matriarch of the family, Nelson Duncan I's wife, Martha, called him in for a family conference. She was aware of his dalliances with other men in Manhattan, which continued even after he married and raised a family. The last family conference like this was when she insisted it was time for him to marry, and she had provided the name and telephone number of the woman he was to court. He had listened to her then, and would listen again.

It was time for him to step up and be a worthy carrier of the Duncan name. The family still had great wealth and the status of name and genetics, but it was slipping. The computer revolution had created a new wave of wealth, and there were now hundreds of new billionaires stepping over the Duncan family in prestige and power. She thought it a shame; many were unworthy of their fortune and status. Her legacy must be making sure that the Duncans won the long game with these pretenders to the throne. Martha needed Nelson to be part of this in some way, even as she was committing most of the family's future prospects to his younger sister Judith.

She told Nelson it was time for him to assume a more appropriate place at the top of the social pyramid. She had found a position for him as the CEO of American Life Insurance. ALI was a major life insurance company located in Hartford, Connecticut, where many of the nation's primary insurance companies had located decades before.

ALI had built a large book of business and assets over the past hundred years in the life insurance business. Part of this was the company's original connections to the trusts of the 1920s and their status as a preferred business. After WWII, they grew their book of business to new heights through their ins with the nation's burgeoning defense industries. Their linkages had much to do with Nelson Duncan II and secret deals with Nazis and the Japanese. Martha still held the chits in hand for these secret deals and was now using them to place Nelson Duncan III where she wanted him.

Martha's advisors shared with her that ALI was a strong enough company and would enjoy moderate and stable growth for years to come. It was the business model for life insurance, after all. If she wanted this to be a game changer to keep the Duncans in the nation's elite status, there was a way to do that too. The idea was to diversify into health insurance under Nelson III.

Health insurance was a growth industry, and the fact that much of this would be under government control should allow them to tilt the playing field to their favor. Martha approved of the business plan for this venture, set up a new board of directors who would be supportive of the plan, and recommended her grandson as the new CEO of ALI.

Nelson III, of course, agreed. He was frustrated that his new home would be Hartford. It was not an exciting place to live, and he wondered whether it had a gay night life. Making this more difficult was part of Martha's plan for him, and he knew it.

Nelson accepted his new role as a divine right that put him above others. He enjoyed telling others what to do, in particular the so-called whiz kids who would bring him reports and proposals for how to implement ALI's addition of a health insurance portfolio to their life insurance platform.

Martha and her advisors were right. Over the course of the 1990s, the health insurance business grew significantly, in clients and dollar value. The government did get far more involved, mostly financially as the source paying for coverage to new enrollees. Even better, government health care agencies, with some prodding from Congress and the lobbyists whispering in its ears, had begun to shift major portions of traditional Medicare and Medicaid business to "private health plans." It was a gold mine, with a main shaft drilled into taxpayers' pockets.

These changes also brought new competitors into the picture. ALI had a leg up in figuring out how to succeed in this environment, but soon the other major traditional insurance carriers headquartered in Hartford built their own new ventures into health care. Some also merged to create a bigger base of effort, hoping they could win by creating near monopoly status in an oligopolistic business.

Soon, hospitals and health care systems also began to believe that they could jump upstream and grab the health care dollar closer to the payor. Those in the insurance world scoffed at the effort of hospitals to do so; most were local, regional at best, and insurance success was all about scale and impersonal national connections that would allow payments for the covered lives to trickle out to policyholders. Sell locally, deny nationally; that was the core business strategy.

These traditional insurers grew more concerned as many hospitals became health systems and began to conglomerate into national enterprises. Most of these still remained too small—even if they covered a number of states—to be serious competitors. But there were a handful that had the national ambitions and lack of scruples to make them serious competitors.

ALI, after fifteen years with Nelson Duncan III at the helm, was not even a contender. Nelson, despite his appetite for making decisions, usually bit on the wrong choices. Those whiz kids had brought him some possible winners, but he had cast them aside. *Why would we create an ancillary health care utilization review capacity that we could use to deny claims? Wouldn't it be easier to just outsource this? Why should we invest in meta-data that would give us the information base to out-analyze our competitors? Shouldn't we be focused on the analysis of our investment portfolios and how we really make money by investing the health care premium dollars we receive?* Bad choices.

The net result was that two decades later ALI found themselves a second-tier player in the health care insurance world. Martha was long gone, having passed on to join Nelson I and his lovers in heaven or hell. Nelson's sister Judith had taken most of the family fortune and name and moved the family legacy forward by taking control of a pharmaceutical company conglomerate. She was now making billions of dollars selling prescription opioids across America, and had little interest in seeing, let alone helping, her dimwitted brother.

ALI itself remained stable enough as an enterprise; its life insurance reserve base provided more than enough financial juice to make it so. There was little risk of a complete downslide, and Nelson held on to that security even as he blamed others for the failures in their health care business line. It might have made more sense to leap out of the business now by selling off what they had to a competitor and either continuing their safe life insurance business enterprise, or investing in some other product line that might have better success.

Nelson preferred the risk-free life that life insurance provided but still felt some manifest destiny to do more than that. He had no acumen for finding an alternative way to do this, so he stuck with the health care insurance pathway set out by his grandmother, and latched on to a proposal brought to him by a business associate to partner with a large health care system by being their insurance partner.

The health care system was HealthMost. HealthMost had grown from being a company originally made up of community hospitals located in midsize American cities across mostly the American West, first by merging with another hospital system that owned hospitals in several larger cities in the West. It had continued its growth with further hospital acquisitions across much of the nation and by acquiring related health care industries that would create a vertical health care delivery power—clinics, nursing homes, rehab hospitals, and diagnostic companies.

HealthMost was very profitable and pressed its advantage of being classified as a not-for-profit organization exempt from most federal taxes and a large portion of state and local obligations. Richard Thrust wanted more—ultimately to be a national health care system with the full vertical line of financing and delivery of health care. To do so, he needed a health insurance capacity, and he saw an opportunity to take ALI's capacity for his own ends.

The partnership agreement was handled by the attorneys for HealthMost and ALI. Nelson was told by his advisors that most of the terms were standard for these types of affiliations and that there was nothing to worry about. There would be significant earnings from getting into bed with a national health care delivery system, and ALI wouldn't have to worry about actually taking care of patients.

Nelson soon learned that the agreement required ALI to provide significant capital to HealthMost for access to their health care delivery system. That ALI had provided the necessary licenses and capacity to be an "insurer" got him a bunch of reports and an award from the HealthMost Foundation. There was a lot of money flowing to ALI for their capital and asset investment, and Nelson II's board remained content enough to let it play out.

It bothered Nelson that he didn't really understand what HealthMost was doing with this capital. He was somewhat used to it, though. He didn't really understand the life insurance business or the investment portfolios managed by his finance executives. These paid out well, and that was all that mattered.

The difference was that the life insurance division addressed him in a manner fitting with his station in life. They were respectful in tone and deed, even subservient to him and his status as a captain of industry. But Richard Thrust, who was charming enough during negotiations, addressed him as if Nelson worked for him. Thrust was rude and short in their dealings, which were mostly by telephone. If they were to meet in person—always short get-togethers—Thrust quickly pushed off any discussions of joint business strategy to consultants or associates he had brought with him to the meeting.

This latest telephone call was just another rude reminder of how much Nelson regretted this new relationship. Thrust had told him that ALI would need to implement some changes to their data management systems in order to comply with electronic data requirements of the federal government. HealthMost would provide the technical requirements through a consulting team they would provide to ALI, and would even pay for half the costs of the upgrade. But the changes would have to be done by the end of next quarter, and Thrust told Nelson that he would be held accountable should the deadline not be met.

Imagine being told by this pompous ass that he had to do anything. Nelson knew Thrust was from New York City, but not from bloodlines like his. No, his family made their way into America in the garment business on the lower Eastside. Richard Thrust had sold towels to make his way through school. He may have become a big shot in the hospital world, but he had no business addressing someone like Nelson in this way.

What would Dad or Grandmother do, he wondered. He flipped through his Rolodex to get the phone number for his vice president for technology. He would get Glen Hines on the HealthMost request. And then it would be his ass on the line if it didn't get done, not his.

Chapter Fifty-Four

Young Irv Gets a Master's Degree

Irv became a degree candidate in the University of Washington Masters of Health Administration program in 1983. It was a two-year program, with a required internship over the summer between the two school years.

Irv enjoyed his time in the MHA program. The instructors were for the most part smart, interesting, and personable. His classmates came from varied and diverse backgrounds, and the study requirements were not so overbearing as to distract from his desire to maintain a life beyond just school and studying. Most of the courses were akin to a liberal arts degree, with a focus on areas of study relating to the unique challenges of managing health care organizations.

He did his internship with Group Health Cooperative of Puget Sound the summer of his first year in the program. Group Health was a staff model health maintenance organization—something of a rarity, looking across the country. This was a health plan that received insurance-like premiums and provided care to enrollees by owning and operating its own health care facilities and staff.

Group Health Cooperative's greater uniqueness was that it was owned by consumers, not investors or even a not-for-profit corporate enterprise. Many of the private insurance companies or enterprises that set up HMOs were controlled by shareholders and presumably held a major profit motive. The way they provided care was reflective of this, using contracts to discharge their obligations to provide care to people.

Group Health was instead organized around a community ownership model of consumers, with a governance approach that made listening to these community voices a core matter for the life of the organization. Irv did his internship in the policy department for Group Health, reviewing various governmental and corporate policy proposals.

The administrative rounds that were part of the internship also gave him his introduction to the administrative operations of the health care system. He became more interested in this career track than the health policy assignment of his internship. He was so fascinated that he accepted a position as an assistant administrator in a small psychiatric hospital outside of Seattle when he graduated from the MHA program in 1985. It was a low-pay job, but it was a start. He liked it—it was interesting and he thought it was a useful thing to be doing. Irv was off and running on a career in health care.

Chapter Fifty-Five

Nelson Duncan III Stews

Nelson Duncan III was still steaming over how Richard Thrust had spoken to him on their phone call earlier in the day. The unmet dreams of his family had chipped away for years at Nelson's ego, and he sensed the family's disappointment in him, at least in some general way, since to really understand it would have driven him to behave differently than he had. He did understand that he was not the captain of industry that men of his social standing were due. There remained a residue of pride, though, and he was angered by the arrogance of Thrust and his ilk, men who were not worthy of their standing speaking to him as if he were a household servant.

He caressed the neck of his lover. Grandmother had made his sexual trysts harder—but not impossible—by relocating him to Hartford. She had no way of knowing that gay attraction was a common thing, and about to become commonly known and sometimes even accepted. Nelson had found it easy to find a new network in Hartford among the bevy of insurance workers. He had several lovers of interest now, and his wife no longer even tried to object to his urges. She had other things and people to do, and as long as he kept his relationships quiet, she wouldn't object.

Frank was one of his favorites. They would get together regularly in Duncan's penthouse apartment in downtown Hartford. Frank was young and hard-bodied and interested in what Nelson had to talk about. Nelson could talk to Frank, who would not only listen but found what he had to say smart and interesting.

Tonight Frank was commiserating over Nelson's treatment on the telephone by Thrust. Nelson normally would leave out many details when telling such stories out of office to his lovers or others, but this time there was little to hide. A business partner in Chicago had ordered him to open his data system so that he could add some of his files to ALI's server. There was some allusion to a data migration process and wanting to secure the files relevant to their joint venture. But that was all it was—a brief reference. Richard Thrust's ask of him was an order, and without any pretense of gratitude or appreciation or even a hint of respect.

"I don't know why you let him treat you like that," shared Frank. "He sounds like such an ass. You deserve so much better. What are you going to do about it?"

Nelson smiled at Frank and expanded his caressing. This was more of what he wanted: deference, care, and respect. Nor had it occurred to him that there was anything he could or should do in response. It was easier to just complain. "Well, what would you have me do?" He thought it a throwaway question that would bring an end to this dialogue so they could move on to other things.

"There has to be something. Do you really care about what is on those files? It sounds like whatever is on them is his problem, not yours. Maybe they should make an appearance to the outside world. That they see some public light should light a fire up that dick's ass."

Nelson chuckled out loud. "Yes, it would, my dear. I'll give it some thought." He already was—he had all he needed, really, from Thrust and his organization—an income stream that was helpful but wouldn't be a fatal problem if it went away. After all, he had reinsured the underlying risk—he did at least know the insurance business. He had also begun to grasp that all Thrust wanted was access to capital and ALI's insurance licenses. The quick shift in Thrust's attitude toward Duncan showed him that he had been used—it was something he had learned over the course of his work life.

Maybe for once he would prove that one did this at one's own peril. He had never promised favors like the data transfer. Besides, what was anyone going to do about it anyway? He was near eligible for early retirement and cared far more about time with Frank and others than the insurance business.

I'll find a way to screw that bastard, thought Nelson as he rolled into Frank's arms.

Chapter Fifty-Six

Irv's Early Health Care Career

Irv's reason for studying health care in the University of Washington MHA Program was to find a way to fix the broken health care system. He knew this was an issue historically—since well before WWI, as documented by the report from the Committee on the Cost of Medical Care.

Much had happened over the years, and some of it very significant, such as the creation of Medicare for seniors and the disabled and the evolution of Medicaid into a program for many lower- and middle-class families in need. But as a system, things were a mess, and maybe even worse because of the conflicting policies adopted over decades of shifting power between Republican and Democratic politicians.

Irv was about to graduate from the University of Washington School of Medicine and was intent on finding a way to do something about this mess as he transitioned from student to worker. His studies verified that it was a very complicated system, with many parts, and that the answers to its failings were elusive. He needed to learn much more about it, practically, if he was going to contribute to a solution.

Security and certainty were not the things he sought in a job; experience and a chance to ultimately make a big difference were his aims. Most of his classmates were accepting positions with hospitals and other organizations intended to give them an anchor from which to safely and linearly grow their careers. They might stay in those positions for three to five years, and then get a promotion. Or make a lateral shift that had more money or power in similar roles elsewhere. That was not for him.

Instead, he looked for short-term engagements that would provide him unique and deep insights into the health care system. He began by accepting the assistant administrator position in a small psychiatric hospital in south Seattle, where he stayed for a couple of years and got his basic grounding as to what it meant to be a hospital administrator and the unique problems of the mental health sector.

Two years later, he saw an opportunity to grow his knowledge at a bigger and far more complex hospital. It was a one-year Administrative Fellowship position at Seattle's major public hospital, Harborview Medical Center, a teaching hospital, a tertiary hospital, and the hospital of last resort for the insured and very sick.

Irv was selected, and the job didn't disappoint. Harborview had every problem known to hospitals across the nation. One of the first things Irv learned was how hard it was to run such a complex hospital—it was a 24-hour-a-day and seven-day-a-week proposition, and this made it harder than anything he had ever encountered. His primary fellowship project was in the Nursing Department helping with scheduling and logistics, and he learned how pivotal nursing was to the care process—and how little power and respect it got as an element within hospital power structures.

For all that Irv learned about regular and routine hospital management at Harborview over that year, he also learned about the challenges of taking care of those who were abandoned by society and the health care system. Community hospitals across the state, and even major tertiary care hospitals in Seattle and Spokane, regularly transferred their most difficult cases to Harborview, through their emergency room. Or at least the ones where there was no obvious source of payment for care. Major and multiple traumas, rare disorders, and a variety of maladies made up a routine day of hospitalizations at Harborview. Just the list of available translation services illustrated the complexity at play—there were over fifty different language interpreters on call to help communicate with non-English-speaking patients.

Irv was offered a position as director of Operations within the Nursing Department at the end of his fellowship. Tempting as it was, he thought it might focus him too narrowly on one aspect of the health care system and away from his true career quest. He had set out to do this differently than most of his classmates, and one year of on-the-job training within a hospital was not enough.

Instead, he took a project job within the local community clinic system. It was a six-month job to develop the operational capacity to accept capitated payments for care at the various clinic sites. These were much like insurance transactions, with the clinic wanting to receive payments for accepting the obligation to care for patients for a set fee. They would take care of the patients, whatever they needed, with that global monthly fee. It was thought that this would shift the incentives in the medical care system away from providing more service to making the patient better so that they don't need as much medical care. It was at the heart of the HMO movement that began in the 1970s, but different in that the clinics largely served an uninsured population.

Irv learned a great deal about community clinics and capitation payment models and what was necessary to make them work successfully. He saw how there were temptations within the model to solve the "too much care" problem by not providing nearly enough. Even in the altruistic culture of the community clinics, this was a clear and present danger of what they were modeling as an idea; just imagine this in the hands of organizations or people whose interest in health care was mostly about how to make a buck.

The complexity of the project extended his engagement another eight months. Again, he was offered a regular position with the community clinic system. Again, he turned it down and searched for another place to learn more truths of the overall health care system.

This time it was as a legislative aide in Olympia. The Senate Health Care Committee was looking for someone with health care knowledge and experience who would be willing to staff committee work when the State Legislature was in session over the winter months. Irv worked on a variety of health care topics from the public policy angle, learning about the system and the legislative process as well.

Since it was by definition part-year work, it provided him the openings in his calendar to take on projects within other parts of the health care system: disaster planning, clinical information systems for a group practice of physicians, a patient safety initiative at the state hospital association, and more. Irv essentially became a part-time legislative aide and part-time consultant. He didn't come close to maximizing his earnings potential, but made enough for Mary Beth and him to enjoy their life together. They also had opportunities to do things outside of regular work, and did—international trips, volunteer engagements, and other adventures.

After seven years of a nomadic career, Irv was starting to feel it was time to set some deeper roots within the system. One of the health care leaders he met in his travels shared with him that his résumé was starting to look as if he couldn't keep a job. This leader told him that he respected him and was even a bit jealous about what he was doing with his wanderings across the system. But if he really intended to be a difference maker in a big way, he would need to settle into a regular position, and soon.

Irv had also seen firsthand what was wrong, and sometimes maddeningly wrong, about health care. The people who worked in the system were generally smart and committed and hardworking. But the systems of care had huge problems. Just as the CCMC Report had identified years ago, there was no overall system, and doing good for patients was achieved more through ad hoc action and heroic creativity than systemic fortitude. It was exactly what he had experienced during his mom's cancer treatment. It was time that he tackled the bigger problem.

He shared his thinking with Mary Beth and Johnny. Both encouraged him. It was especially helpful that Mary Beth was so enthusiastic about it. They had a good thing going, and he didn't want to screw that up.

One reason Mary Beth was so enthusiastic about the idea was that she most enjoyed Irv when he was his inquisitive and motivated self. When things got stale for him before he decided on a health care career, she got a taste of what he was like when he was bored. She loved him regardless, but an engaged Irv was a far better version for her tastes.

She also experienced vicarious thrills from his varied experiences. She would accompany him on work outings and events when she could, to be supportive and get a better idea of his life. Not that she had too much time to do so—she was now busy building her own career.

It was time for both of them to step into their futures in the community. Both privately wondered, and even worried a bit, about how this might affect their relationship. So far, it had been so good. They hoped it would stay that way. First, both had to find their next positions so they could stretch their wings.

Chapter Fifty-Seven

Senator Gibson Meets with Nelson Duncan III

Senator Gibson welcomed Nelson Duncan III into the penthouse suite of his hotel in downtown Hartford, Connecticut, and motioned to a couch in the center of the room. It was a large suite with a separate kitchen in addition to two sleeping rooms, and they walked by it on their way to the living room.

"Can I get you anything to drink, Mr. Duncan? I hope you don't mind if I enjoy a little bourbon. It has been a long day."

"Yes, I will join you, thanks. Rocks, please." Senator Gibson poured a couple of fingers of Jim Beam Black into a glass tumbler filled with ice and handed it to Nelson before they sat down.

"I don't really know why I am here, Senator. I got a phone call from ex-Congressman Bridgewater, and he said you wanted to see me about follow-up questions around hospital practices in emergency rooms. I run a life insurance company and know virtually nothing about this topic."

"You know enough about health care and hospitals to enter into a joint venture with HealthMost, though." Johnny leaned in from his seat on the couch toward Duncan, sending off his first sign that he was not going to let him off easy.

Duncan was already feeling less at ease. "Yes, we do have an arrangement. But all we do is provide some insurance components to HealthMost for a contract with the federal government, along with some capital. All of the actual health care is provided through HealthMost. You would do better to ask them your questions," he countered.

"And yet, you are the one here. So I will start with you, and if I need to go further with you or them, I will get in touch with the legal staff for my committee." Johnny spoke in his best stern voice, and then began to pepper Duncan with all sorts of questions. Questions he knew Nelson could not begin to answer. The goal was not to get answers from him; it was to rattle him enough to provide some possible way to get behind the firewall of ALI's database. Irv was listening to the conversation in one of the bedrooms in the suite, taking notes.

It might take a while to get to the data aspects of the joint venture, but Johnny had time. He was quick on his feet and experienced in getting folks to open up to him. Before the evening was over, Nelson Duncan III would have gotten over his growing fear and instead accepted Johnny as a new friend. Or at he would have gotten comfortable enough to provide a name or something that might give Irv his way into the database.

The inquisition went on for another fifteen minutes. "I don't know" became the most common refrain from Duncan. Each such answer was followed by another series of questions on the topic, answers Duncan would never have. Duncan started to sweat like a porpoise in heat, and the perspiration was soaking into the white shirt underneath his dark tailored suit.

After Johnny unleashed a stream of difficult questions related to whether ALI had knowingly participated in a scheme to dump patients onto hospitals owned by competitors to HealthMost, Duncan put down his drink. "Stop. I told you, I don't know anything about any of this. It was just a way to get an additional revenue stream to supplement our life insurance business." The lines across his face were wrinkling like a cheap suit. "Can I ask you something, Senator?"

"Sure. Go ahead."

"Why aren't there any staff here for this meeting? I was under the impression that I would be meeting with them and you?"

"Well, I just wanted to keep things between you and me to start, Duncan. I've met your partner Thrust, and he is a real prick. I was curious to see what type of man would trust him enough to do a business deal. I wasn't sure what to expect."

"He *is* a prick. See, I can answer a question." He laughed at his attempt at a joke.

Johnny chuckled too. "See, that wasn't so hard. Now tell me, why did you really enter this agreement?"

"It really is what I have been saying. I could get some additional dollars flowing into the company by letting HealthMost use my insurance license and some of our capacities. I was just looking to keep the board off my back for another year or two. I would be just as happy to take early retirement and do something else." Duncan looked to be close to tears as he confessed his unhappiness to the senator.

The silence between them hung like a wet diaper on a clothesline for what seemed to be minutes. It was probably about fifteen seconds. Duncan looked down at the floor, and then up to Johnny, and then back down again.

"Look, I want to help. It is just hard to do so in my current situation. Isn't there some way I could help where no one but you and I know?"

Johnny was stunned that this was where the conversation was going. "Why, yes." He moved in for the kill shot. "We have extensive protections for whistleblowers. Provided, of course, that they haven't committed any crimes and are not at fault for what they are reporting. Is that the case here?"

"Yes, I keep telling you that. I don't know anything about the health care parts of this. I just know the insurance parts of our arrangement, and those are really pretty basic. But maybe there is something in these that might interest you?"

"What do you mean?"

"I have a database of clients—or I should say ALI has one. HealthMost insisted on using part of our database and privacy systems for some of the records associated with this joint venture. I didn't think much about it at the time. Just thought it was standard practice." He thought he should have been more questioning of everything about this deal with Thrust. "A couple of weeks ago, Thrust called me and had me authorize the addition of some new data into that system. He even reminded me that the contract terms included a strict liability provision for anything that might breach the privacy of the database elements of the contract. I understood it to be a threat."

"Nelson, he can't threaten Congress. Or me. You seem to be a good man who is just in with the wrong people." *And made a very bad career choice*, Johnny thought. "You help us see what is in there, and I will do all I can to keep you out of it. I know you think that politicians can't be trusted to keep their word, but I can. As long as you are sincere and accurate in that you had nothing to do with any wrongdoing, this will be a matter just between you and me. I will need to find a way to see the database with the help of someone else, since I don't know shit from shinola about such things. Do we have a deal?"

Duncan thought for a few seconds. "Yes, we do." The two men shook hands. "What do we say about this meeting?"

Johnny leaned back in his seat. "I'll take care of most of that. I will tell Bridgewater that you were an insolent son of a bitch who was entirely uncooperative. And that I am none too pleased with HealthMost because of it. I'll say that while I wish I had something on them, I don't. And that I expect to see Thrust in person at my field hearing in Seattle. Sam will think he is brilliant in getting you in to see me, and you will not even be a second thought to any of them. You just tell them that I was a liberal ass and said bad things about the president. That should get you some friends too."

This time they laughed together. They both stood and shook hands once more. "One last thing," said Johnny. "Give me your private cell phone number. I will find someone who can get expert eyes on the database and have them give you a call. Code word will be NRBQ. If you hear that phrase from them, you will know they are with me. And here is my number—give me a call anytime on this. And when you get out of this shit of an industry, let's get together again."

Chapter Fifty-Eight

Young Mary Beth Builds a Career

Mary Beth had a front row seat watching her beau Irv find his way forward in life through the Theory of Irv. He was now doing good for others and as part of a new form of adventure and learning for him. It wasn't a great surprise to her that this was what he was doing—she had seen some inklings of this thinking on his part even before the revelations from wandering in the desert with Johnny. She thought Irv's decision to lead a life of purpose was more like unwrapping a box when one already knew what was inside it.

What was more of a revelation to her—and him—was that this purpose would be sought through a career in health care. Until their hike, Irv had said little to her about the health care system, or his experiences with it, other than some very limited comments about whatever had occurred when his mother died. Mary Beth knew it was a bad experience.

Irv's plan had a ways to go, but he was now well underway. He was in his second year of school and would soon graduate. Then he would get on-the-job experience, working up to when he would know enough, and have enough standing, to be a leader in creating big change to a defective system.

Mary Beth was thrilled about all of this. She knew he had been struggling before, as she and Johnny had begun to find their own life paths. When Irv and Johnny went off on their desert adventure, Mary Beth had just begun to work part time at Nancy Jones' political consulting firm. This was going to take more hours from her time with Irv, and she had worried that it would put a strain between them. Instead, Irv found ways to fill his own time outside of her.

She was tickled pink that they had so far figured out how to fit their separate lives together. During the worst of Irv's angst, she wondered whether this would be the thing that caused a breakup, as similar conflicts had for her girlfriends. The truth was, Irv was difficult to live with when he lost his spark. She didn't want to break up—she just needed a little space to pursue her dreams and for him to take up the central role of making sure he felt good about himself.

Now it looked like they were more than in a good place. They would undoubtedly have future questions about how to fit their separate lives into their joint one, but she believed this would not be too big a challenge. They had just weathered a major storm, and both were committed to that, and each other.

Mary Beth had the added current challenge of being the breadwinner for the family, at least while Irv was in school. He was going full time, and in-state tuition was not a huge cost. But Irv wasn't able to work at the coffee plant more than fifteen hours a week, and the cost of living in Seattle was rising dramatically. Mary Beth needed to keep her job at the bakery, and the extra money she made working in the evenings with Nancy allowed them to squeak by financially.

Mary Beth had continued to volunteer her time. Her main endeavor was to help develop the bakery owner's idea for a not-for-profit venture. The original idea was to start up a food bank in northern Seattle. The bakery, and other local food producers, would provide food to those in the area in need. They needed someone to manage this, and Mary Beth volunteered.

The owners were generous in allowing her to devote some of her paid time at the bakery on this work, but much of it needed to happen in off hours or weekends. She found it fascinating to be on the ground floor of creating something that mattered and enthusiastically jumped into every aspect of the project.

She had ideas for how to think even bigger about the program. How about if they staffed it with people who needed work, such as the homeless? What if they did so less as working jobs and more as a training ground for people who could then move on to other jobs in Seattle's active restaurant and food industries? There were shortages of trained staff and a demand for such employees, and they would be making an important social match.

She got the green light to build the bigger program and spent much of her free time over the next year doing so, and then managing it. Irv was busy with his second year in the master's program, and he was happy that she had something else to occupy her time. She even took some classes—the owner paid for a series of community college courses on not-for-profit management for Mary Beth.

By the time Irv was approaching graduation from the master's program, Mary Beth had established her own standing in the not-for-profit management world of Seattle—most of it through the bakery's food bank worker training program, but also through contacts she made while working part time for Nancy.

She was pleased when Irv shared he had been offered a position at a hospital in South King County. It was only about a thirty-minute drive south to get there from their Wallingford home. Best of all, she would not have to give up her own career to satisfy his needs. She still loved him, and saw him as a partner, but did not want that to translate back to the unhappy expectations that her parents had placed on her as a young woman.

She was also in on Irv's idea to build his career by moving to different parts of the health care system. They would spend many an evening talking about how screwed up the system was, and his hopes to help really change it. She was proud of him and his ideals and commitment. Nor was she overly concerned with money—they had more than enough now to be happy in their home and life, even if Seattle continued to get more expensive.

Privately, she knew that part of her support for Irv's plan to explore the breadth of the health care system was that he would do this locally. She might have been able to deal with his moving around the state, but feared that his going beyond the state's borders would put the onus on her to follow or give up on the relationship.

Whatever the reasons for their deal over the next decade, it worked, and worked well, between them. They both pursued their careers, developing their skills and experiences. They intertwined these, and grew together, enmeshing each other in every imaginable way into the distinct lives they were leading. They were happy, individually and with each other.

But the drift of continents happens over time, even if slowly, and Irv and MaryBeth found they were not immune. It was the health care system that held the fissure that threatened to rip them apart.

Chapter Fifty-Nine

1990: Beginning of the Age of Health Reform

Chris Jones now believed that the only way to solve the problems with American health care was to push the political system for major and comprehensive reform. For much of his career, and his father's before him, he had tried to play ball within the American predilection for incremental change. This may have been an acceptable model for other American economic sectors—but it wasn't working for health care.

A first and critical step was to diagnose what was wrong with the system as the decade of the 1990s began—and communicate this in a way that might stick within the political world. It was where the Committee on the Cost of Medical Care had begun its work. Chris re-read their report and found that much was the same as back then. He would need to modernize the context and show how things had regressed, even in the light of profound financial investments and incredible advances in health care interventions.

He drafted a comprehensive policy analysis of the American health care system, with the help of other professors and students within Harvard. There was now a plot and lots of data available to support the reform imperative story he was peddling to whoever would listen.

By most accounts, the American health care system had become the most bloated and inefficient endeavor in the world. It was fragmented and complicated beyond most humans' understanding. Even those who worked within the health care system could barely figure out how to make it work for them or their families when they were in need of medical care.

Numbers backed this up. International health rankings placed the United States thirty-seventh in terms of health outcomes, despite costing a quantum leap more than any other national health care system. America's per person health care cost was a third more than the next nation on the list, and double most other industrialized nations.

Chris would argue with those who wanted to quibble over the international health ranking data. They would point to one or another data inconsistency that might affect an outcome measure. Chris would retort that if we accept their criticism, and a host of others, the basic conclusion would be the same. That is, what if the United States was twentieth or even fifteenth in these rankings? The level of our investments in health care should put us at number one in the world, Chris would assert, and it was a crime if we were even in the middle of the pack. Instead, we were near the bottom.

What is even more damning, he would say, is that this is before one even considers the fact that millions of Americans remain without any health coverage for their health care needs, short of showing up at hospital emergency rooms when they are in crisis. Virtually every other nation in the world had some form of universal coverage for its citizens as part of their less expensive systems. Chris didn't view any of these systems as perfect, and several had significant problems in their own right. But they were at least trying to be comprehensive in the scope of their base health care protections to their citizens.

Health care was also beginning to squeeze out the ability to invest in other things, as a nation, within states, and personally. The percent of GNP/GDP had risen to over 12 percent and was projected to exceed 20 percent in a few more decades. The old joke was that there was a limit to the amount of money that health care could take up—100 percent. But 20 percent seemed like an awful lot.

The economic argument was that every dollar inefficiently allocated to health care was at the expense of other investments that a society could make. Education was typically portrayed as the loser in this allocation, but arguments could be made for other sectors too.

What's more, many of the under-invested sectors might have more value to producing health than health care. If the goal of health care is not to provide more care, but more health, Chris pointed to research that showed that social determinants of health were far more valuable than most health care services. These studies suggested that health care represented only 8-10 percent at best of what it took to produce health, while determinants like housing, transportation, nutrition, economics, and individual behavior were the greatest factors.

Chris knew this didn't mean health care was not worthy, and something that was needed and generally good for people. His dad had understood this when he helped diffuse new possibilities for Americans during the Age of More, and it was still the case. There just had to be some reasonable systemic limits on the thinking of how to make investment decisions as a society so that we were building health and not just financing the costly delivery of health care services.

Governments and businesses, as the major payors of health care, were feeling the squeeze and were anxious to do something about this cost problem. One of their favorite solutions was to enable the rising costs of health care to be pushed off to clients or employees. Copayments, in the form of premium sharing, deductibles, co-insurance, or ineligibility for service began to push a substantial part of the financial obligation for the growing cost of care to individuals and families.

Some of this was touted as a good thing—this price sensitivity would enable a more forceful health care consumer. Maybe, thought Chris. But only if the system was intelligible—and actionable—to the average American. It was not. It was only getting more confusing every year.

Business and employee contributions to health benefit plans had also overshot historic tax incentives; costs were so high, and escalating so rapidly, that health care costs had become a major drag on income rise for many Americans. Wages and salaries were stagnating, even as corporate profits rose, and paying for health care seemed a big part of the reason.

The cost problem was clear, though denied by many health provider constituencies. Some would capture the energy for reform when it rose politically and recast the issue around access—or the lack thereof for health coverage or health care services. That it was an issue at all made these efforts to reframe the debate away from the central failing of American health care possible. Previous health care reform efforts, Chris knew, had been hijacked through this shift of focus.

Less obvious to rank and file Americans was that the United States also had serious problems with quality of care within its delivery system. A system with such fragmentation and distortion would expect to see failings in many areas, and ours did.

Avoidable deaths was one quality metric, and one that could capture public attention. It did when the Institute of Medicine released a report called "To Err Is Human," charging that there were over 100,000 avoidable hospital deaths in hospitals each year. Hospital advocates argued the number, and may have been right. But, like with international health rankings, would only 50,000 be an acceptable number?

Some serious quality improvement efforts were now underway, some from within the industry and field. Data was being used to monitor, compare, and analyze care patterns, and consequently force change in the delivery of health care—with major pockets of resistance in the industry, to be sure. Chris knew that more needed to be done, and that one could argue for comprehensive reform just on the basis of quality problems in health care delivery.

A system in such collective crisis needed a comprehensive solution. Chris now believed this was the only way to solve the American health crisis, and he began to search for ways to help stimulate movement toward meaningful big reform.

It was not like this was a completely blank slate of American policy endeavors. The CCMC study in 1927–1932 was exactly about this subject. Occasional waves of reconsideration had occurred throughout the course of the 1900s—within FDR's New Deal, Harry Truman's Post War America, and Johnson's Great Society. All had failed.

Waves of occasional reform energy came and went in subsequent decades. President Jimmy Carter talked of major national health reform, but ultimately shifted his efforts to an attempt to use wage and price controls to stem the nation's health inflation. The industry beat back the proposal and pledged to voluntarily reduce the cost of care. For a year or so, they even did so, long enough for the political pressure to subside, at which point health care inflation blew sky high.

The 1990s brought serious major reform energy to bear across the nation, helped in no small way by Chris's efforts. States' power had become a political theme in the 1990s, and both political parties began to explore how to shift solution-making away from the federal government toward the states. A number of states began to consider major health care system repair; the cost of health care was destroying state budgets, especially their capacity to provide constitutionally mandated education to its citizens. Maybe they could do something about this if the federal government at least stood aside?

Nationally, health care was gaining traction as a political issue, and the presidential election of 1992 raised the prospects that it would finally become a federal priority. The Democratic candidate, Bill Clinton, had even committed to doing something about it.

Candidates in the past had given it lip service as a campaign issue, but would quickly move on to other issues when they assumed power. President Clinton instead made this a priority of his first hundred days in office. He announced a study effort to identify and then pass comprehensive health reform. The effort would be led by First Lady Hillary Clinton. She established a special policy team to devise a proposal to provide health care to all Americans through a set of competing comprehensive health plans.

The effort was bogged down for a number of reasons, technical and political. First Lady Clinton's effort was mired down in the technical complexity of the proposal. It was also tightly controlled and didn't build the broad support needed to garner political support across the Congress. The clock was ticking, and the task force was moving very slow. Instead of fast strike legislation, it bled into an issue for the midterm elections of 1994.

Republicans branded the health care reform proposals from the Clintons as exactly what was wrong with America and used it to take control of the House. That guaranteed comprehensive health care reform would not happen during the Clinton presidency. Nor was President Bush the second about to introduce the notion during his eight years in office.

There were some notable state-based efforts over this time period. One of these was in Washington State, where a comprehensive health care package using the notion of competing comprehensive health plans was passed into law. The state formed a commission to implement the law, but before it went into effect, the law was repealed by the legislature. The main culprit was, again, politics. Republicans took over the state legislature by running candidates who criticized the reform package.

Other states tried similar large reform. A major stumbling block increasingly became the challenge of building state action to resolve a national problem. For example, if Washington State, Tennessee, or any state developed a system whereby all residents would be covered for health, wouldn't uninsured people from other states move there? Especially if they were sick and in need of medical care?

The political failure of these national and state reform efforts fed the new political notion that health care was the third rail of politics and shouldn't be touched. Politicians used the issue in their campaigns, but mostly to raise money and criticize their opponents, not to develop real momentum on a policy effort to pass comprehensive American health policy.

Chris was disappointed by the outcome of these forays into comprehensive health care reform. A few showed real promise, and then were vanquished. Some thought he would be discouraged by this reality.

To the contrary, he was encouraged that the Age of Reform was around the corner. When these reform efforts had begun, it had been said that they were politically foolish. Health care is the third rail of politics, some would say. Touch it and you will get burned, probably fatally.

For sure, there was a political reaction to big solution proposals, even political retribution that killed some of these efforts. But many of the advocates of the effort survived, even under intense criticism and scrutiny. Maybe weakened over the short term but were still in the game.

What was far more important was churning below these policy and political outcomes. The sorry state of American health care was becoming the number one issue for American voters. They wanted change. They may have disagreed on the ideological choices they were being offered, but they very much wanted politicians to come together and find a way to make the health care system practically better. Not doing something about health care had become the actual third rail.

Chris would advise all who would listen that now was the time to double down on efforts to find a comprehensive and major reform of the national health care system. Tackling tough issues is what leaders do, even when it hurts them. Who would step to the table and try?

Turns out it was the first African American president of the nation. Go figure.

Chapter Sixty

Young Johnny Reacts to Political Change

It was a sunny but cold day in Washington, DC, in January 1995. Congressman John Gibson was looking out his window at snowflakes drifting down within a small portico visible through his office window. He had been a congressman for well over a decade now. Remaining an independent had continued to leave him low on the list of preferred House offices. His only real regret about this decision was that he didn't have a very good view.

Today that was not on his mind. He was wondering whether it was time for a change. The last decade of his congressional service had been, he thought, according to theory. He had continued to find a base of adventure and experience and, more important, had found some ways to advance the greater good for his constituents and the people of America. He had grown his constituent support service into an effective operation, while finding practical occasional opportunities to advance bipartisan policy matters in the House and Congress.

He was now wondering whether he would be able to do much good into the future. Just a couple of years ago, he was so optimistic and enthusiastic. President Clinton had come to office and, more important to Johnny, was promising to press for comprehensive health reform. It looked like it had a real chance to pass, and Johnny had done all he could to push it forward. He even engaged his friends—Irv, Mary Beth, and Nancy Jones—to educate him about the issues and policy choices.

Then the process became bogged down. The First Lady's special task force drew much of the blame for that, but Johnny was also discouraged by the lack of a clear legislative strategy to move it forward. Soon enough, the midterm elections arrived. Comprehensive health care reform was the profile issue for Republicans in their congressional races, and they took control of the House of Representatives. There was no chance that health care reform would be back on the agenda for quite a while now.

And things had changed for the worse in the nation's capital—not just in terms of nominal control, though there was a change of political guard of House leadership. Congressman Newt Gingrich was the new speaker of the House. Irv never liked him, which was saying something because he liked almost everyone. More troubling was that he saw how Gingrich was approaching the job—with fire and brimstone. Bipartisanship was being frowned upon, and it seemed like the Gingrich agenda was mostly to resist the Clinton Administration. There were even rumors that the plan was to impeach the president.

Johnny was an independent, so the philosophical matter of party control was not important to him. But the ability of Congress to function was critical. It was hard to pass laws as it was, and rightfully so. To begin to shape Congress as merely a political instrument in the Gingrich way was wrong and would greatly narrow his ability to produce social good.

He was depressed and looking for better answers, so he picked up the telephone and called his good friend Irv. Maybe he would have a more hopeful attitude.

"Irv. Johnny here. It is cold as a witch's tit here in DC and I need a pep talk." He outlined the source of his gloom, hoping Irv could help.

Irv was on his way out the door to his first day at his latest job with a research laboratory, but stopped and sat down at his kitchen table to talk to Johnny. "I hear you, Johnny. The ClintonCare failure was a bummer. Not only there, but here. The Republicans took control of the State Legislature here and are running a bill to repeal the comprehensive reform we passed in 1993." It was in fact why Irv was starting a new job—his previous position was on the staff of the commission created to implement the law, and it was clear this would now be a position without a future.

"So, are you telling me that I should be depressed about all of this? Sounds like you found a way to move on, but I am having a hard time doing so here in DC." Johnny could have a flair for the dramatic, and it was fueling his rare dour mood.

"Whoa, buddy. Yes, it sucks. But you've been through worse. And there may be worse to come. You know—when the going gets tough, the tough get going. Something like that anyway."

Johnny laughed. Irv had a way of calling bullshit on him whenever he went overboard. "You just telling me to man up, Irv?"

"No, I am telling you to do your freaking job."

"What do you mean?"

"You're a congressman, with a ton of seniority and a lot of influence. It would be one thing if you were Joe Schmoe, but you're not. You just need to step back and figure out where and what the opportunities are. There always are, you know."

Johnny sat up, realizing that he needed to adjust his perspective. This was why he called Irv at times like these. Yes, there always were opportunities. He needed to get off his pity parade and figure these out. A minute passed. Johnny was thinking, working through it at his own pace.

Johnny finally spoke. "You make a good point, Mr. Tinsley. I do have ways to help people, even now. I just have to build a new game plan for how to do so. One thing I am thinking is that I want some of this to relate to health and health care. One of my greatest disappointments was that health reform is clearly dead in this town. Maybe there is still something I can do on this front?"

Johnny's mental process was the same as Irv had gone through when it was clear the Washington Health Reform Commission was no more. He had resolved it by accepting a job to decode human DNA at a research laboratory in Seattle, a national leader in this, and succeeding would create great new ways to improve health. He shared this story with Johnny.

"You think it has a chance?" asked Johnny.

"Yes, I do. And if we can determine how disease imprints on our DNA, the way we treat people could revolutionize. Imagine how we might personalize medicine for people if we had that information? It is right out of *Star Trek*." Irv sounded truly excited by this venture.

"Wow. You can fit my knowledge about this in a thimble, and I can still see what you are saying, Irv. Makes me think that I should step back and take a look at the big picture here and find my own way to help advance things." He took another couple of minutes to think, while Irv waited patiently on the other end of the line.

"What if I brought a few of us together to do some brainstorming?" Johnny finally asked.

"Who are you thinking of?"

"You. Me. Nancy. Mary Beth—and I hear she has become quite the facilitator and could help structure our time together. And how about Nancy's dad, Chris? I spent some time with him the last couple of years on health care reform, at Nancy's suggestion. He knows more about this stuff than anyone I've ever met, including you. Anybody else you can think of?"

"Not off the top of my head, but I will think about it. When you want to do this?"

"Well, if it works for you and everyone else, we have a break coming up for President's Day. It is a federal holiday, so maybe you all have the day off? I will be in town for the week, to meet with my constituents and to see Reena and the kids. Maybe we can find a room somewhere and do a bit of brainstorming that day or over the weekend?"

"Sounds like a plan, Johnny. I will ask Mary Beth tonight and make a few phone calls to the others. Sounds like a fun and worthwhile thing to do. But now, I've got to run. Now that you've reinforced that my new job is a worthy one, I should probably get there only a half hour late on my first day."

"Just tell them that you were dealing with a national emergency. And that you can't tell them more or you would have to kill them. By all means, get your ass out of there and to your job. Thanks, buddy. Hope this works out, and see you in just a few weeks."

Johnny hung up the telephone and put his feet on the radiator in front of the window and behind his desk. He put his hands behind his head, interlocked the fingers, and rocked back in his chair. Yes, he thought, there were opportunities out there. He just had to find them. The game was still afoot.

Chapter Sixty-One

Irv and Lance Review the ALI Data

Johnny and Irv agreed that the best way to acquire the ALI data offered by Nelson Duncan was through Johnny's Chief of Staff Lance Givens. Lance was a longtime aide to the senator on his personal staff, not the committee. They went back to his House days, and had become friends. There were only a few people in Washington, DC, who Johnny would trust with anything so important, but Lance was on that list. He also had a background in computer sciences and should be able to deal with system protections within ALI.

Irv briefed Lance on the full particulars of this case, since up to now Johnny had mostly brought him up to speed on only the patient dumping matters at issue. Irv still left out a few of his suspicions in his briefing with Lance. He was beginning to sense that these were deeply troubling, and he thought it would be irresponsible to suggest them to a senatorial aide without more real evidence.

Instead, he told Lance about the corpse and the threat of a pandemic associated with it. Lance would know that it would be imprudent to talk about such matters with anyone, as rumors, in such a case, could indeed kill. If there was something helpful in those files that proved something else was afoot, Lance would soon enough know the full story.

Lance invoked the NRBQ codeword in a telephone call to Duncan and set up a meeting in a Hartford bar where Duncan handed him the goods. Lance was surprised it was only a flash drive, thinking that there would be so much information behind the firewall that he would receive a disk or even a tape. Initial speculation was that HealthMost was using ALI because the amount of information related to the joint venture was massive and they needed the additional analytic capacity of the insurance company. Clearly, that was not the case.

Lance returned to DC to review the contents of the file. Irv took three more vacation days and flew to DC to join in. The two researched the data files in Lance's office, on a secure computer provided to members of Congress that would protect them from outside surveillance.

There were several distinct files stored within the ALI database. One was a record of all of the clients served by the HealthMost-ALI joint venture and, most particularly, those who were enrolled in the special demonstration project with the federal government. There were thousands of names, insurance identification numbers, enrollment dates, and estimated capitation payment amounts, covering residences all across the nation. Many, make that most, of the names were Latino.

This file looked to be a standard client summary to an insurance program, and on its face, it even made sense that it would be found on the ALI server. The only thing notable was that the total of estimated capitation payments amounted to tens of millions of dollars per month. One column in the file did classify "Disposition" through designations of A, U, or D. Whatever those codes meant was a mystery—there was no key. A handful of records had blanks in this column.

A second file was also what might be a standard collection of data from such a joint venture—the monthly financial statements pertaining to the business. For both organizations there would be distinct bookkeeping entries for the impact of the transaction on them individually; this file contained the financial record of the aggregate transaction for the venture. Again, the most revealing thing from it was its scale—tens of millions of dollars in ongoing monthly revenue. There were also entries that spoke to even larger blocs of revenue received from the federal government. Lance and Irv made a note to do some further digging into these revenues.

The third file was the one that seemed most suspicious. It was a listing of names and insurance numbers, with the addition of other personally identifying information such as date of birth and nation of origin. The originating sources for the names in the records were various hospitals and medical centers, mostly from the western United States, and an inordinate number of them from southern states. It was also notable that most of the names were of Latino origin, much like the other files pertaining to the joint venture. The records were flagged with a similar special number to what Irv had found in Phoenix.

They surmised that this must be the full list of patients seen by HealthMost health care facilities across the nation and assigned to their treatment disposition. Was it a special "discharge" as was the case in Westside Medical Center? Perhaps.

They downloaded the data sets onto spreadsheet software so they could do some cross analysis. Lance's background in computer science proved helpful to this process. The first obvious step was to cross link the third file with the first—was this a subset of the full list of clients?

It was a subset to be sure, and nothing like the 90,000 clients in file one. But it still held a sizable number—7,000 names. A cursory review of the sub-record showed that almost all were Latino names, just like the ER list from Phoenix.

They manually created another list—the 117 names from the paper files in Westside Medical Center. There were no numbers available to cross-check these with the third file, so they used the names as their basis for cross-checking the two files. This analysis found ninety-three of the names from Westside Medical Center on the list of 7,000 names. Looking at the names that were not found, they guessed that it was their inability to match precise names in the files that accounted for the gap—the names were common, but some with different or shortened spellings.

Irv looked for Rodrigo Lopez on this list. There he was, including date of birth and county of origin—Panama. The disposition column was blank.

Irv and Lance reviewed the names from the paper system of Westside Medical Center and made notes on additional details provided in the third file for those cases. Most notably, there were two other patients in the Westside records for whom the disposition column was blank in the third electronic file.

The two men pulled back from the computer screen and sat around a worktable in Lance's office. For another hour or so, they sipped coffee and speculated as to what this data might mean. The coffee was needed—they had been at their analysis for over five hours and it was now 2 a.m.

There was something out of the ordinary going on here, but no smoking gun that they could see yet. Most of their general conclusions were similar to the suspicions Irv had when he first saw the paper list—Latino patients being flagged in HealthMost health care facilities for special treatment. Now there were thousands of names at play, not just hundreds. Experience and instinct told them that this special treatment wasn't a good thing for these patients, but they couldn't be sure about that.

They had done all they could that night and needed some rest, so they agreed to meet again the next afternoon, when Johnny would be able to join them for a debriefing. If either thought of anything else in the meantime, they would telephone the other.

They met with Johnny the next evening after other office staff had left, back in Lance's office so that they could use the secure computer if it was needed to show Johnny what was on the files.

Lance and Irv alternated recapping what they had found the night before. Johnny offered his assessment of where things stood when they were done with their report; it was similar to what Irv and Lance had concluded in the wee hours of the previous morning.

"So, we have confirmed that the names on the paper list from Phoenix are clients of this federal demonstration program, served by the joint venture, and were flagged for something special. We can now also see that whatever this is, it goes beyond one hospital and to something broader—over 7,000 patients within the HealthMost system. Nothing obvious as to what this special thing is, and it might not be anything more than their records being flagged in the system. I know it stinks to high heaven, but there isn't enough for us to do something with it yet."

"Agreed," said Lance. "This was exactly where we were last night too. But we've got a bit to add from today that gets us further down the road of showing something wrong is going on. Shall I fill this in, Irv?" he added while looking at his co-conspirator.

"It was your find, so go ahead."

"Okay. I was thinking about this earlier today and was struck again by not just the Latino names but the countries of origin. For one, why this was even a data flag. And that most of the countries were from the southern American hemisphere and matched with the reports we have been getting from the administration of illegal immigration hotspots. I am sure both of you were already processing how curious it was that the names were almost all Hispanic. Senator, I am sure you would have picked up on commonality of countries of origin to immigration of hot spots we have been briefed on.

"So, I had an idea. You will remember last year that we had a big fight with the administration over their enforcement of the border. Members of Congress were being inundated with reports of abuse, certainly on the southern border. Much of this played out in the media, like the stories about family separations. What got a little less media attention was that many offices were getting deluged with constituency requests to follow up on loved ones who went missing in their state. They suspected that ICE was involved but didn't know for sure and were getting no help from ICE or other federal agencies—not even letting them know if their loved one had been detained or arrested or murdered on the streets.

"So much of congressional office work is constituent relations," Lance continued, "and the silence of immigration officials became a real problem—and for members on both sides of the aisle. Really for all offices, but it was those of us that border other nations that were really struggling to give our constituents answers. There was a quiet deal struck to give us some access to help with inquiries. Not for all offices, but those with borders. Most think that this is just about the Mexican border, but, of course, Washington State borders Canada, and we do get these cases too. Not as many, but it is the same vacuum of information from ICE and Border Patrol.

"The solution was to give certain offices access to a database inquiry of people being held by federal officials, and those who were officially deported to their country of origin. Only one individual in each congressional office was given access to this database, and it could only be accessed by a secure federal computer—the one sitting over there next to my desk. And, yes, I am the designee for this office," Lance said.

"Long story a little shorter. I queried a random ten names on the list from file three. All were people who were either in detention or who had officially been deported. I did another ten—same thing. Figured I better be careful about running all seven thousand names through, but my guess is that we will find them all on that list. So it seems like this has a lot to do with immigration, odd as that sounds on its face since we are talking about what a health system is doing."

"Strange indeed," noted Johnny. "And some fantastic research, Lance."

"One more thing. When I shared this with Irv, he asked me to query 'Rodrigo Lopez.' Not to be found in the federal immigration hotlist. I also checked the other two names that had blanks in the 'Disposition' column. Same thing—no record of deportation or detention. Seems like more than coincidence, doesn't it? I was tempted to search the other names on the full file with blank dispositions, but thought it might attract too much attention. But I certainly could if you think it is something we should do."

"How many people are we talking about?" Johnny was more serious in tone than his usual friendly manner. All three of the men were feeling that what they were uncovering was growing in importance by the hour.

"I did a fast review of the file one records—it was a lot of files, so I may not have the exact number. I think it is thirty-seven—thirty-seven names on the full client list where there is no disposition code. I don't know if that is good or bad."

The three digested the grave consequences of what this new information was telling them. It was Irv that finally gave voice to what they were each thinking. "The most likely conclusion is that HealthMost is somehow involved in helping immigration identify and deport people in this country. That is shocking, since it would mean they are doing this to people who come to them for health care. I have barely been able to get my brain around this in the few hours I've been thinking about what Lance found."

Johnny shook his head, breathed in deeply, and felt Irv's pain. He looked out the window of the office, taking in the import of what they had found. It was his turn to give voice to what each of them were thinking. "It is shocking, but the one advantage I have over you is that I've been watching this immigration fever up close and personal for the last decade. That this administration will do all it can to throw people of color out of this nation is no surprise to me. They have even made mention at some of our secure briefings of special programs they are deploying to identify illegals and remove them from our country. They claim national security concerns whenever we press them for details. Maybe, just maybe, the goings-on with HealthMost are part of that."

"That would be politically explosive even if it is not technically illegal, wouldn't it?" asked Irv.

"Yes and no," said Lance. "They have been doing such outrageous things for so long that one more thing on this list is not going to move any political needles, even if it was completely illegal. They've been setting such new norms around these things. It might be some greater embarrassment to HealthMost, but they seem to be a pretty shameless bunch."

"I think Lance is right about both points," noted Johnny. "I will do some quiet digging on the immigration side and try to get a read on how explosive all of this might be and what we might do with it, when. I do think we've got something big and horrible to expose, but we have to be thoughtful on how to do that in this environment. And toward what end."

Irv felt a lot of air go out of the room. He had been on the track of this investigation for two months now. It felt like a big and messy thing from day one, and had only gotten smarmier with his every step. What he thought might be an isolated abuse by one hospital now seemed to be a program run by a major national health system, in contract with the federal government. There appeared to be some type of conspiracy to keep this a secret. And now he was hearing two people he trusted telling him that it might not be enough to do much about it. It was enough to make most optimists see the worst.

"God, I really hope that is not the case," sighed Irv. "You know best what to do on that front. I do have to say that we can't bury the lead on this story yet, though. Rodrigo Lopez is dead, that I can assure you. He is part of this system of whatever it is. Someone linked to the federal government now has his body, but he is still missing in action from your special immigration record system. Two other people seen at Westside are similarly missing. And another thirty-four from across the nation. Maybe figuring out what happened to them is really what we have to do."

It was more stream-of-consciousness pouring out from Irv than anything he had thought through in length. When he said it, its wisdom stuck like Velveeta on macaroni. Johnny and Lance looked at each other and frowned. True that, each said to themselves in silence.

Chapter Sixty-Two

Irv Finds a Leadership Job in Public Health

Irv had spent almost seven years meandering through various jobs within the health care system in Washington State. It had been an interesting and useful journey, but he was now intent on finding the right and very important next stop in his career's journey.

He was convinced that it was time to take a forceful step—to a position that would allow him to push major health system reform. His short-term explorations had been enjoyable, and he had contributed to society at each of these stops. But none had done much to address the bigger problems with the health care system. His personal calling was to do that. *Now*, he thought, *is the time for that.*

But where? There were jobs to be had, but few would offer much in the way of an opportunity to influence big change. He sought counsel from others to help him find the right position. He had met many leaders in health care over the past decade and now searched them out for advice, or better yet, leads.

This networking revealed that a major issue to his quest was geography. There were opportunities across the nation, but a much smaller set in the Seattle area, which had become a preferred destination for young professionals. Irv concluded that leaving Seattle would endanger his future with Mary Beth, who was now settling into her career locally. He decided against a move, for now, leaving limited options.

Positions of major influence were few in the Seattle area. There was little turnover, and even if such positions opened up, his background was unlikely to make him a natural fit. He needed to find a unique opportunity. Advisors suggested he find someone who could create a new position just for him. His skills were unique, and if monetary compensation was not his driving interest, there were local leaders who might be willing to take a chance on him.

It sounded good in concept, but was harder in execution. An additional pressure point was that he was told he must choose carefully. Leaders understood his rationale for moving across the system over the past decade, but told him that his short stays at jobs made him look unstable and unwilling to commit. One more move of short duration might forever cast him as unreliable or even flaky. It would be hard to lead change with that reputation, so he better stay put wherever he landed for a number of years.

He interviewed for several positions over the next few months and was offered a couple of jobs. These were more in line with what he had been doing than what he wanted or needed now—short-term projects rather than a leadership position. He turned them down.

By now, he had left his last job. It gave him a lot more time to look for the right job, though it required him to live off of Mary Beth's earnings. The plan was for him to be patient finding the right job, and she was willing to keep supporting him. The universe would find him when it was ready, much like the other great things that had happened in his life. Even so, he was getting restless when he was still unemployed six months later.

One morning he read in the newspaper that the director of the Seattle-King County Public Health Department had resigned, and a new director had been recruited to take his place. He was coming from Los Angeles, and his background was intriguing—a physician and private philanthropist who had a record of trying to bring major change to the health care system.

Irv decided to make meeting the new director, Torrey Cain, a priority. Realizing that Cain would be very busy once he moved north, Irv requested a meeting with him in Los Angeles. Irv had plenty of time available for a road trip. An appointment was set and Irv drove down to California for the meeting.

The two hit it off immediately. It was reminiscent of his chance meeting with Johnny so many years ago, also in California. Dr. Torrey Cain shared Irv's passion for change in the American health care system.

The Theory of Irv

An African American, he had grown up in Watts, decidedly on the wrong side of the tracks. He had beaten the odds and become a success, attending medical school and then practicing as an emergency room physician. He liked patient care, the adrenaline rush of being an emergency room doc, and giving back to his community as he worked in a hospital on the edge of his original Watts neighborhood.

He also had a hankering to get involved in bigger change possibilities. As he told Irv, "I got tiring of patching people up every day in the emergency room—and then seeing them all over again just a few weeks later."

He got involved in the local medical society and the State Medical Association, and this opened new possibilities for his career. He got a doctorate in Public Health from UCLA and became the chief health officer for Los Angeles County.

His most recent position was as chief strategy officer for a conversion foundation in Los Angeles. A not-for-profit hospital had sold off to a for-profit chain, and $100 million in assets were invested into this foundation as part of the deal, to improve health in California. Most of the work of the foundation was through grants, and Torrey learned much about change process and grant making.

After five years at this, he was ready for his next move, where he could help stimulate bigger health system change. The Seattle-King County public health job looked to be just that to him.

Torrey found Irv's take on the Seattle health care and government scene enormously helpful. He could see that the two of them shared a passion for big change. They also had complementary experiences and talents. Torrey needed allies in his new job, so when Irv intimated he was looking for his next position, Torrey was soon asking whether he would work with him.

"Doing what?" asked Irv.

"I don't know exactly," said Torrey. "Let's create something that will build a real change agenda in the public health department and the local health care community."

They kicked the tires on how they might do that for the rest of their meeting and found that wasn't near enough time to do the topic justice. Torrey cancelled a dinner event so they could continue the conversation into the evening. They talked well into the night, and Irv slept on Torrey's couch rather than going back to his hotel room.

Over breakfast the next morning at Torrey's house, they agreed Irv would go to work for Torrey. They weren't exactly sure of the position. Torrey asked Irv to think more about this and propose something.

They continued their dialogue by the occasional phone call and regular email. Irv suggested he become an assistant director for policy at the Health Department. He would report to the director and manage a portfolio of change projects for him. Irv included a set of potential projects—a collaborative healthy communities planning project, a children's health program seeking to build early learning into a health coverage agenda, an oral health project, and a prescription drug assistance program.

Torrey's counter proposal was that Irv become special assistant to the director. He wanted Irv to have independence from the traditional line authorities within the public health department, which would allow him to be more aggressive in leading and managing change projects. He would be less likely to get distracted by the shorter term political priorities that Torrey would have to spend much of his time on. Irv accepted and started the week after Torrey arrived in Seattle.

He and Torrey were now in partnership as major change agents in the greater Seattle region. Irv's role was to function much like he had for the past ten years—leading discrete projects aimed at helping organizations achieve better health or health care. Now he had much greater authority to design not just the projects, but their ultimate goals. It was wonderful to have a boss who was as insistent as Irv that these include the aim of big change in their goals.

Irv and Torrey Cain hit it off like Ben and Jerry. They made their own flavor in their partnership, a different combination of nuts, chocolate, and marshmallow. More importantly, they began to hit home runs out of the park like Babe Ruth.

Their first project was to convene various local stakeholders around creating a vision of a healthy community. Torrey had experience with such efforts from his time at the foundation, and Irv had studied these as part of a past work project.

Many public health districts had projects working within their local community to improve health, and some did this with the involvement of the medical community. Torrey and Irv did this in partnership by designing their approach consonant with the Healthy Communities movement.

This movement began in the 1990s, somewhat quietly but consistently beginning to shape change in the health system. At a basic level, Healthy Communities was a health system change philosophy that tried to grow leadership for change at the local level by building relationships and practices that would provide enduring action to major health issues faced by people and communities. Its guidebook was a prescription known as the "Seven Patterns of a Healthy Community."

Critically different from other efforts, Healthy Communities was not something to be imposed from above, but rather a true homegrown grassroots effort. Government was a vital partner in many efforts, but could not be a controlling force. Torrey and Irv consulted with some of the leaders of the movement and devised an approach that would allow them to stimulate a local coalition in a shared leadership model. They convened a group of key leaders across the greater Seattle region willing to try this effort.

Early on, the group decided that leadership projects would be essential to building trust and progress. Only then would they be able to really attack systemic problems.

The group decided to address the social determinants of health and invest in housing as a means to promote health. The high and growing cost of housing was a major problem across the region, and they promoted and funded alternative arrangements that would provide preventive health commitments as part of the package. Their success paved the way for the coalition to tackle other issues.

One major endeavor was to assure that all children in the county had health coverage. This involved not just identifying health coverage options, but working with diverse communities across the region. Many new immigrants were unaware or distrusting of private coverage options, and the coalition built a network of allies within these communities. Importantly, the health design of the effort did not end with providing coverage in the event families or individuals needed care. Rather, it was to actively promote health. So, for example, childhood immunizations and other well care treatment protocols were incorporated in the grassroots outreach, and the region attained one of the highest levels of compliance with CDC recommendations in the entire nation.

Next up was an oral health project working with dental organizations in the region. Again, it was not just a matter of connecting people with services, but trying to break down the fragmentation and barriers attendant to oral health. In this case, it involved changing the approach of insurers and the medical care system toward oral health. The body was connected to the mouth, and there was no good reason to isolate these systems. Medical outcomes improved as a result of breaking down these barriers.

This became the pattern of engagement for Torrey and Irv for much of the next three years—working through the Healthy Communities Coalition to identify practical projects that would benefit the health of the community while also yanking down the systemic barriers of the overall health care system.

As time went on, they used their social capital to take on even bigger systemic problems. Trust, within the coalition and with the public, was growing, and they could act more aggressively as a byproduct of each successful project.

Irv had found his dream job. Much of the real leadership that made these projects work came from him. It was by no means a solo effort—Irv's leadership model was to engage their broad coalition on the projects. Torrey was the vital political figure who made it all possible by keeping the work one step removed from opportunistic politicians, while Irv brought the technical, professional, and creative design capacity needed to make the projects a success.

Their portfolio grew, as did their reputations. Torrey and Irv had built a national model for how to use a public health department as a Healthy Communities leadership platform for big health system change. They were regularly invited to speak at public health conferences across the nation, which built even more capacity for Torrey and Irv to leverage change. The possibilities seemed endless.

Nearing the end of their third year of doing so, they decided to take an even bigger bite at the apple of system reform. They were confident, and this made risks seem less ominous. Besides, it was worth it, they said. If they knew how this one would play out, they might have decided otherwise.

Chapter Sixty-Three

Johnny's Friends Give Him Health Care Policy Guidance

Johnny's staff booked the Edgewater Hotel in downtown Seattle for his meeting on President's Day 1995. The story was that the Beatles had once stayed there and taken up the hotel on its advertising claim that one could fish out of the windows of one's room. The Edgewater was on a dock jutting out into Elliott Bay and Puget Sound. Johnny thought about getting a fishing rod and giving it a go, but figured he didn't have enough time.

No, his friends would be here soon enough—Irv, Mary Beth, Nancy, and her dad Chris. Johnny had flown west with Dr. Jones, and they had a long conversation on the plane. He had gone to stay with Nancy at her house for the weekend, while Johnny went to his home outside of Duvall to see Reena and the kids.

The meeting was labeled "Health Reform Debrief" on a sheet of paper taped to the door. That was not its best description. It was not intended to be looking back at what wasn't, but to provide ideas for how Congressman Gibson could proceed with improving health and healthcare in the wake of the demise of comprehensive health reform during the Clinton presidency.

The others soon arrived, and after hugs among longtime friends and a bit of catch-up on life stories, they settled into the comfortable chairs in the hotel suite. They didn't need a formal conference room for this conversation—it was more important to be comfortable. They had a view of the water and the Olympic Mountains across Puget Sound on this partly clear day, and that helped them ease their minds into the job at hand.

Mary Beth had agreed to be their facilitator. She had developed a great talent for leading group dialogues in the not-for-profit world through her part-time work for Nancy. The firm had developed a reputation for creative group processes across the region, and Mary Beth became their resident expert. She had asked for a grease board so they could draw pictures or otherwise document their progress.

She asked Johnny to begin by outlining what he was looking for out of today's meeting. He did so, essentially reciting the recent telephone call with Irv. The good news was that his depression was over. Now he was energized to figure out what he could do next, but he remained at sea over what this should be.

Mary Beth had asked Johnny to come to the meeting with his three most important questions about this and now asked him to share the first of them.

Number one had to do with ClintonCare, and Johnny directed it primarily to Chris Jones. "So much of this legislation was about how to organize and provide health coverage to Americans. The complexity of their model of competing health plans was part of what slowed down the change process. Since, many have questioned whether we would have been better served by advancing a single payor plan with the government as the organizer of this care, not competing insurance companies. But my first question is not this, but whether this should be the focus of what I try to do to improve health and health care in the United States?"

"Great question, Johnny." Chris Jones spoke up quickly. He was a relative newcomer to the group, but was already feeling comfortable with them. "The answer is yes and no."

"Okay," said Johnny. "Now that we have settled that, let's bring in lunch." The group laughed.

Chris chuckled with them. "Let me explain. On the one hand, the need to determine how we provide health coverage to all Americans is a moral and design imperative to fixing the American health care system. So many Americans are left out, especially when they are most in need. So, we do have to fix it for those reasons. But it is my view that even if you don't believe in this moral imperative, as a matter of system design, we won't be able to fully rationalize a new health system without dealing with its consequences. So much time and energy and focus go into this problem, and it will stop our ability to achieve big reform until we have chosen and implemented a method to make sure virtually all Americans have some form of minimal health coverage for at least catastrophic health care needs.

"The other problem with this is that this question ends up taking so much of our energy to solve, and the ideology and money around doing so are where much of the political conflict over the means to this end gets energized. This is why both ClintonCare and the Washington State legislation here ended up with these complicated proposals for using private competition among health plans as the way to provide coverage—it was an attempt to build a coalition of interests to support a hybrid answer. At the end of the day, many interest groups and the Republicans wouldn't bite, and they used this to punish Democrats who had pushed this answer. That is what will take a while to settle out now. Republicans have no ideas for legitimately reforming health care, so we will need the Democrats to get back into the conversation to trigger the next movement for real reform. We know that won't be for at least two years, maybe much longer. All to say that focusing some attention on the core question is important in the months and years to come, but focusing on this would mean that failure is the only option for some time.

"The good news, on the other hand, is that this is probably not the most important issue in, as you framed it, Congressman, figuring out how to improve health and health care in America. We just need to clarify this a little bit by saying that the real objective of our pursuits is to create health for the American people. Health care is an important thing, but it is merely a means to a bigger end. Much of our health care policy, especially since the end of WWII, has been about just creating more health care though. And in one sense, the search for the best way to cover everybody is also about finding a way to get people more health care."

Chris stopped to assess whether the group was keeping up with his argument. So far so good. "What I am suggesting is that our real objective is to find ways to create and promote health for the American people. There are ways to do this outside of health coverage, and they are arguably far more important than coverage in the bigger policy sense."

"What are those then?" asked Johnny.

"The usual lingo for these is the social determinants of health. That is, medical care only contributes somewhere between eight and ten percent to producing health for people, while the rest of the health impact pie consists of issues like education, housing, what we eat, and our own behaviors as people. As the cost of health care has risen dramatically, it has squeezed our financial ability to deal with many of these. Education is a great example of that at the state level. So, more medical care is probably our least effective investment and an opportunity cost as to the other choices we haven't made."

Irv was tracking the professor's logic and chimed in. "So you are saying that Johnny should find ways to improve these other things now, while waiting for the political circumstances to shift on the health coverage question?"

"Exactly," said Chris.

As the group began to accept they had made a major discovery already, Nancy spoke up. "Hold on, Dad. I am a little confused. From the time I was a little girl, you and Granddad were harping about the Committee on the Cost of Medical Care that he worked on in the 1920s. I remember the five recommendations like the Pledge of Allegiance—Medical Service through Organized Groups and Costs Managed on a Group Basis were the two bellwethers you and he would emphasize. They don't sound like the social determinants of health to me. Are you now saying that the committee got it wrong and that these are not the blueprints for fixing the system? You would have washed my mouth out with soap if I had said that in my younger years!"

"Pops would be so pleased that you raise this, Nancy. And yes, we would have. No, I am not saying that they had it wrong. A couple of design things first. Managing costs on a group basis was what they were saying needed to be done about the health coverage issue. They were saying, as I was earlier, that there had to be some social form of protection for Americans, though they were leaving out the insistence that it be insurance in form. Organized groups of practice were in large part trying to make the product of health care better so we can afford to do this. Remember, while costs were far lower then, their perception was that the cost of medical care was a national crisis.

"Remember, there were other recommendations too," Chris continued. "One was to strengthen public health services, and another was to coordinate what was done at the state and local level. These included, in their thinking, an important focus on things outside of medical care that would produce health—the social determinants. They saw these under the domain of what they described as public health and thought they'd best be managed locally, not by the federal government. There was not as much pushback on these recommendations, but they are critical to those of us who saw the whole report as the blueprint for the future.

"It is also fair to say that there was so much more to be learned as time moved on. Back in the 1920s, the primary focus was on finding ways to bring a series of new medical care discoveries and possibilities to the American people without breaking the bank. If they had the knowledge of things we've discovered since, I have no doubt that their recommendations might have different labels and even perhaps some additions. Like the social determinants of health."

"So is it really as simple as Johnny focusing on these social determinants and trying to do something about them?" Irv thought it too simplistic an answer.

Johnny confirmed Irv's thinking. "It doesn't sound so easy to me. I wouldn't know what to do with this answer. I mean, it makes sense; it just doesn't provide me much practical direction."

"I agree completely," said Chris. "My argument was only to get us to understand the greater forces at play as we try to figure out what to do. Finding exactly what to do is the greater challenge, I think, and why we need more dialogue to figure this out."

Mary Beth injected herself so she could manage their time as a group. "So, if we are all in agreement with the basic argument presented by Chris, we can move on to exactly this practical question. Are we all good with this?" She looked around the room, and all nodded or voiced their assent. "Okay then. That seems like progress. Not that this next question seems any easier. Johnny, does moving on to this fit with the other questions you prepared for our meeting?"

Johnny looked at Mary Beth and the group. "Sure enough. I would say my other two questions were practically asking what the heck should I be trying to advance in my health or health care agenda!"

Mary Beth shifted her gaze toward Chris again. "Got any ideas on how to help us deal with this question? It sounds like you have some experience with it."

Chris had thought long and hard about this question and was ready with his answer. "I have worked with a number of groups on this type of thinking. There have been many takes on it, some loaded by the perspective of who they are and what they represent, at least in the political world. But one useful example comes from a health foundation that was approaching this from a broad and, as much as possible, unbiased point of view."

The group looked ready to hear about this.

"To keep it simple, they spent several days in a retreat probing this question so they could build a template for what they would do with their resources toward this end. They summarized it with six action areas. They were trying to boil down the immense complexity into six practical realms of action by them and others.

"They framed the action areas as follows: Increasing Value in Health Care Services; Investing in Prevention; Avoiding Addictions; Protecting Against Injury and Disease; Promoting Community Health; and Taking Personal Responsibility for Health. Underneath, they had action plans and approaches for practically advancing these topics through their work."

"Are you suggesting that I try to do all these things? It sure seems like a lot," said Johnny.

"Not at all, Congressman. I am suggesting we spend some time trying to find whatever area—these or others we might come up with—floats your boat, and see what practical opportunities we can build through your role in Congress. Experience is that these things are so hard to do that it is critical to find passion on the part of the leader of the effort for it. That is you."

It was making sense to all of them, concluded Mary Beth. "Let's spend some time settling on one or more of these areas or another, and then seeing if we can find some discrete things that really float Johnny's boat. Sound like a plan?"

Again, a resounding yes came from the group members. Chris raised his hand though.

"I thought this was your idea, Chris?"

"No, I am not questioning your conclusion. All I wanted to say was that we should keep in mind that at some point, I hope in the not too distant future, we might need to figure out how to advance a full set of thoughts about this. What I mean is that comprehensive health care reform will be back on the political agenda again, and I really hope we can make sure that issues like these are part of what comes next . . . something far more relevant to the big question than what ClintonCare included. Something really in line with the bigger thinking of the Committee on the Cost of Medical Care."

He could see that there were no dissenters in the room, which made him feel good. Pops would have washed his mouth out with soap if he hadn't made this statement.

Chapter Sixty-Four

Irv Plans to Go Undercover

"There has to be another way." Johnny loudly voiced his disagreement to Irv and his Chief of Staff Lance Givens, who were sitting across from him in his congressional office, only a few feet from him on the other side of his large walnut desk. His objection was so loud, they leaned back from his verbal blast, more from surprise than force.

"I appreciate your concern, Johnny. I really do. But I cannot think of any other way to find what we need to know about those missing patients. If we go to anyone in the federal government, there is a pretty big chance that whatever we have uncovered will quickly disappear from public record. Even if we used the whistleblower statutes for the allegations, like Lance suggested. There is little doubt that this would be a huge embarrassment for anyone in power, and they would hide behind immigration laws or patient privacy or something to make sure that this never sees the night of day." Irv was trying to convince Johnny, and himself.

"What about a media play?" asked Johnny.

"Sure, there will be some attention to what is at best a messy and questionable situation. The media might even catch someone lying in a cover-up. That might even lead to some heads rolling, though probably underlings who will be told to take the hit in exchange for some payoff. Whatever the media might do will also surely let it be known to the perpetrators that someone is on to them and it is time to get rid of any evidence. I bet the trail would get very cold if media attention took—if it ever did." Irv had been working through this alternative in his mind and could not see how it would get them much further. Media strategies had disappointed him before.

The Theory of Irv

"I agree," added Lance, "we can probably stop whatever it is from happening anymore, but I doubt it will get us closer to understanding what happened to the thirty-seven patients. I do think that we can make some hay over the arrangement with HealthMost here on Capitol Hill. It stinks to high heaven, and we can play to the public embarrassment. The shock value will be high if we do it right. Even for that play, though, we need to know much more than we do now—most of our case is speculative and will be spun to fit the usual narratives. Headlines will quickly suck these into the usual blather on immigration and health care. My guess is we have to clearly expose what is happening with the thirty-seven patients to take this anywhere—presuming it is something bad and that we have some idea what it is. We've got to get inside, and quietly so we can control and leverage the wrongdoing."

"Isn't there someone else who can do it?" Johnny continued to probe for alternatives.

"What, are you going to do it? Just imagine, a sitting United States Senator going undercover, pretending to be a sick Hispanic patient seeking care at a HealthMost hospital emergency room. A lily-white senator at that. No, I don't think you can do it. I think it has to be one of the three of us. I am the only one who speaks any Spanish, right? And the one who knows how health care and hospitals work." Irv had convinced himself he should ride point.

"All right, all right. It has to be you . . . there is no other way. But I don't have to like it, and pardon me if I worry about you. I imagine we can get you back in the country, eventually, if you are deported. But we don't have any idea of what happened to these thirty-seven patients. It could be even more dangerous than that."

Irv nodded. He might have convinced himself this was the right plan, but he was concerned for his personal safety. "Yes, I do know that. I will be counting on the two of you to watch out for me."

"Where would you go in?" asked Lance. "Phoenix?"

"No, I spent too much time in the Westside Medical Center emergency room. They might remember me there. I don't see any advantage in going to their tertiary hospital downtown either. My thought is to go in at a smaller hospital in a smaller city. HealthMost has a hospital on the south side of Albuquerque. I was born in Albuquerque and lived there till college, so I know a bit about the community and how to blend in. That is where I go in."

"Makes sense. As much as any of this makes sense." Johnny remained concerned over how this industrial espionage might turn out for his friend. "Let's go through the plan in detail. I want to know exactly what you are planning."

The three men spent the rest of the evening outlining just how Irv Tinsley would become an illegal from Panama presenting at an emergency room in New Mexico in cardiac distress, with underlying severe symptoms and an insurance card with HealthMost/ALI. It wouldn't be easy.

Chapter Sixty-Five

A Fissure Grows Between Irv and Mary Beth

Irv and Mary Beth thought they had found their groove. They had th separate careers, both on the upswing, and they kept them in balanc with their togetherness, still living in the small Wallingford home they had moved to over a decade ago.

Irv's was influencing big change in the health care system after almost a decade of job hopping. He had become the special assistant to the director of Public Health in Seattle and King County, and he and his boss, Torrey Cain, were bringing major health system change to the region. Director Cain provided the power base to get the projects on the coalition agenda and Irv the creativity and management expertise required to move them forward. It was a major time commitment, but Irv was having the time of his professional life.

Mary Beth was still working at the bakery. She now only worked a few shifts as a waitress and spent most of her time with the owners managing the bakery. They found she had a great aptitude for business and organization, and exploited her talents when they could. For her part, Mary Beth was happy to get the experience and found great joy when she was able to apply her growing business and leadership knowledge to the food bank project under the bakery's not-for-profit wing.

Mary Beth's time was also occupied with courses at the local community college. She was adding to her knowledge in such fields as accounting, logistics management, and computers, and had a couple of years' worth of courses left between her and a college degree. She knew this credential would be important in order to advance her career and thought there was plenty of time to get the degree. She would be patient.

nce in a while, it irked her that her career was moving forward, while Irv was able to rapidly advance his. She wasn't so much ed with him; it was more that society expected she would be the to make sacrifices around career for the good of the family.

This was the first fissure that began to grow between them—nothing that couldn't be resolved in normal circumstances. They remained in e and faithful to one another, and cracks that might destroy other lationships seemed to be a very small matter to them.

It was health, and the health care system, that stretched the gap into a chasm. Six months after Irv started his new job at the public health department, Mary Beth shared that a routine mammogram spotted a lump in her breast. A biopsy was scheduled for later that month. It was near the Christmas holiday when she got the test done. It was New Year's Eve when she learned that it was breast cancer.

It rocked their world. For Mary Beth it was a first. She had been a model of health during her life. Her only experience with personal loss had been the result of sudden events—a heart attack had taken her dad and an automobile accident one of her childhood friends. Now she had within her something that she couldn't understand—her own cells warring against her and threatening to take over and, maybe, kill her. Reading about the disease didn't help her grasp what was going on, intellectually or emotionally.

Nor did her interactions with the health care system provide much clarity. Her primary care physician was comforting and generally helped make her feel better about what was to happen. Then she was referred to an oncologist. Further testing led to a decision to treat through a combination of surgery and chemotherapy.

Her partial mastectomy turned into an uncoordinated trip through the health care system. She found the pre-surgery instructions and explanations of what was to come far off from the actual experience. The surgery itself was hard but, in its isolated episode, manageable enough. She was sedated and woke to find herself in the recovery room.

Then she was shipped off to a hospital ward. She was to be up and around within twenty-four hours, they said. It ended up being three days because of staffing problems at the hospital. When she got home, she was ready to move on, but that turned out to be a pipe dream—she had contracted a urinary tract infection, likely from the catheter inserted for surgery. She went from feeling uncomfortable to miserable within a day and found herself back in the hospital for a week, dosed with heavy antibiotics. There were a lot of excuses about why this happened. As near as she could tell, the infection was related to inadequate training of a new nurse in the recovery room.

No one apologized about any of this. Mary Beth was happy to go home when she got better enough, realizing that a urinary tract infection was a life-threatening diagnosis in its own right. Her comfort was short-lived, as the follow-up with her surgeon showed that the margins of the cancer excision were not complete. He recommended further surgery, and soon. The immediacy of another surgery and hospital stay was bad enough; far worse was his recommendation to do a full mastectomy and to remove both breasts.

Mary Beth tried to better understand her options for care, but found little information accessible to the average human being. It seemed the only choice was to follow the recommendation of the surgeon. The surgery was scheduled and went as well as such surgeries can go. There were no more infections or other iatrogenic maladies. But less than three months after going to the doctor for a routine physical, she found herself home reflecting on life as a woman without breasts and about to start a regimen of chemotherapy, a treatment that was sure to be difficult and would add hair to her list of lost body parts.

Irv was mostly a good partner to Mary Beth in this bad trip. He knew a lot about the health care system and did all he could to make her journey a better one. He took notes in meetings, knowing she would never remember details of these conversations. He regularly checked her ID bands and treatment plans—he knew simple errors led to many horrible health care outcomes. He hand delivered test results to different offices, even as it shocked him to see how primitive the hospital's "advanced" electronic medical records systems actually were—they couldn't even share a simple CT scan among physician offices. He tried to manage the bills and financial issues associated with her care, though this was something that came months after treatment and continued for years as bills came at them for seemingly forever.

It was hard on him too. It was harder than Mary Beth could understand, as she understandably had her own ghosts to deal with then. For Irv, it was déjà vu all over again going back to his mom's death: the diagnosis, the treatment, and the screw-ups. And ultimately he would experience the suffering and then loss of the person at the center of his life. Mary Beth, and to some extent, Johnny, were the only people that he had fully opened to other than his mom, afraid as he was to be so vulnerable and hurt again. He had opened the gates, and now the health care infidels were moving in for the kill again.

He didn't share his deeper pessimistic thoughts with Mary Beth. She had enough to deal with, and he would soldier up and do his duty. He did, but every night cried himself to sleep, and when he did drift off, it was only to nightmares of fading faces and funerals.

Johnny was doing his thing in DC and was maybe the only shoulder that Irv had to help him confront his ghosts. But there was only so much even he could do given the distance and continuous nature of the tortuous path. Johnny came out to see him and Mary Beth in late February for a few days, and Irv started to feel more optimistic. Johnny's departure a few days later revealed it to be a temporary state of mind.

A complicating factor was the nature of the disease and the support circles that formed around it for Mary Beth. Her oncologist connected Mary Beth to a patient support group, and she found the peer support helpful, not that there were any great answers to be found.

Irv was invited to attend these sessions with her. For breast cancer, these groups were mostly "women's groups" and he felt unwelcome. Few of the women would even look at him, even on the rare occasions when he spoke up. At some level he understood—many of these women's experiences, as patients and in their lives, were made worse by living in a man's world. They applied this bitterness toward him and it was unsettling.

He felt even more alone after these sessions, even as he saw how much good they did for Mary Beth. The treatment was going well now, though Mary Beth had lost all of her hair and was otherwise beaten to shit by the side effects of chemotherapy. Irv found excuses not to attend the peer group meetings; even when he drove her to them, he just waited in the car. Irv retreated more and more to his job as his safety zone.

The Theory of Irv

It was not as if the cancer destroyed their relationship. They were still together and coping together. But it had blown a chunk of their connection away, through no fault of either. It was just a consequence of life's tragedies, with a little salt on the wound courtesy of the health care system.

They might have made it through mostly intact as a couple, if not for one last health care matter. One evening, Mary Beth shared with Irv that she was pregnant. It was nothing they had planned on, nor had they ever decided whether they did or didn't want children. They would have to figure it out now.

Mary Beth was torn. She hadn't really planned on kids, after spending so much of her younger life rejecting the wife and kids future pushed by her parents. That didn't mean she wouldn't want one, or even some. She figured there was more time before they had to decide and was not expecting the decision to come wrapped in a blanket of cancer.

Irv was also of a mixed mind. He had some yearnings to be a dad, but the Theory of Irv didn't say anything about fatherhood. He figured they would have to cross this bridge at some point, but he also thought they had a few more years to do so.

Whatever their desires were about becoming parents, things got more confusing from Mary Beth's cancer treatment. She was about to begin the next several rounds of chemotherapy, including new doses that were showing great promise in actually curing the malady. Her oncologist said that there were risks associated with these treatments, especially for a fetus. It shocked her to hear of the birth defects linked to early clinical trials.

Her instinct was to have the baby, but she could not reconcile it with the risks—not to her, but the baby. And to Irv. She knew that her medical journey had been tough on Irv in its own way, and she thought the prospect of a damaged baby might further hurt him, and them.

Irv was scared of the risks too, for the baby, for Mary Beth, and yes, for himself. But he had also come around to believing that fate was telling them they should be parents. It was not his decision to make, though, he thought. He must support Mary Beth and whatever she chose, even if he did not agree with her conclusion, and was hesitant to share his real thoughts with her.

She finally decided on an abortion. He accompanied her to the procedure and held her hand through most of it. They cried and hugged and talked about trying again. He never told her what he really thought, holding this inside. The crack between them grew some more.

For Mary Beth, life just got worse. The owner of the bakery retired, selling off to a new owner. One of the reasons to get out was the cost of health care. The health insurance coverage for the bakery was already expensive because they were individually rated, and now they would be absorbing the cost of Mary Beth's cancer care. The slim profit of the bakery was now a loss.

Mary Beth felt guilty that her illness had destroyed the business model for the bakery. She also had to figure out what it meant for her own career. She was momentarily hopeful when the new owners decided to focus on the bakery business and spin off the not-for-profit food bank. A new board was created, and they would need to recruit an executive director. Mary Beth, who had essentially created and successfully managed this venture for years, wasn't even qualified to apply for the job because she didn't have an undergraduate degree.

She decided that she had to leave the bakery. She wanted to be an executive director of a not-for-profit organization, for a cause she could believe in. Once she got a clean bill of health, felt better, and had regrown a small smock of hair, she would search for her next job.

To her dismay, she found no opportunities in the Seattle area to become a not-for-profit social service leader. It didn't matter that she had been doing this for much of the past decade, without the title. Over that time, these roles had grown in stature, with a professionalization that said one needed an advanced degree to be the leader of a not-for-profit organization—usually master's level preparation or its equivalent, and most certainly, an undergraduate degree.

It now angered Mary Beth that her missing degree had become a major barrier for her to move on. She could do the work, and very well. She could have easily gotten her degree if she made it a priority over the past decade, but had instead dabbled while helping others build their dreams. It wasn't Irv's fault, but she was jealous of his advanced degree when she didn't even have a college degree. The distance between them kept growing.

She was forced to take a part time job as a waitress, and she also enrolled full time at the community college—she thought it essential now to get an undergraduate degree. It didn't help that she found the courses somewhat useless in helping her understand how to run a not-for-profit. They were teaching how to resolve problems she already had ample experience with, and little to do with how to do so practically. It frustrated her to be going backward in her career.

Mary Beth was regularly scouting for new job opportunities and began to look outside of the Seattle area. Irv was now their breadwinner, and he told her to do whatever she needed to find her way through this. He paid for school and did what he could to be supportive. Privately, he felt them slipping apart and didn't know what to do about it.

Chapter Sixty-Six

2010: Federal Health Reform Happens

The problems of the health care system were mounting, that much was clear as the nation went to vote in the presidential election of November 2008. Doing something about it seemed a remote possibility, as Americans were absorbed in the calamity that was the Great Recession of 2008.

Christopher Jones thought the economic issues were linked to the health care problem. Federal health costs were continuing to balloon, and a new president would need to control health care costs in order to address the major economic issues confronting him or her.

Chris was encouraged that this thinking was flashing among Democratic candidates in the 2008 presidential race, even if it was not being discussed publicly in any great detail. Hillary Clinton, one of these candidates, had been burned by the issue in the early months of her husband's presidency and was hesitant to go all in on the proposition for reform. Another candidate, Senator Barack Obama, spoke only generally about the issue, without making any major commitments.

Quietly though, Chris was pushing their key advisors to understand the importance of dealing with the health care issue. He shared his treatise on health care problems and copies of the Committee on the Cost of Medical Care.

Senator Obama's policy advisors took notice of his arguments and began asking questions. Chris was pleasantly surprised when Senator Obama won the election and made health reform his top domestic priority after economic recovery.

President Obama was willing to use political capital on the issue, and his advisors tried to learn from the mistakes of earlier attempts.

President Obama would be more flexible on the policy answer and instead try to move legislation through politically. Votes, not expert design, would define the policy play so that he might build a proposal with bipartisan support. If even a few Republicans would sign on, then the use of health care reform as a political weapon might temper.

Doing so opened the door to considering a conservative proposal for fixing health care. One of the central features of the Obama reform package was to provide health care coverage to all Americans through different mechanisms, rather than creating one government solution to all circumstances—the great fear of those on the right.

Medicare, Medicaid, employer coverage, union coverage plans, and more would still exist. For those who did not qualify for any of these and needed to get coverage, the Obama plan set up a marketplace of health plan options that Americans could sign up for. Plans for these exchanges had minimal standards but also had flexibility in how they shaped their benefit packages.

Americans would be required to have health coverage and would face financial penalties if they didn't. They could choose health plans during an annual open enrollment period in late fall.

One of the keys to this approach was that it was based on what happened in Massachusetts under Republican Governor Mitt Romney. Its intellectual source was a paper published by the ultra-conservative Heritage Foundation, and it was expected that some Republicans would support the Obama effort because of this.

It was not to be—not a single Republican member of the House or Senate signed on to the final bill. Still, it passed, since Democrats had sufficient majorities to proceed on their own. Some argued why they were using a conservative policy measure to provide coverage absent any conservative political support. A handful of Democrats continued to argue for a single-payor plan, and many suggested that Congress should at least create a public option plan as one of the choices for Americans within the health care exchanges. This was not to happen, though Congress did expand Medicaid so that many more working poor would have a subsidized means of getting health care coverage.

Republican resistance to the new law was immediate and harsh, and included legal challenges. The overall law was upheld, but one lawsuit ended with the United States Supreme Court ruling that the Medicaid expansions could only advance through state-by-state approvals. The first year rollout of the federal marketplace exchange proved difficult, especially the website and online method of getting signed up. Republicans railed against what they labeled Obamacare.

Christopher was more than a casual observer of the Obamacare policy debate; he had fueled it with various ideas. Citing the CCMC Report and using some of its recommendations as a base of proposals, Chris had presented a ten-point plan for an Obama Health Reform Proposal.

A form of universal coverage was part of this, and he shared his program concerns with a single-payor proposal. He also conveyed his concerns of turning over the American health care system to competing private health plans, absent a strong regulatory framework that would hold them accountable and make it hard to abuse their market position.

He accepted the proposition to create the federal marketplace exchange, but cautioned against making it too complicated. The notion was to allow Americans who can't afford health care coverage to buy some baseline protection at a highly affordable price, not to create a national insurance program or drown it in complexity. That was already a problem.

Rather than an independent public option, he suggested using the Medicare program as a simpler means to provide a public alternative to private health plans, to allow younger people and families to simply buy into the Medicare program at the same actuarial cost as senior citizens, paying for the premiums instead of using payroll deductions. This could be for the hospital portion only, or it could include the other services covered under Part B.

Much of Chris's effort was devoted to other elements of the Obama Health Care Reform proposal. He thought that the universal coverage feature was intended, in large part, to allow policymakers to move on to the even bigger problem of the health system, including cost and quality and outcomes.

Chris was encouraged by the early receptivity of the Obama advisors to address these other health care system issues. Throughout the political effort to craft and pass legislation, they remained receptive to ideas to do more than just address coverage.

The final bill passed by Congress included some important features. For example, the legislation included a major funding commitment to a public health fund through a National Public Health fund. This could be a game-changing investment in public health consistent with the CCMC recommendations.

The president and his advisors understood that cost had become a major problem with American health care, and they were committed to doing something about it. Many of Chris's ideas were about how to do this—based on extensive evidence over the past thirty years that showed what worked and what didn't.

Over the course of the political debate, the need to bring on providers and insurers to secure votes led to a constriction in the cost containment provisions. The proven ideas for how to put a lid on costs were replaced with a series of pilot projects and research by the government into what might work. In essence, they pushed the question of how to force cost reductions on the system to a future time and political fight.

One important element that Chris supported was an investment in hospital quality improvement. The federal government would provide grants to support a collective hospital effort to use data to improve key quality of care problems. This gave funding traction to a movement within the industry and, for the first time, built a power base within the hospital field in support of quality of care.

Despite all of this, Obamacare became a major bone of contention between the two major political parties. Importantly, it sustained through the reelection of President Obama in 2012. Republicans were able to take over Congress, making them hostile to further implementation of the Act. Hundreds of symbolic votes were taken to express their dissatisfaction—not enough to override a filibuster by Democrats in the Senate, and thankfully so to many Republicans, who otherwise would have to think more seriously about replacement policies.

Chris's verdict on the ACA was ultimately mixed. He thought that the access improvements were good and useful. Certainly to those in need, such as low wage adults with major health issues and who did not have health coverage and would now be eligible for Medicaid in many states. That people could buy coverage through the exchanges was generally a good thing, though Chris blanched at the clumsiness and complexity of the federal exchange marketplace.

The Public Health Fund also got more dollars flowing to underfunded state and local health districts, and that was a good thing. Many had been struggling from decades of underfunding at the state level and had been starting to ignore their fundamental role of disease surveillance and detection as they accepted funding for specific projects.

Chris would have preferred that the fund be used to do more than that though. His suggestion was that Congress include the adoption of a simple and quantifiable set of national health goals that would guide the use of the funding and other health decision making by the federal government. The federal government, and whoever it relied on to achieve these goals, could then be held accountable for achieving these goals. Health could be improved in a big way.

The cost control and system design parts of the Act were Chris's major disappointment. Some of the thinking within it was not terrible; it was just far too hesitant in asserting the need for action to slow down and even reduce the national price tag for health care. Indeed, Chris thought it should be the first of the National Health Goals—to hold the national cost of health care within some established limit set by Congress.

Without such bold action, he expected the system to continue to move along as it had for the past ninety years: adapting to new opportunities, but growing consistent with the incentives to do more and to find marketplace opportunities that would enrich many. America needed something far bolder than Obamacare; Chris was sure that at best this law was only a somewhat bigger incremental step toward major health care reform.

The surprise election of Donald Trump to the presidency only made sure that this was the case. Candidate Trump had greatly criticized Obamacare, without specifics. With a Republican Congress in place, one of his early efforts as president was to repeal the Affordable Care Act. The original plan was to announce the repeal on the day of his Inauguration, January 20th.

Supporters of the law rallied, in particular hospitals across America. Their initial effort was to assert that just repealing the law would create a health care crisis. Any such effort must also include a sensible "replacement" of the law.

President Trump and congressional allies were forced to respond to this caution. They took some of the ideas that had been voted on in Congress back when there was no chance they would pass out for a spin.

When viewed through the lens of potential real American health policy, they were found wanting by the health care field, by many consumers of health care, even by many Republicans. Even attempts to repeal the Medicaid expansions, which had been a centerpiece of Republican efforts across the states, was beaten back—millions of Americans in both parties were reaping the benefits of health coverage through Medicaid.

When the House switched back to Democrat control in the 2018 midterm election, the effort to repeal the Affordable Health Care Act was effectively suspended. Health care would, again, be a major issue in the 2020 presidential election—early polls were showing that it was the number one concern of American voters. The outcome of the election would do much to shape the politics and ideology around the next iteration of American health care policy. And Chris was intent on finding a way to shape this policy.

Chapter Sixty-Seven

Mary Beth Moves to Shelton

The petri dish of life had gone bad for Mary Beth. She was attracting bad mojo like honey did flies. Cancer was a horror in its own right, even if she was making a full recovery. Losing her job was almost as bad, especially when it revealed to her that time spent functioning as a business manager got her no credit for being capable of doing the same job elsewhere. On top of everything else, things weren't good at home. Irv was spending most of his time at work in his new job. It made her jealous, even though she hated to admit it. There was no denying she was unhappy.

There were plenty of not-for-profit executive director positions available within greater Seattle, but Mary Beth couldn't even get an interview because she did not have an undergraduate degree. She spread her search to other communities in Western Washington, hoping that things might be more flexible in other parts of the state.

One day she spotted a listing on the electronic job board for the Olympic Peninsula. It sounded right up her alley—a new organization that needed someone to build it from the ground up, like she had with the bakery's food bank venture. Better yet, there were no degree requirements for candidates.

The job had its own limitations, to be sure. To start with, there seemed to be a big question mark in terms of longevity. It sounded like a three-month venture, with a remote chance for an extension. Any continuance would be measured in weeks and months. It didn't pay much. The benefits sucked. Still, it excited Mary Beth that there was something out there that might revitalize her career.

It troubled her—and Irv—that the geography would be problematic. The organization was located in Shelton in southwest Washington just north of Olympia, a roughly two-hour commute from their home in Seattle on a good day—the commute would be much longer when freeway or ferry delays might add an hour or two to the trip. Mary Beth was almost ready to say no to the job, but Irv insisted she apply. She was offered the position.

Their deal that allowed her to accept was that she find a place to stay during the week, and they would get together on weekends, in Seattle, Shelton, or wherever. They would remain a couple and try to manage their conflicting vectors.

Mary Beth was secretly relieved to have some space between her and Irv. As much as she still loved him, things were difficult. Their relationship was complicated, and she didn't fault him—or herself—for anything. But it was clear that their life together was in question until one or more likely both of them got in a better space.

So, Mary Beth took the job. She and Irv moved on. It wasn't technically a split; it was described to friends as a temporary move by Mary Beth for a job that probably would not last all that long. Their times together became more occasional as time ticked on; they were never totally apart, but were not totally together as before.

They knew but never stated out loud to each other that it was also a convenient time to build this distance between them. Mary Beth focused on her new job, hoping things would work out with it and her personal confusion. Irv hoped to rekindle his life with Mary Beth, but wasn't sure it was possible. He also would focus on his career, at least for now.

Chapter Sixty-Eight

Irv Goes Undercover

Irv listened to the loud whine of the ambulance siren as it sped through the streets of south Albuquerque, headed to the emergency room at HealthMost's Promise Hospital, with him on a stretcher in the back.

It had taken a couple of weeks to implement his plan to infiltrate the hospital. The first step was to arrange for more vacation time from his job, and again, Director Welch was all too pleased to get Irv further out of sight and mind. The next step was to fly to Albuquerque, where he would make his final preparations for his journey into the medical care system.

Irv stayed with his father and his stepmother at their house on the east side of Albuquerque. It was his first visit in a couple of years to see his dad. They had drifted apart once his mom had passed. It wasn't a hostile relationship between the two, just distant.

For whatever reason, Irv and his dad found time on this trip for some of their better conversations in recent years. It pleased Irv immensely that this was the case, but it couldn't distract from the reality that was first and foremost a business trip.

His dad's place offered an excellent cover for it. Irv stayed in a garage next to the house that had been converted into separate living quarters. He could stay there as long as he wanted without any observation or concern from anyone. No one other than his dad might wonder about his whereabouts when he went into the hospital, and he told him that he was going camping for a few days. It was as close to a lie as Irv had ever told him, but it was for Dad's protection.

It was partly true—for all he knew, presenting at a HealthMost emergency room as an undocumented immigrant from Panama might just turn into a camping trip. If he somehow went missing for an extended time, Irv gave his father a contact number. Dad wondered why it was the chief of staff for a United States senator, but left well enough alone. It was enough that Irv had visited him and that they had found some good moments. He didn't want to risk any friction that might discourage future trips.

Irv spent two days in the garage apartment assembling supplies. He had bought some used clothing in a Seattle Goodwill store: old jeans, a T-shirt, sweatshirt, and sneakers. In Albuquerque he found a makeup kit that allowed him to darken his skin to a color closer to an itinerant fieldworker. He had let his hair grow out and had not shaved over the past week. When he stopped at a roadside crop stand just south of the Albuquerque airport after landing, he bought some peppers and other vegetables that he put in a paper bag with his used clothes, aromatizing his costume.

The most important part of his preparation was the papers brought with him from Seattle. He went to a physician friend and asked her to help him with a public health investigation. Irv said he couldn't disclose details, but mentioned it had to with allegations of patient dumping. He asked for medical documents that would indicate medical symptoms requiring hospital treatment. His physician friend knew better than to ask questions and agreed to help out.

Irv came to Albuquerque with fake papers that presented him as Roberto Hernandez, an undocumented worker from Panama, with coverage through HealthMost's joint venture with ALI. There were several similar names in the ALI client file, enough that inquiries about his identity should find a match. There wasn't a need to prove the details of his new identity—that was the lot in life for an itinerant worker illegally within the United States. It would be more suspicious if there were details.

What was needed, though, were medical documents that would steer his course of treatment in the right direction. These needed to mimic Rodrigo Lopez's, just in case the treatment protocols at the hospital were diagnosis specific. It was unlikely, he thought, but possible.

Irv explained the conditions he wanted to test. His physician friend confirmed that the medical diagnostics of such a case would indicate a patient in grave condition—a candidate for a major heart attack, or someone who had already had one. He added there was no way that a patient presenting with these symptoms would ever be considered stabilized and ready for discharge—it would be a violation of the law on its face to do anything other than at least admit the patient into a hospital for further evaluation.

Irv asked his friend to put together documents that would mirror this condition. Irv had brought blank, generic medical forms to use as the base of the invented medical record. They also discussed the medications that might trigger indications similar to this condition. He was curious whether there were drugs that might mimic these symptoms and justify a hospital transfer or discharge.

The reason for this question was that Irv wanted to enter the emergency room with more than a trail of medical records—he wanted to present with actual symptoms. The drugs would quicken a pulse to seemingly dangerous levels. His hope was that this symptom, along with the records, the clothing, and sweating profusely in the Albuquerque heat, would lead HealthMost to process him as they did Rodrigo Lopez in Phoenix.

The plan was not without risk. It was hard to fathom that HealthMost might be murdering these patients. Still, Irv assumed that he would be in danger if discovered. The drugs also had dangerous potential side effects beyond elevating his pulse. Nor could he be completely sure of the pharmacologic origins of what he was taking—he got the drugs in the black market through a contact he had made during one of his investigations.

It was now Sunday evening and time to put the plan into action. Irv took a cab from his dad's house to a KOA campground on the south side of the city, paying cash so he did not have any information on him that would identify him as other than Roberto Hernandez. He left his wallet, phone, and anything other than his disguise in Dad's garage. He felt guilty about shading the truth with his dad and even revised the plan so he actually spent part of the night camping.

Arriving at the campground around 4 p.m., Irv changed into his costume behind some bushes, threw away the clothes he was wearing, walked around in the ninety-degree temperature to build up a sweat, popped his pills, and lay on the ground waiting for the pharmaceuticals to kick in. A few hours later, at what he guessed to be around midnight, he walked to the pay phone in the campground. The phone was one of the key features of his choosing this location, and he used it to place a 911 call. He faked observing a man in distress, speaking a mix of Spanish and English, and hung up once he was sure they knew the location. Then he lay back down on the ground near the entrance of the campground and waited for an ambulance.

It came shortly after the call, and now he was on his way to Promise Hospital. He knew that ambulances in Albuquerque were required to take patients to the closest hospital, and from this campground, Promise Hospital was ten miles closer than any other facility. His heart raced as he was placed in the ambulance, from the drugs and his nervousness about stepping into harm's way.

The ambulance pulled up to the Promise Hospital after a fifteen-minute drive. The EMTs wheeled him into the emergency room, and hospital staff immediately assessed him. It was a busy night in the ER, and Irv had chosen the night shift on a Sunday for his trip so that staffing would be at its lowest level. They wouldn't have much time to dig into his case; there was too much going on otherwise. But his symptoms were so severe that it would force them to evaluate and triage him soon.

He pretended not to understand English, making it difficult for the EMTs or hospital staff to get details of what was wrong from him. A practitioner who spoke Spanish tried to interview him, and Irv feigned disorientation. The truth was, he was a little dizzy from the medications and the heat. They took his pulse and noted it was quite high; a blood pressure reading was similarly in a danger zone. Since they couldn't get anything useful from talking to him, they looked for identification and found his fake medical information.

For a couple of hours, he remained on a stretcher in an evaluation room, hooked to a heart monitor. Every so often, ER staff would walk by and glance at the monitor and him, and then move on. There was a big clock on the wall, and Irv could see it was now 3 a.m. Things were slowing down in the ER, and staff were circling back to resolve the cases that had presented earlier in the night, including his.

A person he thought to be a physician entered his stall, with a nurse and a person in street clothes holding a clipboard. "Looks like he has stabilized somewhat; pulse is down a bit but still elevated to dangerous levels. From reviewing the medical notes that he was carrying with him, my bet is that he is in need of a major cardiac intervention. We could contact the cardiologist on call to take a closer look. What do you think, Brenda?" He looked at the woman in a nurse's uniform.

"Normally I would agree," said the nurse, "but Anita tells me that her registration inquiry has flagged this as one of those patients we send out."

Anita, the woman with the clipboard, spoke up. "Yes, he was flagged by the patient registration system. They usually get here in about two to three hours to take away the patient."

"I don't get it," objected the physician. "Shouldn't we be doing more than that? I know I am just out of my residency training, but I thought we were legally required to stabilize patients like this before moving them out?"

"No—we have to do as instructed by administration," insisted the nurse. "They have been clear that we are to call this number and wait for transport, only doing things necessary to make sure that they don't die or get sicker in the emergency room. They said that because the patient is staying within our health system, we are complying with the law. Not sure I really, fully believe that, but I do know that a nurse on the evening shift didn't follow these orders a couple of months ago and was fired the next day. I don't think I want to test this, do you?"

The physician frowned at the nurse. "It's not right. But I've got plenty of other cases to deal with tonight. This sure isn't what I thought I was signing up for when I applied to medical school."

"It's too late anyway, Doctor. I've made the call. The transport team is likely to get here before the cardiologist on call even if we called him now. I'll keep an eye on him and wait for the transport crew to get here." With that, they all left the room, leaving Irv to ponder the conversation and the clock on the wall.

At 5:20, a large man dressed in jeans and a surgical scrub shirt came into the room with Anita, took the medical notes beside the bed, put them under his arms, and wheeled Irv's gurney out to the dock where Irv had entered the ER four hours before. There was another vehicle waiting, more a van than an ambulance. Irv looked at the license plate and tried to memorize it as they picked him up and slid the gurney into the vehicle. They hooked up oxygen and strapped his hands down to the stretcher. Then it was off down the road. Irv could not hear anything up front but a radio playing old country western songs.

They were moving at a fast pace; the sounds of cars and trucks passing in both directions suggested they were on a major freeway. At first Irv was alert to every sound and movement, but seconds became minutes and then a couple of hours of monotonous transit. He couldn't pull himself up to look out the window because of the restraints on his arms attached to the stretcher.

Eventually they pulled off the freeway, traveling on quiet streets for about ten minutes. Then they stopped and the engine turned off. Soon, there were voices outside of the van, but they were too muffled to make out any details. He thought they were speaking Spanish. The back door opened and the attendant who picked him up at the ER jumped in back with him. He poked at Irv, seemingly to see if he was still alive or awake. Irv mumbled to make sure that he knew both were true. The attendant didn't seem to care one way or the other. He crouched over Irv and reached around his head. Irv was confused by this at first, and then realized that the attendant was putting a blindfold over his eyes.

It looked like his research had gotten him what he wanted. But would he live to tell anyone what he had found? He strained to learn more with his ears and nose as his trip continued by wheeled gurney. Out of the van. Wheeled into a building. Rolling down a hallway. A door opening. Into a room. Spanish voices, speaking in hushed tones. Smells—there were others in the room with him. The door closed. They seemed to have just left him here, alone on the stretcher. The blindfold wasn't coming off, and he couldn't move his hands.

Irv waited, eventually drifting off to sleep. Was this a nightmare or real? Either way, he was nervous.

Chapter Sixty-Nine

Mary Beth and the Mason Health Foundation

Mary Beth found a small cottage for rent in Shelton and began her new job at Mason Health Foundation. The day of the move found her with mixed emotions—the excitement of a new job and a chance to get her career on track mixed with the sadness of leaving Irv and Seattle. The demands of her new job quickly pushed aside time to dwell on her choice, and she got to the task at hand.

She was now the executive director of the Mason Health Foundation. From the interview process, she knew it was a newly formed organization with little shape. It was doing nothing other than waiting for someone to arrive and chart a course. That was the attraction—a clean slate of possibility. Mary Beth was literally and metaphorically all in on that proposition.

The roots of the Mason Health Foundation was a transfer of assets from a community clinic that had provided health care across Mason County for twenty-five years. The clinic was a not-for-profit organization, but was sold off as a consequence of a new managed care contracting program instituted by the Washington State Medicaid agency.

Seeking cost savings, the state contracted with a national health plan, agreeing to pay a bulk rate for taking care of Medicaid clients across the state. It was a major reduction in state costs for the program, and in exchange for the cost reduction, the state gave the national health plan great leeway in setting its provider network. Their business plan was to force price reductions on providers by limiting participation in their network. If providers did not agree to contract for greatly reduced prices, they would not be part of the plan's network.

The clinic thought its role as the only primary care option in Mason County gave them leverage to negotiate higher prices, and they were surprised when they were summarily cut out of their plan. Medicaid patients across the southeastern Olympic Peninsula were told they must get their health care from providers under contract in Seattle, Tacoma, or Olympia.

This was the beginning of the end for the clinic. Through an agreement with the federal government, thousands of Medicare patients in Mason County with dual eligibility for Medicaid were also assigned to this plan. The state employee coverage plan soon followed suit. Government made up most of the economy in this region, and there weren't enough local patients left to make up for the financial loss to the clinic from these lost government clients.

The local hospital had figured out how to make things work on the margin, but the physicians in the clinic left town in search of more stable practices. After a year of appealing the government decision and being denied a solution, the clinic gave up. It closed its doors and sold off its assets, which by then was mostly a building in downtown Shelton worth a little over $180,000. By law, the proceeds of its sale had to be transferred to a not-for-profit beneficiary.

The leaders on the clinic board were disappointed by the lack of local political support to save the clinic and wanted to send a message of the need for greater local control over Mason County's health care system. They encouraged a retired business executive who had a vacation home in the area to form a new not-for-profit organization, and then transferred the proceeds of $183,000 from their closure to the newly formed Mason Health Foundation.

The new board members included the retired business executive, Fred Hays—a local physician formerly employed by the clinic who chose to keep Mason County as his home—and a nurse who worked at the hospital. They had a general sense of the health problems of their community, but not many ideas for resolving them. They soon discovered it would take time and energy to put together a plan, let alone implement one. The $183,000 was helpful but not much in the greater scheme of things. They needed someone who could grow and run the organization.

They found a few local candidates who could perhaps have been capable managers of the foundation, but no one who knocked their socks off in terms of ability to create something new. What they heard from these local candidates was that they could provide a few grants and hold a health fair.

The clinic needed a candidate who could propose something more. It might not work out, but they were willing to take a flyer rather than make a safe choice that would do little to change the local scene. Odds were that Mason Health Foundation would only be able to make a short-term political statement about loss of local access to health care and control anyway.

They opened up the position across the larger region. The $50,000 salary was attractive to locals, but not to the greater swath of potential candidates in more urban areas. There were few benefits. The job had little definition, and it would take a lot of work to succeed. Nor was there much job security—they would likely run out of money within the next year, or even months.

Mary Beth was the only candidate who excited them. She saw possibilities in their situation. Check. They wanted someone who had created a new not-for-profit organization before. Check. Someone willing to take risks and organize all the functions of the organization, without much in the way of resources to help. Check. Someone willing to relocate to the Shelton area. Check.

She had additional attributes too. While she didn't have a degree, she was close to having one through coursework focused specifically on management and organization. She had volunteered at a number of not-for-profit organizations and knew something about the field. Her optimism seemed to be matched with a willingness to work hard, oftentimes in ambiguity. She was likable and easygoing.

She accepted their offer and began the new job the next week. Her first day on the job entailed a long meeting with the new board. She asked them for three months' time to research and recommend a way forward. They agreed; they had no better plan for how to proceed, and this seemed to make sense.

Her three months of research culminated in a day-long meeting with the three board members. They convened on a Saturday at a restaurant just outside of Shelton. Mary Beth began with an overview of what she had been doing over the past three months—meetings, reading, and thinking. She made a presentation of things they knew but needed to be focused on as they considered what to do—a chamber of commerce analysis of the county's business picture, a county health needs assessment, and a relational environmental assessment constructed through interviews with key leaders in the area.

She described a local economy in transition from its logging roots to tourism and government services, but with unique and valuable natural resources in its boundaries or in close proximity. Health needs related to growing chronic disease problems, made more difficult by lack of access to health care service, especially local services. A range of organizations and leaders in the area who had skepticism as to what MHF might do, some jealous or even angry that the clinic had given them the money and not them. The community was friendly enough, but had a *go it alone* culture with limited collaborative mentality.

This information set up an extensive conversation among the board members. Mary Beth thought it critical that the board be partners in the quest rather than just be judge or jury to her ideas, a technique she learned working in Nancy's consulting shop—it was called flattening a meeting so everyone in it felt that they had something major to contribute to its outcome.

She also deployed another one of these group process techniques by asking them to vision MHF's future in the region by identifying an animal that captured how they saw this. It got the board members out of their traditional boxes and thinking bigger. They had a lofty discussion of ways that the Mason Health Foundation might catalyze a new way of health and life in the area.

Ideas were popping, but not enough to set a program agenda for the organization. Mary Beth could see that many more discoveries were needed before they could get granular. Instead of pushing these before their time, she captured the collective energy of the group up to then and focused them toward a set of limited next steps for development.

One important agreement was to set a mission for MHF of "improving the health of Mason County." Another was to consider the elephant in the room—the lack of resources to do much of anything for very long.

Mary Beth had an idea for how to address this: add a proposition to the fall ballot to form a "public hospital district in northern Mason County" that would provide a forum for needed services and programs consistent with their mission. Importantly, approval would mean access to property tax receipts arising from the county's primary asset—land and natural resources.

A second step was to build support for this ballot proposition not through hollow promises but by engaging in a real dialogue with the people and leaders across the county as to their needs and visions for the future with respect to health. MHF would do this through community meetings in every town across the county over the next seven months.

The election would tell them what they should do next, if anything. Mary Beth asked the board to invest $100,000 to get the proposition on the ballot and hold the local meetings. With her salary, rent on a small office, and this $100,000 expense, the Mason Health Foundation would be pretty much broke by Election Day. They would find a way forward through this plan, or die trying.

The board members had come to the meeting expecting something edgy but not a walk on the edge of the cliff. But the plan fit with their bigger instincts about MHF. It was why they hired Mary Beth and not a manager with a track record of running things. Go for broke. They approved the plan.

It was left to Mary Beth to do almost all of it. She was tired, excited, and scared, but also optimistic. She couldn't wait to share the news with Irv and Johnny—she had promised to call them both that evening with whatever came out of her meeting. They would be so proud of her!

Chapter Seventy

Irv Wakes Up in Limbo

Irv awoke to noise within the room. He was still lying bound and blinded on the stretcher where he had been left some time ago. He could hear voices speaking Spanish, more voices and louder than when he was wheeled into the room. He couldn't fully understand all that was being said, but thought he made out several pleas for help. There were responses of "*un momento,*" and he heard footsteps moving across the floor. There were odors too—food and body. It was the unmistakable smell of a hospital unit, a combination of antiseptic solution and body wastes fighting for dominance in the air.

Fifteen minutes later, he was still lying on the stretcher with his blindfold in place. All he could do was listen and wait. Then he sensed someone moving closer to him. Hands touched his shoulder and made their way to his head. They were undoing his blindfold.

It took a couple of minutes to clear his vision when the blindfold was removed. The lights in the room were bright, and Irv squinted as the ceiling lights shone in his face. In twenty seconds, he was able to make out the basic features of a face looking over him: a middle-aged woman wearing a nurse's uniform. She had a flat affect, neither smiling or frowning, and kept alternating between looking at him and the contents of a medical chart hooked to the stretcher.

"I don't know why they insist on these blindfolds when they bring you in here. We can take it off now though. *Comprende inglés?*" she asked Irv.

"Si," he responded. There was no longer a need to obfuscate the situation—he needed to figure out where he was and what was going on. The sooner the better.

"Good. Most of your roommates don't."

Irv, with his vision clearing, twisted his head up and peeked to the left. He was in a large, rectangular room, about a hundred feet long and fifty feet wide, with twenty hospital beds, ten on each side. All but two were filled, and it seemed as if they were almost all men. Irv's stretcher was in an alcove at the front of the room by a door, and near a desk that seemed to serve as the nurse's station. There was a small storeroom behind the desk, and he saw IV poles, stretchers, and wheelchairs. Irv recognized the architecture as that of the 1930s, when hospital wards held multiple patients, not like today where most new patient rooms were private, at least for those who had insurance.

"My name is Maria. You were admitted to our medical facility late last night. We are going to take you off this stretcher and put you on one of these beds as soon as I get some help. Then I am going to give you a couple of sedatives in an IV solution and put you on oxygen. If you are hungry, I can offer you a light breakfast. The physician will be by sometime this morning to take a look at you. If you need anything, ring the call light next to your bed. I will be there as soon as I can. But as you can see, I've got a lot of you to take care of, so be patient. Understand? Any questions?"

Irv nodded his head. He wanted to know a lot more, not just about his care but his whereabouts. "Where am I?" he asked in his best version of a broken Spanish accent.

"All I can tell you is that you are in a health care facility in the southern United States. You will remain confined in this unit, but even if you weren't, you would find that there is nowhere to go. So I wouldn't worry about where you are. Our job is to get you healthy enough so that we can send you back home. I don't know much of what happens after you leave from here, but I am not allowed to tell you more than that. So I hope you don't have any more questions, because I don't have any more answers."

With that, she shuffled off to take care of her next patient. Half an hour later, a male orderly came into the room, and the nurse joined him a few minutes later. They helped Irv on to his hospital bed on the right side of the room, three beds from the nurses' station. They released the wrist restraints so that he could move off the stretcher, but immediately reattached them to the hospital bed after changing him into a hospital gown. They put his clothes in a bag taped to his bed. Confinement and restraint were the two clear patient care directives he discerned from the start of his time in this unit.

Looking around some more, he wasn't even sure this was a hospital. The oxygen and other medical supplies were provided by portable machines and plugged into standard wall sockets. The more Irv focused on the room, the more he suspected it might be a TB hospital or nursing home. That would be odd in its own right as patients as sick as he presumably would not be candidates for such a placement.

He could see that the other patients looked quite sick. Some were moaning, many were semi-conscious, and few looked like they were on the road to recovery. There were fifteen men, he thought, age running from their twenties to maybe their fifties. He saw three women too—all looked to be well beyond middle age. His instincts from many years of working in a hospital told him that the patients looked more like candidates for an ICU, not a residential setting where mostly custodial care would be provided.

Still, this room was a better alternative than some of the possibilities he had imagined in the scenarios played in his mind over the last week. He had imagined an ICE detention facility, being caged like an animal behind a chain-link fence, with no medical care and sleeping on a cot on the floor. He had remembered last summer's discovery of a Phoenix office building that was home for a floor of illegals, a hundred people sharing one bathroom with no food or other facilities, locked in together during the sweltering heat of summer. He even thought it possible that he might be dropped off in the middle of a desert or the mountains, simply left to die.

He felt the drugs kicking in once Maria started his IV. He deduced it was likely some anti-anxiety medications to make him more compliant. His mind was clouding over, but he fought it, trying to keep his faculties alert enough to plot his next steps. An edge of fear creeped in as the drugs overtook his intentions, and he struggled to release himself from the restraints. He knew he was at great personal risk, certainly if his fraud was discovered, but even without that.

It was getting hard to maintain his focus. The drugs were winning the battle with its allies of the monotony of the situation and his tired state. Maria made occasional patient rounds. Few of the patients rang their call buttons or moved or said much; they lay in their beds with monitors occasionally bleeping. Most slept. Maria spent much of her time sitting at the nurse's desk, sometimes filling out forms but otherwise checking her cell phone and reading magazines.

There wasn't a clock in the room, which only further disoriented Irv. There were no windows out to the day; what had once been upper transoms were now closed off by pieces of plywood screwed into place near the ceiling. Irv would have to figure out his own method for counting time.

Several hours after he had been put into bed, he guessed, food trays were brought in, holding a bad version of hospital food. Irv had no appetite, and what was offered didn't tempt him, so he ignored his tray of food. Lunchtime, he thought, must be around noon.

Perhaps a couple of hours later, a short man in a lab coat came into the room. He had a stethoscope around his neck and conducted himself with an air of indifference. Irv watched him move around the room with Maria in tow, looking at the patients, then picking up the charts and making notes on them. Presumably, he was the unit doctor and Maria was providing her nursing report verbally as he made his rounds.

Irv couldn't hear much of what they were saying, until they got close to his bed. Even then, it was hard to make out exactly what was being said. Nor was there a lot; this was a cursory attempt at patient care. He heard Maria say, "He is close to ready for discharge" as they looked at a patient on his side of the room, three beds down.

When they got to his bed, he waited for the physician to speak to him. He was obviously awake, one of the few patients in the room to be so. The doctor pulled back the blanket covering Irv and opened up the hospital gown. He scanned him, more like he was looking for a ripe tomato in a supermarket than in some caring evaluation. When the doctor shifted his attention to the chart attached to his bed, Irv asked the physician why he was here. The physician ignored his question, made a note on the chart, and began to move away. Irv pleaded for an answer, any answer. "*Por favor, dónde estoy?* Please, sir, where am I?"

The physician ignored Irv. "Curious fellow, isn't he? Suggest we up his meds a bit. It will make it easier for all if we calm him down. It looks like he will be with us for at least a day until we can get a handle on that heartbeat, so we better put in a catheter too." With that, Maria and the physician continued their patient rounds.

Irv started to realize that his only hope of learning more was with Maria. After the physician left, he rang his call button several times. When she would come over, he would express some medical or personal comfort need and then try to get her to talk with him. She was a reluctant conversationalist.

Their longest interchange was when she came by to insert his catheter. The humiliation of the experience for him encouraged her to be a bit more civil. It was an uncomfortable insertion and made it hard for him to focus on any meaningful questions. But at least they had a moment that might help to open things up later. No pun intended, Irv thought. And nothing useful did she have to say.

More time passed and Irv guessed that evening was approaching. Confirmation was the arrival of the dinner meal tray, even less appealing than the lunchtime fare. After the trays were collected and wheeled out of the room, Maria took a swing around the room to observe each patient. She again ignored Irv's attempt to talk to her.

She moved back to the desk, grabbed a purse, and lowered the lights in the room. Waving at Irv, she unlocked the door with a key and went through it. Irv was left with eighteen other patients in the room, attached to his hospital bed with a patient restraint. He presumed that an evening or night nurse might soon arrive and maybe he would have better luck with them in learning more about his situation.

He waited, and waited some more. Every couple of hours, or so, less as time moved on through the night, a person would enter the room, take a fast walk around, and leave. They could have been a nurse or doctor, but seemed to be more of a prison guard in their dress and demeanor.

Irv fought the meds to stay awake and observe events through the night. He would doze off, but awoke regularly from the occasional rounds, a moan from a roommate, or the bleep of a monitor alarm. It would be a restless night for Irv—of that much he was sure. He wondered whether a new day would bring any clarity as to what he should do next. For now, he had no idea.

Chapter Seventy-One

A Public Hospital District Is Approved

The Mason County Public Hospital District was approved by voters in the fall, with over 80 percent of support across the county. It was a remarkable success that voters would approve a property tax increase that would bring $350,000 a year into this new special-purpose local government. The three board members of the Mason Health Foundation became the first new board of the new local "PHD," and Mary Beth was appointed its first executive director.

It was thought that the Mason Health Foundation would fade into the background as the new special-purpose government came into being, but the old moniker proved sticky, and anything with government in its name carried some message baggage. The Mason Health Foundation became the practical name of the new local government.

Mary Beth had organized the campaign for the ballot proposition, with help from her three board members and consulting assistance from Nancy Jones. One important step that Nancy suggested was getting the local hospital to support the proposal. The board approached the hospital's leadership and promised the allocation of $100,000 of the property tax receipts to them. This neutralized one source of potential opposition and resulted in several hospital leaders even speaking in favor of the idea.

There was opposition from some businesses and older leaders in the county—the former with a point of view that any property tax increase was a bad idea; the latter that if there was a need for such a thing, they would have done it long ago. Mary Beth used her charm to keep the opposition civil and respectful. She welcomed discussions of the proposal and listened to what everyone had to say. Ultimately, she insisted, this was a question for the people of Mason County, and her job was to make sure they had the information needed to make the best choice.

The campaign was fueled by the second action of the board adopted at their retreat—a series of community dialogues on health in every town across the county. The idea was to demonstrate what it meant to have an organization like MHF in place.

Nancy helped Mary Beth develop a structure for the meetings. The common agenda was a facilitated dialogue that made sure the meetings were respectful conversations and not bitch sessions that pulled on old disagreements. Health care was a divisive topic, a byproduct of the noise from the two major political parties. MHF was not wanting to wallow in that, but to find instead points of agreement by the people of Mason County. They would do this by identifying common values.

Mary Beth relied on local leaders and organizations to organize and bring together the attendees. MHF would pay for facilities and snacks and run the meetings, but it was up to each area to organize based on its own community.

Each meeting opened with a video produced by Nancy that served as the ice-breaker to the dialogue and set objectives and context. Mary Beth facilitated every meeting, through a structured dialogue. An early agenda item was to frame local problems with health or health care. Importantly, no one could dominate or load the agenda—once a problem was identified by a community member, only new problems could be added to the list.

The structured process allowed Mary Beth as moderator to stop multiple stump speeches that frequently took community meetings down a rabbit hole. It also left much more time for the problem-solving phase of the dialogue. While specific solutions to problems were discussed, the outcome of the meeting was to brainstorm values that would guide future efforts to improve health in the community.

Political insiders and some established leaders initially criticized the approach. Mary Beth and the board stuck to their guns, believing it critical to show they would operate in a new and inclusive way. They found great support over the first conversations, and the naysayers began to quiet down.

Mary Beth was encouraged when the reviews of the meetings showed that attendees felt that MHF was genuinely interested in listening to what folks had to say. That was the most critical thing to do. Many participants shared they had attended other forums on health care problems, but that these were usually organized by politicians, government, or health care organizations that were far more interested in telling them what the problems were and why they should support their solutions.

The MHF approach was so different and well received that some participants asked whether county or even state leaders would listen to what they had to say as well. They appreciated that MHF was asking and listening, but questioned whether those in power cared at all about this. Mary Beth told the group she couldn't promise that anyone would listen—honesty was a value she held dearly and wanted the foundation to hold too. She would give county and state leaders every opportunity to listen by committing to organize a summit for local leaders to share the results of all the local dialogues.

Surprisingly, this summit was well-attended by both local leaders and a representative smattering of statewide officials. Candidates for public office were invited, but were told that this was a listening meeting for them, not an opportunity to make campaign speeches. Mary Beth presented a draft set of values at the meeting; community members had essentially proposed ten such values in their local dialogue sessions.

The ideas were shared and sharpened at the summit. At the end of the day, a draft set of ten values were presented, and the assembly used an electronic voting method to prioritize them. At the top of the list was a fundamental value of fairness, closely followed by local control and shared decision making.

Attendees were given an opportunity to personally or organizationally endorse the values. These were folded into a draft statement of health and beliefs for Mason County based on the structure of the Declaration of Independence. Over a hundred people signed on, including almost all of the political candidates in attendance.

Mary Beth was thrilled with the success of the local and community-wide meetings. They showed a real thirst across the county for trying to do better in terms of health and health care, and finding positive ways to do this together. She had carved a leadership opportunity for Mason Health Foundation to do so out of thin air.

The positive reaction to the meetings translated to great support at the ballot box for the public hospital district proposal. Mason Health Foundation now not only had positive energy and a set of commonly held values for health across the county, but a funding source that would provide the resources to give it a go!

The Theory of Irv

The first eight months of Mary Beth's time as executive director had been busy ones—three months of research followed by five months of convening local dialogues and managing a ballot campaign. This made it hard for her to get to Seattle on weekends to see Irv, and he would come to Shelton a couple of times a month. Less as time went on.

Maybe now that this work was concluded, she would be able to figure out where things stood with him. Whether she was ready to face this or not, she discovered her responsibilities with MHF were only growing. She now had to complete the process of bringing the new public hospital district into existence—a governance process, financial controls, personnel policies and procedures, and legal agreements.

It was imperative to fast-track these so they would qualify for property tax payments the next year. Most of the $183,000 originally awarded by the clinic was spent, and time was of the essence to get new dollars into the organization. Mary Beth also sensed that it would be important for MHF to quickly deliver tangible expressions of what their mission and the values meant—program, policies, and other activities evidencing that the faith of the county's people was well-placed, in her and MHF.

There would be no rest for the weary—not that MaryBeth was tired. She saw this as an opportunity of a lifetime. The opportunity cost would sometimes nag at her, and she did her best to push Irv out of mind and body.

Chapter Seventy-Two

Irv In Limbo 2

Irv heard a rustling at the door of his antiquated hospital ward, and it soon opened. Maria was here. It must be the start of the day shift, which was usually 7 a.m. at health care facilities, but it was possible it was earlier or later in this unique place. Maria dropped her personal belongings at the desk and then moved around the room, checking patients and records. As needed, she emptied catheter bags and adjusted IV bags. Occasionally, she would take a temperature or check someone's blood pressure.

She stopped at Irv's bed and took his pulse, comparing it with what was recorded on the monitor. She was again dismissive of Irv's attempt to engage in conversation with her.

Now twenty-four hours into his stay, Irv knew the routine, such as it was. The only new and different thing on Day Two was that his bedmate three slots over was taken away. This began by the physician making a note on his chart when he made his rounds, followed by Maria making a telephone call from her desk.

An hour or so later, an orderly came in, accompanied by the ambulance driver who had picked Irv up at Promise Hospital. They went to the bed, removed the patient restraints, and helped the man in the bed to his feet. They helped him remove his hospital gown and put on what must have been the clothing he wore when he first sought health care. He looked healthy enough now—a little unsteady on his feet, but that would be expected after days lying around medicated in a hospital bed. They put him in a wheelchair and took him out the door—after putting a blindfold on him. That was that. Maria cleaned up the bed and area.

Irv imagined what leaving meant. His faculties were getting clearer, largely because he detached his IV when Maria wasn't looking by using his teeth. He didn't really need the IV since his symptoms were made up—and he didn't want the drugs in him. He would let the line drip into his mattress so as not to alert her that he was non-medicating, and reattach when she made her rounds.

His guess was that Patient X was about to be deported. His hypothesis: HealthMost flagged certain seriously ill patients in their emergency rooms and housed them in places like this until their dangerous conditions stabilized enough to discharge them to their country of origin.

Otherwise, there was probably a risk that the effort to deport them might hit a snag, including possible referrals to well-meaning support organizations. What he was thinking was monstrously wrong—it would mean that there was a secret mass deportation effort, using health care facilities to identify illegals and remove them from the country when they sought treatment at HealthMost facilities. Most were probably not seriously ill and could be immediately sent home. But, on occasion, very sick patients would need some other approach—and this was it.

If they were really trying to heal these patients, there would be a lot more care going on in this unit than what Irv saw. His symptoms merited a consultation with a cardiologist and a range of specific tests of his heart and circulatory system. That seemed unlikely to happen.

No, this unit looked to be all about just getting people to the point where they could move back into the deportation system. Irv imagined it was probably a low and loose standard; maybe just that they had to be able to walk and not look to be at death's door. He also figured this was where he was headed shortly—the drugs he swallowed at the campground had surely begun to wear off, and his pulse rate and blood pressure were probably already near normal. He guessed that was why Maria had taken a manual pulse, testing whether the reduction in his pulse was accurate.

He didn't think there was much for him to learn from actually being deported, other than to confirm his theory. That wasn't the goal of this clandestine research—it was to figure out what happened to patients like Rodrigo Lopez. He needed to know what happened to the ones who were presumably too sick, or dead, and couldn't be stabilized and deported. Regardless, he didn't have much more time in this unit one way or the other. He would have to do something soon or likely he'd be on his way to the border and Panama by tomorrow.

He waited until Maria left for the night and made his move. During the day, he had hidden a knife from his meal tray in his bedding, using his teeth to provision it away. The restraints had been slack enough to allow him to eat, and this gave him just enough wiggle room to get the knife in his hand at an angle that allowed him to slice into the restraints. It wasn't the sharpest knife in the world, but nor were the restraints that sturdy. The major confinement strategy in the ward was drugs, and they weren't expecting someone like him—healthy and sober and intent on getting away. It took over an hour to saw his way through the first restraint, and once he had a free hand, he needed only seconds to release himself from the second.

He detached the tape securing the IV on his clothing, and the leads to the heart monitor. Swinging his legs out to the side, he got out of bed, slung his catheter bag over a hook on the IV pole, and pushed it around with him as he searched the room, listening carefully for any activity at the door. He guessed it would be an hour or two before the night watch made its rounds.

Irv searched the nurse's desk. There wasn't much in it, just some medical supplies and stationery. This wasn't much of a medical facility, that was for sure. He moved on to the supply closet behind the desk. Most of its contents were the essentials for custodial treatment of patients—IVs, catheter bags and needles and such.

Irv looked around the front desk area for anything else that might be of use to his investigation—there was little, and probably intentionally so. The telephone was attached to the wall, with a small bulletin board next to it. There wasn't much on the board, not even the usual labor notices. There were a series of phone numbers. One was labeled "Mortality Management," so he used a Magic Marker to write down the number, using his leg as stationery.

He moved around the room to get a better look at his fellow patients. Most were heavily drugged and non-responsive; only a couple even noticed him. The charts on their beds indicated all had serious medical conditions. All had Hispanic names and Mexico or various South

American countries of origin noted on their chart. Many of their serious conditions were cardiac or neurological in nature; a couple related to their renal systems. There was no care plan laid out in the charts—more evidence that the goal was merely to stabilize them enough to get them across the border to their countries of origin. Their health would have to be dealt with, or not, on the other side.

The patient on the other end of his side of the room caught his eye. As he got closer, he could see that he was a small man, probably in his fifties. On closer look, he realized that he was not just in an unresponsive, drugged state. He was dead. He likely had passed after Maria's shift change. Irv had little time to process the loss of life he had found; this was hardly a moment for reverence. Rather, he assessed the opportunity in the situation.

This was the goal—to see where a patient like this went. You can't transport dead people across the border using the deportation system; even that has its limits in inhumanity. Irv looked at the medical record. Jose Rodriguez was very likely one of those "U" patients in the computer file—and there had to be a way for Irv to track what happened to him next.

He looked around the room a second time, searching the desk more thoroughly. If only there was a cell phone or beeper or some electronic device. There was none. He then moved to the supply closet again, at first seeing nothing of use. Then he spotted the shrouds on the bottom shelf.

His plan formed quickly. There was a good chance that Jose's death wouldn't even be noticed until Maria's return tomorrow. Once she arrived there was probably little Irv could do, other than try to overpower her and anyone who came to her aid. He took her at her word that they were in the middle of nowhere. Even if he got off the unit, where could he go? And how could he possibly track what happened to Jose?

No, he had to force an opportunity to see what was going on. The answer was in the shrouds or, more to the point, him in a shroud, with Jose. The nursing staff presumably had some responsibility for getting dead bodies prepared for transport—that was why the shrouds were in the storeroom.

It was now or never. He yanked the catheter and his IV out and put on the clothes stored in the bag taped to his bed. He used his gown and some unused pillows to fluff up the empty bed to make it look like he was still in bed asleep. He knew from watching rounds that the night watch was not very vigilant. Maria would discover the ruse quickly when she arrived in the morning, but not before working her way around the room to all the other patients first. By then Irv planned to be long gone.

He searched through the shrouds in the closet and pulled out an extra-large kit. His mind briefly wandered to one of his first assignments as a hospital administration intern—researching shroud sizes. That hospital had only small versions on hand, and it resulted in dead limbs sticking out as bodies were wheeled down the hall, spooking visitors. He had no time for that memory—for now, it was useful to know something about standard shroud sizes.

He eyeballed the shroud for actual size and then carried it down to the dead man's bed. He detached Jose's hookups and finagled him into the bag. He then picked up the bagged body and put it on a stretcher rolled down from the front area. He left the shroud unzipped for the moment. The small man took up less than half of the bag, since it was made for very large, deceased patients. Irv was counting on this.

He went to the telephone in the room and called the number next to "Mortality Management." "Yeah," the voice on the other end of the line answered. Irv was hoping someone would answer.

"We got one," said Irv, in clear as white English. "We want to get it out of here ASAP because we've got some VIPs touring later this morning, so the sooner the better." He was making it up as he went along, hoping that a combination of laziness and bureaucratic fear might make his plan succeed.

"All right. But what are you doing up there this time of night? John came by about an hour ago and said all was quiet on the ward."

Irv had no idea who John was, but guessed he was one of the sentries who did rounds during the night. "That's right. I got a call from the boss about this VIP tour, and he said that I should come in and make sure we got things covered for tomorrow." Irv had no idea who the boss was but hoped that was enough to get the man on the other end of the line moving. "He seemed pretty amped up about this, so you better come and get the body out of here, and gone, before he gets pissed."

"Okay. I got it. Keep your pants on." Irv almost chuckled, still feeling the sting of where he had pulled out the catheter and wishing that he had kept his pants on. "I'll be up in a few minutes."

"Good. He's all bagged up; I will leave the chart on top." Irv hung up.

He grabbed the medical records from Jose's bed and put them on top of the stretcher with the shroud, then rolled all to the front of the room by the door. There was one more thing—he took a straw from the supply closet and used a pen to make a small hole in the bottom side of the shroud that contained the dead man. He inserted the straw flush to the hole and taped it down so that it could let air into the bag without being easily seen. He put the pen in his pocket.

Then there was just one last thing to do, distasteful as it was. He crawled onto the gurney and slipped in, legs first, next to the dead man, pulling the small body next to him. There was barely enough room for him to fit, though he would have to count on indifference to the obvious question of how a man who weighed barely a hundred pounds now weighed almost three hundred.

It was creepy squeezing in next to the dead man. Irv had come so far, and so it seemed like this was one small distasteful step after a bunch of crazy big ones. He made sure the medical records were still on top of the shroud, and then twisted his arm through to zip up the bag as much as possible. He got as comfortable as he could, found the straw taped to the bag, put it in his mouth, and breathed.

About ten minutes later, he heard the door unlock and open. Footsteps moved to and then around the gurney. Whoever had come to get the body started to wheel it out of the room. He—or she—farted loudly. Irv almost laughed, but this was serious business and he was not out of danger.

He was wheeled down a couple of hallways, presumably the same ones he was wheeled through after his midnight transfer from Promise Hospital. A chill soon told him that he was outside, confirmed when he heard an engine start and a vehicle approach the gurney. It sounded like a diesel engine, and the sliding door opening sounded more like a small utility truck than a van or an ambulance. Four arms grabbed hold of the shroud and placed it in the vehicle.

He heard, "These stiffs sure get heavy. He's in. Get 'im out of here," followed by "I'll swing by on my way back from the airport. Shift should be just about up by then. Maybe we could go grab a drink at that bar just over the border."

It had worked. Irv was on his way out of this place, with evidence. They were headed to an airport—that much he now knew. Which one, he had no idea. It was close to the border. Where might it head and what would happen next? Maybe, he thought, he was on his way to Moses Lake? He felt an odd sense of accomplishment with that conclusion, and even a twinge of hope.

The hope was short-lived. A more balanced view of his situation was that he was now stuffed in a bag with a dead man and about to be transported to who knows where by the type of people who seemed to care little about murder and other crimes. He had no identity and no one else had any idea of his whereabouts.

His prospects seemed bleak. *Too late to do anything about that,* he thought. *I signed up for this. Maybe one of these days I will choose the easy path through life. No, that never happens. Better to keep thinking like Johnny that most things work out for the best.* Irv prayed that this would be so in this situation. He remembered Johnny's objection to him taking on this undercover project. Even the great optimist had his doubts about this one.

Chapter Seventy-Three

Mason Health Foundation Grows

In three months, the Mason County Public Hospital District—AKA the Mason Health Foundation—was up, running, and funded. Mary Beth and the new commissioners had checked all the boxes on the formation of the new hospital district and received the first installation of property tax receipts for the year—a governance structure, a set of organization policy and procedures that would generally guide their operations, and several volunteers in place to help with the doing. They had bank accounts, an attorney, and a financial service to manage the books.

The staff remained a core of one—Mary Beth. She secured a small office in a shopping mall in downtown Shelton that was flanked by a community bank on one side and a furniture store on the other. A grocery store, coffee shop, and tire store filled out the mall, and the coffee shop proved to be a convenient spot for meetings.

The board asked Mary Beth to arrange an open house in early April to celebrate the official creation. Mary Beth didn't crave the attention that would come from this but knew the symbolism was important. The board surprised her that evening by presenting her a special leadership award. Local leaders praised what she had achieved with Mason Health Foundation.

Mary Beth appreciated the recognition, but was a bit embarrassed by the attention. Part of it was her innate shyness, but even more was she didn't think they had done much yet. The celebration was largely about a funding source for MHF's activities, as if this was the objective. She cringed at the thought that her legacy in Mason County might prove to be her authorship of a property tax increase.

The real challenge was to make a positive difference for the people who lived in Mason County. The property tax dollars were nothing more than fuel to pursue the organization's mission to improve health. Even as she worked on the creation of the district, she was pondering how they might do this.

The set of values derived from the local meetings seemed a great place to start. She was proud of these—they offered a guiding light to blaze their path into the future. While these values could shape their actions, she also knew that the "what" of their next play must be concrete and tangible organization outputs.

She suggested to the board that their first program action be to provide small grants to organizations across the county for health improvement activities. The community meetings had exposed a county-wide resource shortage for health improvement. Mary Beth thought that these communities had more assets than they typically knew about. Yes, money was short but every place had health activities going on that others in the community knew little to nothing about. She advised the board that if they used their funding to resource health action, their model should emphasize building local collaboration so they just didn't add more unknown actions to the mix.

She reminded the board how quickly hospital leadership had changed their mind about the public hospital district proposal once they offered to let them share in the property tax receipts. The hospital then even agreed to coordinate their activities with the foundation and others across the county. Perhaps MHF could similarly use some of their property tax receipts to make small grants to groups across the county for collaborative health improvement?

Mary Beth did not have any experience in grant making and joined a statewide association of grant makers to get advice on the idea. Its membership included large and small foundations, some government, others not-for-profit organizations, and still others trusts held by private and family foundations. All one had to do to be eligible for membership was to make grant awards in some way. MHF was doing exactly that through the award to the local hospital, so it was eligible.

She found an immediate benefit in meeting peers who were doing work in the same field. It was not so much any specific advice that she liked; it was just nice to have people to share the experience with. She realized in retrospect how busy and lonely her first year in Mason County had been.

Most of the ideas she found in the association for grant making didn't really fit MHF's needs. The best practices reflected more the needs of large grants made by wealthy organizations. These had the time, resources, and inclination to undertake complicated programs, and incorporated such things as proven outcomes, data-based decision making, and sustainability plans for when the grant ended. None of these seemed particularly relevant to her situation.

She did find one small foundation that instead thought of grants as an asset to be used not in terms of specific programs and outcomes but toward relationships that leveraged local assets. This notion of "social capital building" was an interesting one. It resonated with what she heard in the local meetings across Mason County. The executive director walked her through how they built their grant program using these alternative principles.

The final program approved by the board was Mary Beth's adaptation of the approach. It involved very small grants, $1000 to no more than $2500. Applicants would need to explain how they would generally use the funds, not in terms of a project, but in terms of working with others in the community. MHF would not ask for long and traditional grant applications, but a one-page statement of intent. Mary Beth would then visit the community to test the potential of the award to build local social capital. Deliverables would not be project reports but assessment of working relations with others in the community. Importantly, awards would not be limited to the usual one, two, or three years. Rather, MHF was offering an ongoing funding source that would allow long-term commitments to collaborate on local health improvement.

The board found great interest in this funding across the county, and it became MHF's first program success. They funded a total of thirty-five local grants in their first year of the program. Applicants were excited when they were awarded the dollars and appreciated how easy it was to work with MHF. Most of the grants broke down silos in the community. MHF rewarded them by continuing or even growing their funding the next year. Anecdotally, it seemed health improvement was happening across the county, though MHF wasn't able to evaluate this in any scientific way.

A collateral impact of this grant approach was that it also built a strong reserve of trust between MHF and local community leaders. MHF was starting from a good place because of the local meetings; this grant process only added to this reservoir.

Most of Mary Beth's second year of work was building this grant program. The balance of her time was spent developing ideas for their next program initiative. Important as the grant program was, the board also wanted to act more collectively as a county. The summit held after the local meetings showed that there was interest in this and found consensus around values. Could this energy somehow be harnessed to improve health in a bigger way?

The board explored this potential by convening breakfast meetings with local leaders. The agendas were structured around the values adopted in the resolution from the summit, and consisted of brainstorming how these areas of agreement might be translated to tangible action.

Many ideas came forward from these meetings. Most did not seem actionable by MHF because the "action" was a thing that some other organization was already doing. For MHF to step in would build on fault lines of conflict across the county. MHF's strength was that it could transcend the history and friction of others, and intruding on others' roles would work against this. This greatly limited what MHF could do programmatically.

Mary Beth saw an opportunity within one of the values identified in the community meetings; it spoke to the need for people to accept personal responsibility to improve their own health through taking actions under their control. This had triggered a contentious debate at the summit, as it overlapped with the decades-long ideologic division within the American health care system.

The debate typically fell into two opposing frames—those who believed that the government should be responsible for financing and managing health care, and those who believed it should be decentralized to markets and individuals. Irv had explained to her how the tension was underneath the failure of the nation to ever adopt a national health care policy—this ideologic difference had over time been accentuated by the two political parties as a central feature of their political disagreement.

What came from the summit was interesting in that this polemic was shot down by participants, as it had been in the community meetings where it had first come up. Rather, almost all noted that at its heart, health improvement required an individual responsibility and a collective responsibility. The real question was the actual degree of each to be applied, and almost all felt that there was room for both to flourish. There was also a great frustration expressed as to how the political parties made it impossible to have a rational conversation about the right blend.

The program idea Mary Beth proposed was for MHF to become a platform for helping various organizations and people tap in to their contribution to health improvement in both responsibility realms. MHF would create a way for people and organizations to record what they were doing to improve health across the county. MHF could do this simply and cheaply through a website that would use game theory to make this a fun endeavor, more a health challenge than an inventory.

Most of what MHF provided was recognition and a sense of being part of something bigger than oneself. Organizations would post their collective health action areas, and people could get credit for being part of these efforts by liking the activity on MHF's website. This earned organizations recognition and MHF even more participants.

MHF also built a series of simple health trackers that allowed individuals to record what they were doing around such things as physical activity, weight loss, and hydration. They could even get credit for answering a weekly health improvement quiz.

Using game theory, MHF made the tracking a fun and competitive endeavor. Special challenge months would make their focus energy during key times of the year. Successes would be celebrated through articles on the MHF website or in local newspaper or radio coverage.

People and organizations valued the positive attention brought to them by the foundation. Every month, those who had obtained a minimum number of credits for health improvement on the website game page were entered into a drawing for prizes.

No one had ever seen anything like it. And it worked, by all available program measures for such a creative endeavor. Importantly to MHF, it was an inexpensive program innovation. The initial website development cost only $35,000 as Mary Beth found students at the local community college who developed the site as part of their degree requirements. Ongoing costs to the website, awards, and public recognition materials cost about $25,000 per year.

The Mason County Healthiest Community Challenge, as it became known, also provided MHF with an extensive list of email addresses of people and organizations interested in health improvement across Mason County. At the time, there was little intent to the acquisition—it was a practical need to be able to communicate with participants about the challenge.

The new world of digital communications was just beginning to reveal itself as a force that could be used for good or evil. For now, it was sufficient that MHF had an affordable way to directly communicate with people on its extensive email list. In the very near future, it would also become another critical flank of MHF action. Years later, Mary Beth would reflect on the happenstance of how in a matter of months these email addresses became an essential tool for finally fixing the American health care system.

Chapter Seventy-Four

Irv and Jose on a Plane

The vehicle transporting a dead Jose and a live Irv traveled a short distance; Irv guessed about five miles. There were few sounds to be heard other than the vehicle itself and an occasional thud from the bounce of the road—it was an uneven track they were driving on, maybe even a dirt road. The ride then smoothed out and they soon stopped. A door slid open. The shroud was lifted from the vehicle and placed on the cold ground. The door shut and the truck drove off. Then Irv heard two propeller engines start up—they must be at an airport. Irv figured they would soon be in flight, on their way to parts unknown.

Sure enough. The shroud was moved into its next travel spot, and soon, Irv could hear a take-off. When they were airborne, he carefully jiggled the zipper on the shroud loose and opened the container bag just enough to look out, carefully, making sure he would not be discovered. There was not much to see. He was in the back of a four-passenger propeller plane. There were no passengers, only a pilot in front. Irv could not make him out in any detail as a red net was hanging between the baggage and the passenger areas and blocked much of his line of sight. He didn't want to move about and draw attention.

It was cool and he was thirsty, so when he saw a box of water near the shroud, he slowly reached over and grabbed a bottle. He took turns sipping water and breathing; the straw had worked to help him breathe in the shroud, but it wasn't like he was drowning in air. The radio in the front of the plane occasionally barked out garbled words.

Irv lay back down and waited. There was not much else to be done at the moment. He also figured that such a small plane would not translate to a very long trip. An hour and a half later, he was proved right when the plane lowered altitude, in preparation for landing, Irv thought. They hadn't gone far. A plane like this wasn't all that fast, and it was a short flight, nowhere near far enough to get to Moses Lake. Irv thought of major cities within a few hundred miles of southern New Mexico. He couldn't be sure that they would be landing at a major airport, or even that they even started this trip in New Mexico.

As the plane landed, he drew back into his plastic cocoon, bringing the half-empty water bottle with him. The plane hit ground with a bang and a bounce, tossing Irv slightly upward. He landed on Jose's bony and cold elbow.

It was a short taxi from the runway to the parking spot for the plane. With the engines off, Irv could hear other vehicles and planes nearby—it was a busy airport. Maybe it was the Albuquerque airport? Irv reviewed the list of potential cities in his head again.

He kept still as the shroud was pulled out of the plane and put into what he surmised, from peeking out a small hole he had left in the top of the shroud, was a hangar. He thought about trying to make a run for it, but he could hear voices in the hangar and knew he wasn't alone. There was no telling whether they were friend or foe; the only reasonable choice under the circumstances was to assume the latter.

Irv debated whether to change his mind. Any chance to do so went away when workers came over and put the shroud on a transport cart, along with other baggage. The cart motored out to another plane, and Irv saw through his eyehole that it was a much larger jet. The shroud was placed on a conveyor plate that slid up to a storage compartment. More hands inserted him and Jose into the compartment. Soon, the door to the compartment area shut and the engine on the plane roared to life. Jose remained unmoved by his change in venue.

As the plane took off, Irv opened up the shroud. He confirmed that he was alone with a peek out of the bag. The only light came from a red light on the far wall, which didn't exactly fill up the compartment with light but provided enough for Irv to survey the storage area. It was closed off from the rest of the plane.

Comforted by the privacy, he slid completely out of the shroud, leaving it open and accessible should he need to quickly slide in again. He stretched his arms and legs and opened his back. Hiding in a shroud was not good for the spine.

THE THEORY OF IRV

He saw a small door at the far end of the compartment, presumably leading to the passenger area or another general storage area on the plane. It was locked and he concluded that this small area would be his home for the next leg of their journey. Before long it got cold—there was no climate control. The air was cooling and getting thin as the plane continued to climb. Probably a long flight, thought Irv. He was happy to put distance between him and where they had come from, and pondered how he could stay warm.

He looked around the compartment, but most of what was around him was of little use: cases of household cleaning supplies, prefab storage units still in separate pieces and shrink wrapped on a skid, even a generator. Digging into boxes in one corner, he found several cases of dog food. It disgusted him, but he had not eaten in two days. He opened up a can with a pull top and used his fingers to gobble up a few bites. It was not that different from the hospital food at his last stop, he thought.

Irv continued to survey the compartment. There were no standard passenger suitcases in the bin, meaning that there probably weren't any normal passengers on this flight. It was likely a cargo plane, and the contents suggested it might be headed to a remote location. The hold contained the types of things that one would find on a cargo flight from Seattle up to Alaska. Though he thought it likely the supplies were headed off the normal grid, he couldn't be sure that this flight itself was going directly to somewhere remote.

Before long, he had crawled around the entirety of the storage room and taken a gander at everything in it, the dog food already churning uncomfortably in his stomach. He looked about the walls of the unit for something else that might help.

There was an emergency raft, a hatchet, and a first aid kit attached to a wall. If he needed any of these, things would be going from bad to worse. For a moment he thought about removing the hatchet and bringing it into the shroud with him, should it come to that. For as bad as this situation was, he had so far been quite fortunate, but he wasn't sure luck would stay on his side.

Then he spotted something of interest on the far end of the unit, near the locked door to the innards of the plane. It was only dimly lit by the red light, so he crawled over several skids to get a closer look: blue overalls, used and hanging on a hook, probably something that a worker put on to help load or unload the plane. Maybe they were even used by crew who were now onboard the flight, in the more comfortable quarters on the other side of the door.

The overalls were scratchy and didn't fit him all that well, but they provided him warmth and he was glad to have it. He buttoned them to the top to retain his own body heat as much as possible. Maybe he should try to get some sleep—at least a short nap. He had been up for most of the past two nights and was tired and needed to clear his head. It could be a problem if he didn't wake up on landing, but Irv was a light sleeper. *Never could sleep on planes*, he thought. Maybe this would be the exception.

He curled into a ball around some boxes, sliding his hands into the two deep pockets on the overalls for warmth. There were some things in the pocket, and he pushed a little deeper, seeking more warmth.

Then he felt it. Not warmth, but something else. There was no mistaking what it was. It was a cell phone. Not a fancy new iPhone, but one of the old basic flip models that were standard fare in the early 1990s.

Irv pulled it out of the pocket and took a better look. It had power; the dials and screen lit up. It even provided a little more light within the cargo hold. He held up the light from the phone and looked around again. Nothing worth seeing better, but the phone itself was another story. He saw a "no signal" indicator, and knew that they were too high and remote to connect to a cell tower. For now, at least. He went to the settings section and found some basic information—number, provider, and the like. There were no saved numbers or contacts listed. The call history showed only a handful of numbers that had been called in the last month.

Sleep was now out of the question. This phone was something he could use. But how? He leaned back on a crate, sipping on the water left in his bottle stolen from the previous flight. He had heartburn and gas. There was no time to worry about that, so he fought through the discomfort.

A plan formed, and he went into action. First, he pulled out the pen that he had taken from the nurses' desk and wrote down all of the telephone numbers and other numbers and information he could find on the phone—twice, once on a piece of cardboard that he then folded up and put in his pants pocket, and then on his thigh. He wanted to make sure this information was preserved, as the phone would be going on without him.

Once he had transcribed the numbers, he moved on to the next phase of his plan, which he could not fully initiate until there was cell service again. But he could get a head start. Service might not come until landing, depending on where they were headed. This would create a risk, but it was essential to the plan that he be ready to move quickly.

Irv climbed back next to the shroud and unzipped it so that he could get better access to Jose's body. Opening up the dead man's shirt, he probed with his fingers around the stomach, just below the ribs. He arched the body so that the stomach area stuck out a bit higher than the rest of the corpse.

Then he moved over to the emergency first aid kit on the wall. As expected, it included an assortment of medical supplies. He was looking for two things in particular—a small knife or scalpel, and some suture material. There they were. A small Swiss army knife with several blades and catgut 2. He took both out and put the kit back on the wall. Better things look untouched in the hold, just in case someone was paying attention, he thought.

He sat down next to Jose and waited for his moment. He might have to work quickly and he wasn't sure how long each step might take. Every few minutes he flipped open the phone to see if cell coverage had been found.

Time passed . . . a lot of time. Irv was sleepy now, but dared not doze off. He realized that the phone had a clock and saw that it was now 7 a.m., time zone uncertain. Another hour passed. He thought that the plane was beginning to descend and checked for service every minute or so.

There it was. One bar, intermittently. Now, two bars. Even three. He pressed the call button and listened for a dial tone. Bingo. He entered a number, one that he had committed to memory before heading to Albuquerque for his investigation. He was hoping there would be an answer on the other end, but he knew that if not, it would go to voicemail, which would be checked regularly.

The number was the hotline that Lance had created for him. It was part of how they got Johnny to agree to his undercover project. This secure line, obtained through US Capitol Police, would be where he would call if he got to a phone with an outside line. The telephone in the nursing unit didn't have one; he had tried, but it only connected to inside extensions. The cell phone offered the access he needed.

No one answered, and he left a message, speaking loudly to make sure his voice was heard through the roar of the plane engine, and then repeating it to be sure that it got through. "Lance. I am in a cargo plane. I do not know where I am headed. But it is essential that you track this cell phone. Here is the telephone number in case you get disconnected. This is the identifier number for the phone: Track it through both. I am okay and have much to report. Will contact you as soon as I can."

With that, he put down the phone, leaving it flipped open after he ended the call. He thought they would be able to track the phone through its digital chip, but just to be sure, he would keep the phone active to provide a backup way to see where it went. There was no reason to assume an immediate loss of cell service if they were landing in a populated area.

He turned to his next task. A bit more gruesome than the rest of the plan, but necessary. He took the knife and pulled out its largest blade. Feeling underneath Jose's ribs, he probed with his fingers for a soft opening free from bones or fast hardening dead organs. He found what he thought was a good spot and cut a six-inch slash through the stiff flesh. He stuck the knife deep into the slash and repeated his cut, opening the hole in the body deeper and wider. He compared the size of the opening to the open cell phone, added another couple of inches in length in both directions, and then reached inside the cut and scooped out with two fingers as much bodily goo as he could. He tossed the glob of stuff toward a corner of the cargo area. He looked in at the open wound and dug out some more. *Good enough*, he thought.

Taking the still open and live phone, he inserted it carefully into the opening on the body. The last third of the insertion was difficult, requiring him to give the phone a firm shove into the cavity. Irv got down low and peered in as best he could to check the phone's screen. It was a little hard to see, but it looked like the call was still active. He took a strand of the catgut, tied one end on the needle that came with the kit, and used it to crudely sew up the wound. Not many juices were flowing out of the body by now. No surprise, he thought. His suturing didn't need to be pretty. The point of this step was to make it look like there was a medical procedure done on the body, nothing out of the ordinary.

It was as good as he could do, and he closed up Jose's shirt, stuffed him back into the shroud, and zipped it up. It was time to leave his travel partner. *Peace be with you,* he prayed over the corpse.

The plane was landing. There was plenty of time left for the next part of his plan, but it was essential that he not be seen until the time was right. Irv crawled to the other side of the compartment, still wearing the overalls, and hid behind the generator, crouching down behind its wood pallet. It was the largest object in the storage unit, on the far side of the plane from the exit door, and offered good cover.

The plane slid to a landing and then taxied for a few minutes. The engine cut off. The time was getting near.

When the cargo door slid open, Irv could see a man in blue overalls reaching into the breach, securing the open lid with a cord. A conveyor belt was pushed into the storage compartment. Irv could see daylight through the opening, staying hidden as best he could. It was not time yet.

The man climbed into the compartment and began to take small items in the cargo hold and place them on the belt, which brought them down to a transport cart at ground level. One of the last of the smaller items to go down the belt was the shroud. *Until we meet again, mi compadre.*

The conveyor belt was pulled out of the opening and soon replaced with the forks of what looked to be a power lift. The man opened the door to the compartment a bit wider to accommodate the lift and then began to remove larger and heavier items from the hold using the lift. A path was being cleared to the generator, which the man was looking at and guiding the forks toward now. Irv waited to see which side of the generator the man moved toward—he had to pick a side to try to fasten the lift. The man moved to the right, and Irv slid to the left.

"Can I help with that?" he belted out.

The man looked up, startled. "Where the hell did you come from? And who the hell are you?" he asked.

"Joe Devlin. First day on the job. Just got my paperwork done and they told me to come out here and help you with this load. Guess you didn't see me."

"New guy? What happened to Frank?"

"Got me. The boss man just said to get my ass out here and help if I want to get paid."

"They never tell me shit around here," lamented the cargo attendant. "Don't just stand there—grab an end. We are going to need to push this a few feet over this way to get the fork on it and get it out of here."

Irv followed his orders. He had to maintain his cover and at his first chance make a break for it. His plan was to calmly walk away and into the hangar and airport—unless Frank showed up looking for his overalls and phone. Then it was time to run like hell.

They lifted the generator out of the storage area and placed it on the ground next to the airplane. They loaded up more supplies on a cart, probably to transport them into the hangar about fifty yards away. Irv saw a man about two hundred feet away, talking with another member of the ground crew. The man kept glancing over as Irv packed the cart, and now was beginning to slowly saunter over. Probably Frank, ready to help . . . oh, sorry, is all the work done now?

Irv wasn't going to stick around and let this scene play out. He jumped behind the steering wheel of the transport cart and pushed the gas pedal, heading as fast as he could toward the open hangar. He wasn't sure that this was where things went, but it didn't matter. It was an open door, and he could see that the airport concourse was behind it about another hundred yards away.

Security was really tight getting into airports. Irv hoped not so much on getting out. Once inside the hangar, he stopped the cart and ran outside through the far door, looking for an open door into the concourse. After a couple of false steps, he found one. He yanked it open and discovered it opened it to a hallway. Just to his right was an airport security guard sitting at a desk. He looked at Irv.

"End of shift?" he asked.

"Sure enough," said Irv. "Have a good one," he mumbled toward the guard, striding past him with his head lowered, toward a sign pointing to an exit from the gates. Once he got past the guard, he quickened his pace, almost running, while hoping no one was following.

He was safely inside the concourse now, and regular passengers were milling about, checking baggage and getting ready to move through security to their gates. It wasn't super busy. Irv was relieved to be back among civilization. *The more people the better now*, he thought.

He looked behind him. There was no one following. He let out a big breath, winded as he was from his sprint down the hallway. *Where the hell am I?* he wondered.

He looked around the concourse and saw a convenience store a stone's throw away, so he walked over and took a look at the newspapers sitting on a table just inside. *The Sioux City Journal*. He was in Rapid City, South Dakota.

There was food on display on another counter just a few feet away. He was hungry and tired, and he should eat something while it was in front of him. But when he reached for his pocket, immediately he realized that he was still wearing Frank's overalls. Underneath it was his hospital costume, sans wallet. He had two dollars left in cash in his pants pocket—the change from his cab ride to the campground in Albuquerque. It was enough for a candy bar and a bottle of water.

The eagle had landed, and he was alive. He was a bit worse for the wear, but far better than his pal Jose. Tired as he was, Irv was anxious to learn where Jose went. Frank's phone should tell them. He smiled. *I made it.* It was time to call Lance on the pay phone just a few feet away.

Chapter Seventy-Five

Johnny Finds His Way in Congress

Congressman John Gibson had built a solid political career in Congress through the 1980s and 1990s and into the early new millennium. While he was flattered by the attention he found for being a longstanding incumbent, he was most proud of making a difference for people in practical ways.

Johnny had come into the role wanting to continue his adventuring, by using the office as a perch to explore people and life. Soon, he had questioned whether this was enough reason to continue doing so and discovered that he also needed to contribute to the public good while living his adventure.

He also decided to remain an independent who would vote his judgment and conscience on the issues before him, rather than follow the edicts of either of the major political parties. Instead of spending over half his time fundraising for campaigns, he prioritized meeting with those who shared his intent to make a positive difference. This was how he set his daily meeting schedule, not on the basis of the need for money or political connections.

Sometimes his pursuit of good would intersect with the opportunity of major public policy initiatives. Buoyed by his experience with the patient dumping issue of 1986, he learned how to look for these openings. He was best when his vote really mattered to the outcome, as this gave him political leverage to help shape the solution.

Since these legislative opportunities were so rare, he focused on the benefits he could offer more regularly through constituent relations. Early on, he was surprised by how much influence an inquiry from a congressman, or even his or her office, could have on others. It was common sense to use this power to help, and he made sure this was something his office staff did very well.

After his personal revelation in Utah, Johnny concluded that he should build an even stronger process for handling constituent relations in his office. He hired staff for their ability to investigate and solve constituent problems, and built a reputation as one of the best problem solvers for people in the Capitol. It was one person or family at a time for most interventions, but it was effective. Added together over time, he had helped thousands over the course of his congressional career.

Whatever he was doing also got him reelected—without much competition. The longer he was around, the more he was building power to help people. Soon, he was in a position where he, in theory, should also be able to force more big public policy initiatives that could help even more people and for a longer period of time.

One early example of this, he thought, was the effort to pursue comprehensive health care reform at the start of the Clinton presidency. Johnny thought this was going somewhere, and put energy into moving it forward. But it had bogged down and was politically dead as a topic until the political winds substantially shifted.

Johnny had looked for another way then to affect policy in a broad way, bringing his closest friends and advisors to help him find a path to do this. Their meeting had focused on the social determinants of health and a series of practical action areas that he might adopt as his own.

It is too much for any one congressman, he thought. *We need to whittle this down in some way.* One option was to adopt a single area and devote himself to it, or even a few limited issues within an action area. But he wanted to reinforce the importance of all the action areas. He asked whether there was some way to touch upon them all through some other filter that might still focus his energy?

Chris Jones, father of his political consultant Nancy Jones, had one such idea. What he shared was simple enough, in a damning sort of way. He explained that virtually all of the action areas and the specific health problems shared one trait—that there were health disparities. Minority groups across society fared much worse than the dominant white population, and these gaps were most pronounced when examined through the filters of race and ethnicity.

Johnny's group discussed these health disparities at length. Most were shocked by how stark the differences were, and how little policymakers and the public knew about them. It would be of major service to highlight this issue for all to see. If Johnny could also pass legislation that would attack disparities, even better.

This became Johnny's focus as a congressman after the Clinton reform failure. His aim was to elevate the existence of the health disparities and the need to eliminate them. There were some opportunities for specific policy interventions over the years and Johnny would press hard to pass them into law.

For example, he was able to add a requirement that all hospitals identify race as part of their publicly mandated patient information systems and disclosures. Many hospitals didn't even know the racial profile of their patients, which was part of their ignorance of systemic racial barriers within their institutions. Johnny had heard several hospital CEOs claim that "what gets counted is what gets done" in health care, and he called their bluff with respect to disparities and care.

Another example was Johnny's work with the Native American community across the nation to make reforms to the Indian Health Service. He worked to bring more resources to tribes outside of the limitations of this agency, through recognition of tribes as sovereign nations within America's borders.

Johnny knew these legislative improvements were small and incremental steps and that far more would need to be done before there was a remote chance that health disparities would be eliminated. But these policies were a start, and helped raise the issue as a matter of serious national concern. His advisors also encouraged him to keep an eye out for the moment when broader health reform might be a viable topic in Congress. Then he could help push this, while also trying to insert bigger ideas for eliminating health disparities into any such legislation.

Surprisingly, such an opportunity arose in 2008. Barack Obama had won the election, and notwithstanding a major recession hitting the country at the end of his predecessor's term, there was hope and possibility in the nation's capital. President Obama seemed intent on trying to get a national health reform proposal passed into law in his first term.

Johnny could see it was going to be a contentious battle to get major health reform passed into law. The Democrats would need every vote they could find, including Johnny's. Republicans had pledged their opposition and would fight it with everything they had.

Johnny knew this was the case when the Republicans rejected the administration's proposal to build their bill around a Massachusetts plan implemented by then Republican Governor Mitt Romney. The plan essentially relied on private health plans to provide an almost universal access to health coverage for the people of that state, rather than a government-run system like Canada or Britain.

This point became almost irrelevant to the Republican opposition campaign. The proposal was described as a government takeover of health care and translated into scare messages. Public opinion for and against the proposal was soon formed through ideologic campaigns spread by conservatives and liberals, with no common ground in between.

Most of the public fight was about health coverage—who had it, who didn't, and how it might be provided to them. Johnny now knew that the problems with health care were much more than that. And he wanted the legislation to specifically address the issue of health disparities.

Johnny's major suggestion was to have Congress set annual health goals for the nation. The idea was taken from his acquaintance with Harvard's health policy director and father to his campaign manager Nancy Jones, Christopher Jones. The goals would establish national accountability and simple quantitative metrics for achieving these goals; congressional health spending would focus on them, and bureaucrats and politicians would not be able to hide from the fundamental question of whether these investments were making a difference.

Johnny argued that one of these goals must relate to health disparities—documenting their existence in data and requiring their closing over time, toward elimination.

Much to Johnny's great disappointment, his idea was not included in the final proposal passed by Congress. The bill did pass Congress, with Johnny's positive vote. This vote was needed, but was not enough to change the provisions he found problematic.

Implementation of the new law was slow, especially in light of aggressive Republican opposition, which was immediate, strong, and effective, and so began the health wars of the next decade.

Johnny was disappointed. The final Obamacare product was, on balance, a marginal improvement but hardly what he was looking for—major and effective change of the American health care system that would make a positive difference in American lives. An opportunity was lost.

There had to be a better way of creating change—and a better change—in general and with respect to health care. He was determined to find it and implement it. He was also getting more and more impatient with the slow pace of real change.

Much of this was driven by a personal tragedy that showed him problems that were very real for people, also within the realm of one of the Action Areas suggested by his friends years ago—Avoiding Addictions. If only he had taken on this as his priority, perhaps his loss could been avoided.

It was drug abuse that reared its ugly head. The issue was not illegal drugs, but prescription drugs. Johnny did not have the addiction gene. While he would on occasion use various substances for personal entertainment or medical reasons, he would not get hooked, and would go months, or even years, without them.

His wife was not wired the same way. The two were happily enough married, though the reality was that Johnny only saw Reena occasionally. She refused to move to DC, and Johnny was there or traveling much of the time. She was tethered to home with her two children, but when they grew up and went off to college, she struggled to find new ways to occupy her time.

One new endeavor was skiing. Reena was an avid skier in her youth and enjoyed finding that she still had a talent for it. Then she hurt her knee on the slopes and needed surgery. It was a painful injury, and her physician prescribed opioids as part of her recovery. He ordered fifty pills for her, when she really only needed enough for two or three days—more like ten pills.

She took them all and got hooked. The pain itself had subsided, but she needed more painkillers and figured out how to get them. First she did so through other doctors, and then through the black market. Johnny was in DC when this took root, and he did not realize how deeply she had slipped into this chasm. He thought something was amiss when he talked to her on the phone but could not figure out what.

Before he was able to get home and intervene, Reena overdosed and died. Johnny struggled to understand what had happened. At first, he blamed himself, but the more he dug, the more he discovered that this was an all too common problem across America.

He had always figured things would work out for the best. Now they hadn't. He desperately wanted to do something about this and struggled to identify what it could be. He was no longer certain it should be as a congressman. Maybe it was time to stop living his adventure and approach life more like others. But how?

Chapter Seventy-Six

HealthMost Managers Meeting

Sam Bridgewater stepped off the elevator and ambled over to a reception desk that was at least fifty feet wide, shimmering in polished dark walnut, with a single receptionist. She looked tiny behind the massive piece of furniture and the similarly massive HealthMost logo painted on the wall behind her.

Sam had been to HealthMost Corporate Headquarters many times and was confronted as a stranger each and every time. Other than board members and VIPs, everyone was greeted the same at HealthMost Headquarters—as a potential enemy.

He told the receptionist that he was there for a meeting with the executive staff and Mr. Thrust. The receptionist checked the schedule on her computer and Bridgewater's driver's license. Once his identity was confirmed, her hesitant attitude toward him shifted immediately, and she offered coffee and a comfortable seat in the reception area while he waited for an escort into the internal sanctum.

John Mayweather, administrative intern for HealthMost for the year, was assigned to escort Bridgewater to the board conference room. He bantered with Bridgewater along the way, asking about Sam's background and talking up his own experience. Sam was brief in his responses. He wasn't here to network with underlings, but to find out if he had any new assignments from the boss. The HealthMost contract had become the bulk of his client base and revenues, so much so that his status as a lead partner at the lobbying firm was tied to its success or failure. The partners had wanted to create a diversified client base, but the riches from representing HealthMost had derailed that plan.

Normally, internal meetings were held in smaller conference rooms far less ornate than the one Sam walked into. The view of the lake and city below was spectacular, but would be a temptation to avoid with Thrust in attendance. Sam chose a seat with the worst view to the outside.

There were about twenty-five people in attendance—a larger crowd than normal, and probably why this room was booked for it. John introduced Sam to attendees, many of whom he had never met. He realized that today's meeting included not just the executive team and vice presidents for HealthMost but a number of director-level positions.

Chief Operating Officer Lane Stevens called the group to order, and all took their seats around the large table. Stevens sat at one corner of the rectangular table on the lake window side. Noticeably vacant was the head seat immediately next to him. Bridgewater knew this was Thrust's chair and that, at a minimum, he would not appear until at least five minutes had passed.

This time it was longer than that. COO Stevens told the group this was an annual review of HealthMost's national business strategy and then overviewed the plan. He used a large map on the wall to identify all of HealthMost's business holdings—hospitals, nursing homes, clinics, pharmacies, and more across the nation, more in the West than the East. The different assets were color coded, and if a particular holding was discussed, its light would flash on the map. Stevens also outlined the corporation's core business strategy cutting across all lines of business—aggregation, horizontal and vertical control, and price maximization.

There were a few questions from the attendees, which Stevens fielded with the help of Chief Financial Officer Haynes Dickson. Most came from staff who likely knew the answer, but were trying to get noticed by the executives. Sam knew that this would end once Thrust appeared. Favorable impressions were made only through performance and success, and it was a dangerous career move to speak unless spoken to.

One new hire asked a question about HealthMost's not-for-profit status and the implications of recent congressional action on this and their business strategy. It was something about the need for local community benefit plans and coordinated planning with local political jurisdictions. Sam knew generally of the origins of this question—he had gotten an amendment inserted into the proposed legislation that took all the regulatory enforcement teeth out of the notion, and he knew it was now just a paper exercise.

Stevens asked the director of Community Benefit to provide a brief answer to this question. She did, while most of the people around the table seemed to find humor in the notion of their business planning including consideration of their community obligations.

A couple of minutes into her answer, Richard Thrust entered the room and took his seat at the head of the table. The director of Community Benefit stopped in mid-sentence. Any smiles or table conversations ended the second he strode in. Everyone sat up in their seat a little straighter and kept their eyes focused on Thrust.

As usual, Richard Thrust got right to the point—meaning *his* point, and whatever point he wanted to get out of the meeting. "I assume Mr. Stevens has briefed you on the corporate business plan. There are really no changes from the strategy we reviewed last year, with the exception of our new joint venture with ALI Insurance. We will brief you on that at the end of this meeting.

"Now, what I want are some explanations with regard to failures in some of our regions. That is why we have invited our regional directors to this meeting. Most of these failures are unacceptable, and I want to know what we are going to do to fix matters. We will do this by region, starting with the Northeast Division."

With that, Bridgewater sat through four hours of review of business failures identified by Thrust and the executive team, an array of poor outcomes or in some cases blunders. The staff in the room were attentive to each one, most likely from fear that something in their sphere of responsibility would be flagged. Bridgewater noticed how granular many of the infractions were and how much Thrust knew about each of them. He was a smart cookie, of that there could be no doubt. And controlling seemed to be too fuzzy a description of his total command of his health care empire.

Sam was there to identify anything that might need lobbying help or special assistance in DC. Thankfully, there were not too many of these today. There was some special state funding that would need greasing of state legislators, a court decision that would need to be overturned, and a member of Congress who would need a stern lecture. It was hard to pay attention to the rest of the criticisms with such little action of direct interest to his world. He was anxious for the meeting to end so he could be out of physical contact and in view of Thrust.

Sam paid closer attention when communities in key congressional districts were highlighted, and his recent interventions in Washington State made the topic of HealthMost's Shelton Community Hospital jump out at him. Thrust was leading the summary of the problem in this case. It was a community hospital that they had bought last year, with a plan to close it in favor of patient referrals to their larger and far more profitable hospital in Tacoma.

SCH was still open, and its margins were dropping. It lost money from operations last year, but had a small net profit because of property tax proceeds. The company financial projections had noted an anticipated major reduction in the property tax receipts this year, and Thrust wanted to know what was being done to preserve corporate profits. The regional director for the Pacific Northwest noted that the Shelton Hospital had been purchased as part of a larger strategy of reducing the number of rural hospitals across the state. It was a Certificate of Need state, which required new hospitals to get state approval from regulators before opening, and the longer plan was to raise prices across the state once the number of hospitals had been reduced. They could control the Certificate of Need process and become price makers once competition had been eliminated.

"Yes, I know the strategy—I developed it," interrupted Thrust. "That does not excuse any losses. I insist on profits from all of our business units, and if we can't get them from the people in charge of these units, then we will find new people who can."

The quiet room got even quieter. Thrust had blown up a few times over the course of the meeting, but this was the first time he had stated the obvious—those not playing his game would be shot.

"In reading your report, I noted that the property tax receipts come from a special purpose government—a special purpose of a 'hospital district,'" Thrust continued. "Yet, I also see that the funds from these taxes are shared with another entity, and they get over $250,000. How can that be?"

The regional director explained as quickly and clearly as he could that the public hospital district levy was created by this other entity, the Mason Health Foundation, and it had given the local hospital its share as a way to build community unity. The transaction had occurred before

HealthMost's takeover, though the hospital leaders involved described it as a positive and generous gesture by the foundation.

Thrust was having none of this. "Bullshit. What fools. That money should be ours. All of it. Under any circumstances. But if you expect me to sit here and accept that local idiocy and your incompetence to allow it to be stolen by others, that is not going to happen when the hospital operation itself is projected to be in the red this year."

The regional director knew he was in deep trouble. "Is there something in particular you want me to do, Mr. Thrust?"

"Well, first, fire the hospital administrator. I don't need anyone in place who is so stupid that they couldn't see that this was an unacceptable situation. And change out our community board. They don't have any say about what we do, but it will be a good lesson for them. It will also make it easier when we get to the point of closing their hospital. I doubt they even see that coming, but let's make sure they know who is in control."

"Yes, sir."

"And while you are at it, I want you to do something about this Mason Health Foundation. Get me a report on the money they get and what they do with it. More importantly, I want to know what happens if they go out of business. I would assume that their property tax receipts would go to our hospital. Confirm that is the case, or figure out how to make sure it is. And then, do what you must to get them out of the way."

"You mean work a deal to integrate them within our operations in the area?"

"No, I mean shut them down. And I don't care if you have to take out ten nuns and a pack of Girl Scouts to do it. It is our money and I want it where it belongs."

"Yes, sir."

Bridgewater had been listening closely to Thrust's attack. It amazed him that a couple of hundred thousand dollars would be such a flashpoint for a corporation reaping hundreds of millions in profits each year. Thrust alone probably made that much himself each day. But he also knew that Thrust was as vicious over controlling expenses as revenues, and Sam's first priority was to preserve his hefty lobbying contract. That was worth a couple of hundred thousand each month and more.

"One more thing. We will be out there after Labor Day for a special congressional hearing. Bridgewater is working on that for us. I want this local property tax situation fixed by then, or consider yourself terminated. Do I make myself clear?"

"Yes," answered the regional director. It was time to do something, anything Thrust commanded—or look for new work.

The meeting went on to the dissection of failures at other corporate sites, until wrapping up with a presentation, as promised, on the HealthMost-ALI joint venture. There was not much to that presentation, mostly an overview of what was described as the integration of an insurance function into part of their business operations. The main point in bringing it up was drilled through a number of times to attendees—if anything related to ALI and this joint venture came up in their areas or regions, they were to report it immediately to Chief Operating Officer Stevens. They should do so no matter how seemingly insignificant it was.

The message had been delivered on all of Thrust's intended fronts, and the meeting was adjourned. Sam thought there might be some further sub-conversations arising from the meeting, especially with regard to the handful of assignments with his name attached. He was having none of that though. He wanted to get the hell out of Dodge. He had suffered enough for one day to earn his substantial keep. They could find him by telephone, where he could pretend that he wasn't as deeply attached to the devil as he knew he was.

Chapter Seventy-Seven

Irv Makes His Escape in Rapid City

Irv placed a collect call to the telephone number Lance Givens had provided him. Lance answered, accepting the charges. *Who did that anymore?* wondered Irv. It was another thing lost to the advance of technology and cell phones.

"Irv, so good to hear your voice. As soon as I got your message, I've been waiting by the telephone for what I hoped would be your call. Where the heck are you? How are you? What did you learn?"

"Whoa, Lance! You are moving a little too fast for my tired brain. It's been a long and crazy few days. Happy to tell you that I am calling from the airport in Rapid City, South Dakota. It looks like it is about 11:30 in the morning here, and I think it is Wednesday. Is that right?"

"Yes. It is 1:30 here in DC. How did you get there?"

"First things first. Did you track the numbers I left you?"

"Yes. I pulled in one of our interns who has a tech background, and he showed me how to do it. I told him it had to do with a national security matter, so I couldn't tell him why I needed it. We got a signal to the phone number and the ID for the phone, and are tracking both as we speak. Right now, it is still in Rapid City, and at the airport, apparently near you."

"Great. We've got to keep track of this every step of the way; do not let it out of your sight, Lance. Are you sure this is a secure line? If so, I will tell you some more about what happened and what I learned."

"Yes, completely secure; Capitol Police assured me that no one could monitor our call without it being known by us. Tell me all you can and then let's figure out how to get you back to DC so we can talk with the senator."

THE THEORY OF IRV

Irv shared the highlights of his journey over the past few days, leaving out a few details in the interest of brevity and wanting to cut to the chase of why they must track the cell phone. He experienced a surge of adrenaline as he recounted the story and started to get emotional, remembering the great danger of the past few days. He found the energy to give Lance a necessary report, but he could also tell that he was getting very tired.

"Unbelievable, Irv. You know, it is what we thought might be going on when we reviewed the files, but it seemed too crazy to be true. But it is. Anything else you need to make sure I know for now? If not, I suggest we figure out how to get you out of there—and let me find the senator and update him. He has been asking about you and will be relieved to know you are okay."

"No, that should be enough to get things moving. And I need to get moving too. It is not safe for me to stay here too long. It is going to take something for me to get back there, or anywhere. I don't have any money, credit cards, or even identification."

"How about if we come to you, then?"

"Probably a better play. But let's not do it in Rapid City. No need to create a trail to you if they figure out my deception. And I would rather be one more step away from these people. How about I find a way to get to Denver, and you two fly there. Then you can get me to Albuquerque. I should probably let my dad know that I am alive—he must be wondering why I am not back from my camping trip yet."

"Deal. Let's meet at the downtown Hilton in Denver. I will book a room for you using a fake name. Just in case you get there before us. Ask at the desk for me—I will tell them that we are expecting you. Call me or the senator's cell phone if we are not already there. Anything else you need?"

"Just a fake name. How about Jose Upurass? This is just what we are going to do once we figure out where my friend Jose goes to next."

"Roger that. I will get us a flight out to Denver this afternoon."

They hung up and Irv looked around the concourse. He had one last task before he could finally get some sleep. *I need a ride to Denver.* He remembered he still had on the blue overalls and was dressed as an airline worker. No one would think much about it if he wandered down to the cargo area outside of security and waited there for a truck transporting air cargo. He would catch a ride to the central shipping depot, and then find one to Denver with a freight shipment. There should be plenty.

It should work, he thought. If not, he would have to hitchhike to Denver, and he wasn't sure he could stay awake long enough to get a ride. He chuckled to himself. *Sure hope I don't end up in some truck with Jose again!*

Chapter Seventy-Eight

Congressman Gibson Wonders about the Senate

For most of the decade following the passage of Obamacare in 2010, John Gibson remained a congressman, working toward public good in this role much as he had for the past twenty years. When the Congress flipped control in 2012—and again as a political consequence of comprehensive health care reform—his opportunities to do so in the arena of health care shifted to the agencies implementing the law more than Congress.

The election of the most recent president in 2016 had taken that option away. Indeed, it made doing much of anything close to impossible, even Johnny's new passion to do something about prescription drug abuse and the opioid crisis. It was a rude awakening. As much as Johnny and many others had been quick to criticize government processes and politicians in the recent past, there was an entirely new level of incoherence, incompetence, and insanity under way in the halls of government.

Johnny reflected on where things stood, then and now. It had been a good ride for twenty-five years. He had chosen his vocation well, and felt that, so far, he had done a decent enough job of being useful as a politician—especially as an independent politician in a nation where party affiliation defined the ground rules. He had figured out how to help constituents in smaller and more tactical ways. His constituent service in particular had helped thousands of Washingtonians, and others, to navigate the landmines of the federal and state government. And, occasionally, he was even able to advance policy change.

Still, the Theory of Irv told him there was more to be done. His wife's death was gnawing at him. This yearning to do more took flight with the resignation of the senior United States senator for Washington State. Senator Lute Johansen was nearing eighty, and plans were already afoot to anoint his successor within Democratic political circles.

These plans had accelerated with revelations that the senator was prone to grope female staff when he had a few too many at legislative receptions. Once, this was standard fare in the nation's capital and hardly worthy of attention. Reporters, who knew of reputations and even explicit cases of abuse, would not disclose back in the day. It was considered a personal and private subject and would remain that way in the old political culture of DC, and most state capitals, for some time.

Thankfully, a combination of decency and opportunism by new entrants to the news world took the walls of secrecy down around these abuses. Senator Johansen was suddenly facing criticism around his longtime behavior and only made it worse by arguing it was not important to his job. Criticism turned quickly into pressure to resign, and he relented in a tearful press conference.

A special election for his Senate seat was put on the fall ballot in 2018. It was but a few months out and Democrat leaders thought that this short timeline would make it hard for Republicans to field a competitive candidate. Predictions were that it would be a low turnout election, with no presidential race and no juicy public initiatives that would get a lot of people to the ballot box. These operatives believed their chosen candidate would win, and then have time to establish the advantage of incumbency in preparation for a full reelection campaign in another two years.

Johnny checked in with his campaign consultant and friend Nancy Jones to see what she thought about the Senate race. Nancy promised to do some fast research and get back with him. They met in her office near the Pike Place Market on a Saturday morning. Both were dressed casually for their weekend meeting, Johnny in shorts and a short sleeve shirt and Nancy in shorts and a golf shirt.

Nancy greeted Johnny at the door of her office suite and gave him a big hug. "Come on in, my friend." She pointed him to a couch in the large waiting room. There was no one else in the office today, so they could meet in the most comfortable spot.

"Thanks, Nancy. Always good to see you. How's sis?"

"Oh, she's doing great. She was excited that I was meeting with you today. You really won her over by joining her team for the Breast Cancer Run last summer."

"I was happy to do it—and she was so enthusiastic. Some of my best friends lost women in their lives to the big C. But that race—it almost killed me. I had to walk the last couple of miles."

"My family and friends too, Congressman."

Johnny wasn't sure if she was referring to cancer or the race, but decided to let it pass. He had something important in mind and wanted to get to it.

"So, maybe that is a good place to begin, Nancy. You helped me get started in this political business, and I probably wouldn't have gotten past first base without your help. You never really asked me why I wanted to run when I started."

"It was never all that important to me, Johnny. You had a good heart, and that is what I look for in my clients. Or, at the least, the ones who can't pay me very well."

"That's just it, Nancy. It is starting to matter to me that I didn't really have an answer then. Don't get me wrong—I got one after. But then, I just thought it would be a great way to meet people and experience life. It was a job, even a career, that floated my boat in terms of being with people."

"Better answer than I get from 90 percent of my clients, Johnny. Usually they think they are god's gift to humankind. And covet power and ego massages. That's what I mean about a good heart—without that too, these political jobs are more a breeding ground for narcissists."

Johnny got up and looked out Nancy's office window. She was on the fourth floor, looking out over the city streets. It was getting busy out there; a sunny spring day in Seattle would bring out everybody.

"You remember the trip that Irv and I took a number of years back—the Utah hike."

"How could I forget? You two not only survived, but helped to bring to justice some ornery characters who were robbing and killing tourists across the Four Corners area. We even used it in one of your campaign ads. It was great stuff. Of course, I had to leave out the part about the magic mushroom ride you two were on."

"Did you notice any change back then?"

"Of course. Who wouldn't be changed by almost dying and walking seventy-five miles across the middle of nowhere?"

"I didn't just mean by coming close to our end. Toward the end of it, when we thought it really was the end for us, we both reached some conclusions about what we should be doing with our lives."

"Yes, I could tell something happened out there. To Irv too. You were both reluctant to talk much about that part of the hike, though you did tell me a little of the tale. Mary Beth was really the one who spotted the big change. She said that both of you had more of an edge. Not in a bad way, and you were both still the same—looking for adventure in all the wrong and right places. She said it was more that the two of you now had a purpose in life. After she described it that way to me, it became very evident as I watched you."

"Funny thing, I don't think either one of us ever thought much about how people might see us after that. We both sort of thought that it was just an inside karma shift that no one else would understand. So much for that!"

Johnny continued. "The important thing for today's chat is to know that this is what is driving me to ask the question about the Senate seat. I've done some good things since the hike. I can see that—probably far more than I had ever done before then. It also doesn't seem enough now. Reena's death is part of this. Some might think that being a congressman would be a great way to make things happen, but after a decade, I mostly see what I *can't* do. What I couldn't do for even my own wife. When I look at the Senate, and that vacant seat, I think there might be much more to be done."

"John, I won't argue with you about that. But you should know how much you have done for good in your House role. More than almost any of my other clients. Now, the reality of the situation is that the Senate—and this Senate seat at this time—offers some additional possibilities.

"Let's talk politics and tactics—that's what you asked me to take a look at," Nancy continued. "The short of it is that you have a chance, a small chance, of winning a Senate race. At least this Senate race. You've got great name recognition in your district and across much of western

Washington. But not so much in the eastern side of the state. It's not negative—you are just not known. There won't be a huge turnout for the election, and presuming you will have two other opponents, one D and one R, you will have to get a chunk of this eastern demographic if you expect to win."

"Could I?"

"Again, the theoretical answer is yes. We did some testing with focus groups and you played pretty well. Being independent helped with some of them, but the real difference maker is that you seem so different from a regular politician. A chunk of voters would cross their party identification to give you a chance, and there might be enough in a low turnout election to just get you over the finish line."

"I hear a big 'but' coming."

"For sure. The election is only a couple of months away, and you don't have much time to make an impression. What's worse, you don't have the resources to do this, at least in the traditional way."

"You mean ads, especially on TV."

"Correct. It would take millions to buy the time, and the other reality is that the Rs and Ds have bought up most of the available time already."

"So is that a no?"

"It is a big 'it depends.' You have always been an atypical client of mine. You've even humored me by allowing me to try out some creative ways to do political campaigns into the twenty-first century." Nancy was referring to her interest in building a state-of-the-art capacity to run campaigns through digital technology. They had deployed test runs of this in Johnny's reelection campaigns for the past decade.

"Sure. It made sense, and it was also fun. Are you saying we need more of that this time?"

"I am saying that is all we can do. These digital campaigns can be relatively inexpensive, and quick to deploy. But they are really untested, other than in presidential campaigns. Whether they can work in a race like this is just a guess. Most of my colleagues think it is a foolish idea."

"What do you think?" asked Johnny.

"I think it could work, if one had the right product. That would be you. And the product was okay with taking a flyer on such an approach."

Johnny had sat down in his chair while she was talking. He got back up. "Nancy, this product is willing to fly if you are."

Nancy got up and hugged him. "Ooh, I am so happy you are saying that. I thought you would. I've got some stuff to show you. We need to move quickly, so I hope you like it."

Johnny and Nancy stood up and moved to her office so he could look at several draft political ads Nancy had on her computer. "Just one thing, Nancy. If I should crash, do you have any other ideas for what I can do next?"

She laughed. "A topic for another day, my dear. And let's face it, the odds are high that you will eventually crash in this venture. The real question is when."

Chapter Seventy-Nine

Irv Meets His Friends in Denver

Irv's plan to hitch a ride by truck to Denver worked like a charm. He got a ride to the freight depot outside the Rapid City airport and soon found a truck taking a shipment of grain to the Denver stockyards, departing Rapid City midafternoon.

The truck ride was a long one, and Irv made his way to the Denver Hilton from the freight yard about midnight. He had tossed his overalls in the garbage at the truck depot, and was looking pretty rough in his soiled jeans and T-shirt. He smelled awful, a combination of sweat, grime, and grease. He hoped hotel security would let him in—looking at his reflection in the glass door of its entrance, and sniffing under his armpits, he wasn't sure he would if roles were reversed.

He had no trouble, though. The doorman was on alert that he might be arriving and had instructions to immediately usher him to registration. The night clerk was also ready for him and placed a call on his telephone. Johnny and Lance were there and expecting him in the penthouse suite as soon as he arrived. The doorman guided him up to the suite, asking if he had any luggage. "I don't think so." Irv laughed.

The elevator took him up twenty floors, and when the doors opened, he could see Lance waiting by the open door to the suite. They shook hands, and Lance led him into the large space. Pacing around with a phone to his ear was Johnny, standing in the middle of a plush living room. Seeing Irv, he put down the phone and gave his friend a big hug. Irv could see he was crying. Only then did Irv realize just how crazy this whole mission was, and how grateful he was that it was over.

Johnny grabbed him by his shoulders, looking down at him from his six-foot, five-inch frame. "Don't do that again, brother," he exclaimed. "I can't believe I went along with this nutty plan. You could have been killed."

"There were more than a few times over the last several days that I was thinking the same thing! But I learned how to make the best of it from a master. You!"

They both laughed. "Come on in, get comfortable. We brought in a bunch of food for you in case you are hungry. Or a drink. Or sleep. Or whatever you want."

"I had a short nap on the truck ride here. But I really could use a trip to the bathroom. I've got some Alpo to get out of my system."

Lance and Johnny looked at him curiously; this was a detail he had left out of his report to Lance.

"And I really am hungry. Let me get cleaned up a bit and then let's catch up. I've got a lot to tell you, and I am really hoping that you've got an update on Jose."

They pointed toward the bathroom. Irv strode in and used the toilet, and then eyeballed a large walk-in shower across the room. He turned on the water, undressed, and got in, letting the water run extra hot while standing underneath the showerhead. The hot water was refreshing as it ran across his dirty hair and beard. *God, this feels good*, he thought.

He toweled off and put on a fancy robe hanging on a hook in the wall next to the shower. Walking back out to the living room, he beat a straight line to the food in the small kitchen. "Don't mind if I help myself to some of this." He grabbed a plate and filled it with cheeses, crackers, vegetables, and fruit. The plate was overflowing with food as he moved toward a table in front of the couch and placed it down.

"Now, where is that minibar?" he asked.

"No, my friend, we are not screwing around with the minibar. I stopped off and got you this bottle of bourbon when we arrived. Isn't this your favorite?" Johnny pointed to a bottle of Woodford, oat grain.

"Yes, it is. Except for Pappy's of course. Gee, I thought you cared about me and would get me a bottle of that!"

"Let's not get crazy, Irv. A senator can only do so much."

Irv poured himself a large glass of bourbon over two ice cubes. Johnny and Lance joined him in a drink, and they toasted. "To conspiracies uncovered," offered Johnny.

The Theory of Irv

"Here, here," said Irv and Lance in unison.

They sat down on the couch and a side chair next to it. It was time to provide an in-person report about his field trip. Irv slowly reviewed the events of the past several days, trying to remember every detail this time around. Johnny and Lance would occasionally interrupt him with questions, helping him to recall even more details. It was time to be thorough.

"And then I hitched a ride to Denver and found you in this hotel. Now you know it all. What else happened while I was gone?"

"Well, the Seahawks won their Monday night game. But you are probably more curious about anything on our little case here. Lance has a bit of an update for you."

Lance offered up what he had. "So, one thing I did was check on the name Jose Rodriguez in the ALI files and our special setup from immigration. I did find a reference to him in the ALI network, actually a bunch of them since it is such a common name. But one did have a 'U' code. It might be him. On the immigration data network, I found a number of Jose Rodriguezes who had been deported over the past year, but none over the past month. All that seems in sync with what we have been theorizing since we first went through the data. I was going to do a search for your alias, but thought better about it since it might have tipped off someone that we are connected to you."

"Good call," said Irv. "I think we know we will find me in the system, and where. I am hoping you've got an update on Jose's whereabouts?"

"Yes, let me get the latest." Lance looked at his cell phone and tapped a few keys. "Like I shared before, we tracked the body leaving the Rapid City airport about 11 p.m. It has been in flight for most of the night. What is it, about three in the morning here now? About fifteen minutes ago, it landed. Surprise, surprise—in Moses Lake, Washington."

"Bingo. This is really starting to fit together now," said Irv. "And now we can learn what I couldn't that night outside of that airport—where the bodies go from there."

"So far, I can't tell you much. It is still at the airport, or maybe just right outside of it now that I look a little closer." Lance was expanding the size of the image on his cell phone screen. "Probably at the storage unit outside of the airport, getting sprayed with a hint of potato derivatives. And some agent that would mimic severe flu symptoms like the presence of a virus that causes lesions."

Johnny could see that his friend was wearing down and needed some sleep. "I don't think there is much more for us to figure out tonight—until we know where Jose goes next. Probably good for all of us to get a little sleep and noodle this over tomorrow with a little more information and rested brains."

"Getting more sleep sounds like a good idea to me," said Irv, realizing that the adrenaline rush of seeing his friends was wearing thin. "I am starting to crash again. For all that time I spent lying around a bed the last few days, I didn't seem to get a lot of rest. I have heard that about hospitals. Guess it's true. So, which room is mine?"

"Oh, my friend, you get the master suite. Nothing but the best for our master detective." Johnny pointed toward a doorway adjacent to the living room. "Let's pick it up tomorrow, whenever you get up. I will also let Mary Beth know you are okay—she has been texting me every day since you left for Albuquerque, wondering what was up and where you are. I think that girl still has a thing for you."

"I sure hope so. See you in the morning." Irv saluted Johnny and Lance and moved to his room, settling into the plush king-size bed. It felt good—really good. But hearing how much Mary Beth had fretted over his whereabouts felt even better.

Chapter Eighty

Johnny Runs for the Senate

Johnny announced his candidacy for the vacant Washington State Senate seat as an independent and got his name listed on the official ballot along with the Democrat and Republican candidates. Nancy, true to her word, unleashed one of the more atypical Senate campaigns in the history of American politics.

She figured the Democrats would in particular go after him. To counter whatever bad press they might generate, they repurposed the set of Rainier Beer-like ads they had run in the 1980s, making fun of politics and putting Johnny in a starring role. They came up with another ad parlaying his name "Gibson" and the quality of these guitars as just what Washington State needed to make beautiful music in the nation's capital. They didn't actually pay to run many of these ads, instead hoping that their cleverness would end up with free air time and viral spread on the Internet.

On the issues, Johnny ran a populist campaign emphasizing his role as a champion for regular people encountering government problems. He talked of finding bipartisan solutions to major problems, including health care, and questioned whether any Republican or Democrat could do the same in these divided times.

He was open about the passing of his wife and his intent to do something about opioid abuse. It was a most personal message that communicated his heart to voters who did not know him. It moved many.

The real campaign was the digital networking undertaken by Nancy and her staff. They based their network on those she knew could be counted on to be passionately supportive of Johnny—those who had been helped through his constituent services. She was right—it made him thousands of friends; friends who were willing to go vote in an otherwise unexciting election year and tell their friends and family to do the same.

The election came in a blink. It was a close race. Name recognition and his positive general reputation got Johnny a lot of votes, and others liked and remembered the clever and funny ads when they went to the ballot box. Many more were recruited by the passionate social network supporting Johnny through digital word of mouth and friend sharing. The prospect of a low turnout turned out to be right, but it was Johnny, not the Democrat, who benefitted. He was voted the next senator of Washington State.

Chapter Eighty-One

Irv's New Investigation Plan Forms

Irv awoke from his deep slumber in the main bedroom of the Denver Hilton penthouse suite. It took him a few seconds to remember where he was, as scenes from his several sleepless nights were flashing through his brain. He gathered himself, recognizing that he was now out of danger—at least the immediate kind.

The clock said 4 a.m. He was surprised that he had awoken so early. It had only been a couple of hours ago that he had closed his initial debrief with Johnny and Lance so he could go to bed. It was not too surprising though, since he was generally an early riser. He opened up the curtains and winced at the bright sun pouring into his room from the east. It was already high in the sky. These were the longest days of sunshine of the year, and there were no clouds to be seen on the horizon over the cityscape.

He found new boxer shirts, slacks, and a golf shirt on the dresser, probably compliments of Johnny, and put them on. He was ready to venture out to find coffee and get his thoughts together. It had been quite a few days, and there was much to figure out. First, he really had to pee—a lot, it turned out. He took so long that he moved through the central events of the past few days. He wondered whether the tracking device he had inserted into Jose Rodriguez had reached its final destination by now.

He opened the door of the bedroom and walked a short way to the living room and the adjacent kitchen. To his surprise, Johnny and Lance were already up and dressed, seated at the table in the kitchen and drinking coffee.

"Good morning, sunshine." Johnny beamed. "Good to see you up and about. We were a little worried about you."

"What the hell," offered Irv. "It has only been a few hours. I am kind of surprised to see you two up so early."

Johnny and Lance looked at each other and laughed. "Well, first of all," Lance said, "we are on East Coast time, so it is really six in the morning for us. We are usually knee deep in capital affairs by this time back there."

"That would be burying the headline, though, Irv. You, my friend, slept through all of yesterday. Twenty-five hours of consecutive sleep by our count. We thought we might have to get a cattle prod to arouse you from your slumber. We were just debating whether we should go down to the stockyards and get one."

"No!" exclaimed Irv. "A whole frigging day?" He couldn't believe it. He shifted his gaze to the television in the living room. There was no sound, but the date was splashed across the screen. Sure enough, he had missed a day.

He poured a cup of coffee and sat down at the table between Johnny and Lance. "Amazing. Guess I was kind of tired. What have you two been doing while I've been playing Sleeping Beauty?"

"Oh, there is always something for a senator and his chief of staff to do to keep occupied. Lots of phone calls and emails and texts. Tell you the truth, it was kind of nice to hang out here without any official obligations." Johnny looked pretty relaxed, thought Irv, but then again, he almost always did.

"We also had a lot of time to talk about what to do next with this HealthMost thing," added Lance.

"And what did you figure out?" asked Irv.

"You sure you are ready to dive into that?" asked Johnny.

"What, do you think I need a nap? You two talk and I will find a little something to eat while you catch me up on your thinking." Irv moved to the counter, where he found a couple of hardboiled eggs and more cheese and fruit.

Johnny and Lance filled Irv in on the developments over the last day. There was not a lot to report, but what there was surprised and disturbed him. The tracker in Jose had continued sending its signal as it moved west across Washington State, until finally settling in a spot near the Olympic Mountains, a hundred miles or so short of the Pacific Ocean, as a crow would fly.

All that was at about 10 a.m. yesterday. It didn't move for another two hours, and then went completely dead. Whether the phone ran out of battery juice, or stopped for some other reason, they did not know.

They did a thorough search of the media, traditional and underground, to see if they could pick up any noise about Irv's activities across New Mexico and South Dakota. It was dark; nothing at all to be found. They even contacted a friend with the Federal Aviation Administration to try to get a record of any midnight flights from airports across the Southwest to Rapid City, and then Rapid City to Moses Lake. Nothing. It was like those planes didn't exist. Somebody had friends in high places.

They downloaded a detailed map of Washington State and homed in on the final coordinates of the phone—about five miles east of the small town of Union, on Hood Canal. It didn't seem like there was much there, only a forest road and what looked to be an old dumpsite. As they spoke, Irv was able to vaguely remember this road; he had driven by it several times on the highway north through the Olympic Peninsula when he visited Mary Beth in Shelton.

Oh yes, Mary Beth. Johnny had checked in with her to make sure she knew Irv was okay. He told her part of the story—leaving out the parts that would have made her worry. Irv would have to tell that part himself. Johnny did, however, share that they had tracked another potential body to a site near her and gave her the coordinates.

Johnny asked if she was willing to do a little sleuthing for them. "Of course," said Mary Beth.

"Be really careful," said Johnny.

"Don't talk to me like a girl," said Mary Beth. Off she went to find what there was to see at the dumpsite.

They would need her report to fully evaluate where they were in terms of the investigation of the body. It was essential—this was their only hard evidence of wrongdoing and they couldn't lose it.

Johnny and Lance had done some other research as well. They caught Irv up with what they had learned so far. There were some promising leads, but they would have to wait for additional information.

It was time for all of them to get back to their respective homes and wait for their traplines to get pulled to shore. Once they had these, they would talk by telephone. The evil plan was coming into focus, but they thought themselves still far away from having enough evidence in hand to do very much about it.

Chapter Eighty-Two

Mason Health Foundation Faces Money Troubles

The first two and a half years of the Mason Health Foundation were viewed as a success by most people in Mason County, including the MHF board and Mary Beth. Its programs were successful and were perceived positively by most across the county.

Providing resources to others—cash, recognition, and opportunities to work with others to advance their agendas—helped greatly. Some thought their efforts more valuable than others who also got grants, and occasionally argued they should get more, but relations weren't fractured because of it.

MHF's bigger strength was that it achieved a strong standing with the people of Mason County. The Mason County Healthy Communities Challenge was a big part of that.

Trust also grew from Mary Beth's regular travels across the county. She met hundreds of people through these trips—and most went out of their way to express their gratitude to her and MHF for their approach. They liked that MHF was standing shoulder to shoulder with them in trying to make a difference, rather than being more standoffish like many other organizations.

There was also great benefit from another new program they had started—a Personal Health Navigator service. Mary Beth had taken the idea from Johnny and his constituent relations service in his congressional office. Johnny's staff shared how they had done this, and two members left to join MHF to become Mary Beth's staff.

Their job was to provide caseworker assistance to anyone looking to navigate the complexities of the health care system. They spent much of their time helping partner organizations and people across the county navigate the American health care scene. There were barriers everywhere, and many were nonsensical.

A major area of confusion for many of their clients was their private health coverage options. They just weren't sure what they should sign up for, notwithstanding the online support provided by the federal government. Others were confused around whether they were eligible for government coverage programs. Still others had insurance coverage but were nonplussed as to how to access their benefits. Hundreds of people were using the Navigator Service within months of its startup.

Storm clouds for the Mason Health Foundation were rising in the distance though. The local hospital was one cloud. Appreciation for the $100,000 in property tax receipts had faded, especially after the sale of the hospital to new owners. It was the same system that owned a major tertiary hospital in Tacoma, and it was already clear that the parent corporation, HealthMost, was looking at the local hospital and its tax revenues through a new filter. It wasn't a friendly one.

The local health district also had some jealousy toward MHF. Many in public health believed they were the trusted health partner across the county—or should be—and if they weren't it was because the foundation had stolen their birthright. Mary Beth was blunt with them in sharing what she had heard—many did trust them, but just as many in this rural and conservative county found their government status to be of concern.

The biggest threat to MHF, though, was financial. Downturns had hurt the local economy. Two logging companies declared bankruptcy and shut down their operations in Shelton. Property tax values and those that paid the larger bills were declining, and it translated to major reductions in county tax receipts. The Mason County Public Hospital District lost over $50,000 in annual tax receipts its second year—and more cuts were possible, even likely. The state legislature was considering a massive overhaul of property taxes that would redirect property taxes to the state and especially those of special-purpose governments like public hospital districts.

Mary Beth advised the board there was a real possibility that they would run out of resources to keep doing their work. The property taxes were their sole source of revenue, and the original donated funds that started the foundation were long gone. The reduction of $50,000 had already forced them to cut back the size of their grant program. Further reductions presented the grave possibility that they would not be able to sustain it. Initial county budget projections for next year's tax receipts would mean they could no longer afford their two caseworkers.

Organizational demise wasn't imminent, she shared, but foreseeable. It was probably even predictable if the current reality was projected forward a year or two. She believed their best chance to survive was to act before it was too late to do anything about it. That meant finding a new way to generate revenue, and soon. To a person, the board agreed, and they asked Mary Beth to identify some options.

Several board members asked about government funding and grants from private funders. She explained that in the best of circumstances, these were difficult resources to access. It was even harder now, as they would have to compete against other local organizations seeking the same funds, which could threaten their unique positioning of goodwill across the county.

Others asked about private donations. She said this was conceivable—there were individuals with great wealth who vacationed in the county and might eventually see themselves as "angels" who might want to fund MHF. The problem was that it would likely take several years to find such angels. It was better than a prayer, but not much different in odds.

Mary Beth presented them with an idea. It was critical, she said, to build on something they could do and do well. It also seemed essential that the endeavor be entrepreneurial in its nature—asking for others to just give them money was little more than a prayer.

The idea came to her when she was reviewing health insurance policies. MHF was now providing health coverage to her and her two staff, and it was time to consider which insurer to use for the next year. She was reviewing several complicated and costly proposals, and it was frustrating. Her first thought was to consult with her two caseworkers to help figure it out—they had unique knowledge in navigating the conundrum. She wondered momentarily whether MHF could charge for this type of assistance. She laughed out loud—most folks across Mason County barely had the resources to pay for health care or insurance and would be hard pressed to pay MHF on top of that!

Irv happened to be in town for a visit that weekend. When she told him the story, he told her she could get paid by those who sold the product. All she had to do was become an insurance broker.

She had heard of insurance brokers, but had little idea of what they did or how they made their money. Irv filled in what he knew—insurance brokers operated in different lines of insurance business and helped customers figure out what to buy. Sometimes it was because organizations hired them to provide advice for consulting fees. In other cases, though, their payment came from the insurer chosen—a commission because the broker's individual or organizational client had chosen that health plan's product.

Mary Beth wondered whether a not-for-profit organization like hers could become a broker. Her research didn't find anything that said they couldn't, although there was not much out there on the topic. The role seemed to be rife with conflicts of interest, but apparently, it was done all the time, at least by those who wanted to make money.

Brokers were an important part of the Washington health care scene. More were now agents of larger firms and were being paid consultant fees by providing recommendations to larger organizations on how to structure and make their health insurance decisions. No one was doing anything like this in Mason County, at least for individuals and small businesses. *We could do this,* she thought, *and with our expertise could even do more to be of real value.*

Mary Beth worked with MHF's banker and legal counsel to develop a proposal for the board. Commissions would be small in amount, but repetitive. Once one became the broker of record for a client, and presuming they had a broker agreement with the health insurer selected, they would receive a small commission, perhaps as low as $10 or $15. But it was a monthly commission that would continue until the person dropped or changed their coverage, and it could add up, and for months and years into the future, as health premiums rose. With enough clients, MHF could theoretically make enough money to pay for the costs of becoming a broker and generate a margin that would replace the property tax receipts. It wouldn't be a windfall, but enough for the purposes of MHF.

It was critical that the commissions would come from the health plans, not the individual clients. It was not as if an individual or family or business could save money on health coverage by not using a broker. No, the rates for this coverage were approved by the insurance commissioner. If someone made a choice without using a broker, the health plan just kept the difference. Who couldn't get behind the notion of taking money from large health insurance companies and doing some good with it? Mary Beth also recommended that they take all who wanted the service, whether there were commissions involved or not.

What really intrigued her was that it could be a fabulous mission fit for the organization. Much of what her caseworker staff was already doing was close to the broker role. They would need a bit more training to become insurance agents and would have to get licensed by the state. But it was a small gap to fill—they probably already knew more about the health insurance choices than general insurance agents who had built their business with knowledge of only auto or life coverage. MHF would have to add some business capacity to manage the transactional elements of being a broker, but it was not rocket science.

And there was another whole level of possibility in terms of the organization's capacity to help. She learned that most health insurance brokers, even at the larger firms, knew little about health care other than how to compare insurance plans. Some barely understood Medicare or Medicaid and how this interacted with the choice of private coverage.

They knew little about matters beyond insurance—like how to actually get care, especially for the particular health care problems encountered by people and families, or how to build in prevention outside of financial health coverage. There was another new level of service related to the foundation's role to improve health for the people of the county that was possible with imagination and the higher calling of their mission.

Mary Beth presented her proposal to the board. Financial forecasts showed it would likely take a year or two to build the business to break-even, largely because they would build the business one individual or family client at a time. But by year three they were likely to have enough clients and commissions to generate somewhere between $100,000 to $300,000 in annual operating margin to support MHF . . . possibly even $500,000.

It struck the board that this was a shot worth taking. They still had property tax receipts coming in, and would next year. Probably even a year or two after that. While the amount had dropped to below $200,000, and would likely drop more, they could generate small amounts of new revenue as soon as they got commissions from new clients.

The board unanimously passed a motion authorizing Mary Beth to create and implement the program by the fall open enrollment period. The danger to MHF wasn't gone—there was no assurance that this idea would work—but it had a chance, and a chance to do a lot of good. Perhaps MHF had a longer and fuller life as an organization than anyone thought.

Chapter Eighty-Three

Irv's Public Health Job Goes Awry

Irv had found his ideal place to press for major health system reform. It was not through the political system, but its home was within government—the Seattle King County Public Health Department. It was not traditional government policy setting or even regulatory enforcement. Instead, it was using the principles of distributive and local leadership of the national Healthy Communities movement to create reform through practical projects that broke down systemic barriers.

Irv practically led the effort, in partnership with his boss, Director of Public Health Torrey Cain. Torrey created the leadership space within the department and with key community leaders and politicians. Irv provided the creative project design and management expertise.

With a number of successful projects in hand over the past few years, Torrey and Irv pondered what should come next. They regularly discussed new projects. The coalition counted on them to provide new opportunities for consideration. It seemed time to expand the long-term change proposition within their portfolio.

Irv recommended they pursue a creative prescription drug assistance program, an idea brought up when he first met Torrey. The time was not ripe for it then, but was now, with some even bigger change features added to what it was then.

The core of it, explained Irv, was to provide support to people who could not afford pharmaceutical interventions essential to their health. The cost of prescription drugs had been growing dramatically over the last twenty years. All sorts of drugs were available now to treat people, but the cost had gone through the roof. Even if people were insured, the copayment amounts frequently were beyond the capacity of many people and families to get the medications.

Irv outlined how most pharmaceutical companies had their own company-specific programs to provide support to clients who couldn't afford the drugs or copays. The companies would issue the medicines in their programs based on financial need—in large part to develop goodwill and to curry political favor that would stall governmental efforts to hold down their prices through regulation.

They also had cash to burn in rolling out these programs, since they were now prohibited from providing inducements to doctors to prescribe their drugs. Destination resort conferences and gifts were now a thing of the past, and the pharmaceutical company budgets needed to be redeployed.

Irv proposed building a coordinated public health program where local residents in need would check in through the public health department, rather than the individual Pharma companies, to see if they were eligible for financial help from these pharmaceutical company programs. The companies would get public credit for participating. If they chose not to, Irv suggested Public Health would find a legal way to limit their marketing in the Seattle area.

Public Health could also ask foundations and other donors to contribute to a fund for the needy so that it wasn't only dependent on the pharmaceutical company support. Torrey and Irv had been very successful in engaging local philanthropists in other projects, and Irv thought that they could bring millions of dollars to bear to scale up the drug assistance program. It would be one of the biggest in the nation.

Torrey liked the idea. He saw it as a practical way to help people through engagement with disparate parts of the health care system. This was usually the core of the projects that he and Irv would advance as a practical benefit to people through the Public Health Department.

Less clear to Torrey was the bigger change hook to the project. This was the other element they always tried to build in. Irv outlined the rest of the program—the prescription assistance was only one aspect of the overall project.

Accompanying the drug assistance program would be a requirement that the companies work with the public health department to attack the growing problem of prescription drug abuse. People were regularly overusing prescription drugs, or redirecting them for recreational use. This had become a major local problem and was rapidly escalating into a national crisis. Irv mentioned that one of his motivations on the issue was the death of his friend Johnny's wife Reena from an opioid overdose the year before.

Torrey was aware of the overall problem and even Congressman Gibson's loss. Torrey had tried a couple of modest efforts to tackle this problem when he was in Los Angeles at a foundation. It was a hard one to solve. Part of the issue was that pharmaceuticals had become so readily available, and in particular pain medications, where it was a regular practice for physicians to prescribe twenty-five or more pills to a patient who might need a day's supply after a surgery or other medical intervention. To solve it, one needed to tamp down the supply of drugs by limiting the enthusiasm of the drug companies and altering the sloppy ordering habits of many physicians.

On the other hand, these medications were of great benefit if used correctly and in moderation. Just banning them, or choking off their use too tightly, raised a set of problems relating to improper pain management. What was needed was a way to find the sweet spot in between. This invoked a role for the government.

Usually, this type of issue had consisted of thinking of the problem as a criminal enforcement issue, or substituting government for clinical judgment in prescribing and ordering. Neither was what Irv was thinking. Rather, they would develop a social marketing approach to moderate demand, while linking a clinical intervention program to those suffering from abuse.

For many years, this abuse was not even recognized as a health problem. It started to get some attention when college kids began to host pharmaceutical parties. They would bring random pills from the family medicine cabinet to a party and put them in a bowl. Partygoers would randomly pick out a pill from the bowl and take it. Bad outcomes were the obvious result, and this practice started to get public attention—college kids dying suddenly attracted bad headlines.

What really blew the public lid off this problem was wide-scale opioid abuse. These pain medications were just one aspect of the overall problem of prescription drug abuse, although they were stronger and far more addictive than most of the other medications, and capable of being manufactured and distributed profitably through a black market.

Opioids were a regular source of tragedies, far more than the occasional college party story. People would become addicted to the opioids, abuse them, and, far too frequently, die. This was exactly what had happened to Senator Gibson's wife.

Reena may have been more prominent than other victims, but she was part of the reality that these drug problems, unlike heroin and other illegal drugs, happened not just in racially diverse inner cities, but among white populations. It was a problem that Republican legislators couldn't ignore, and they were not able to use their normal playbook to ignore it. It was okay to use mass incarceration as a solution when it was Black victims, but quite another to do so for victims who looked more like them.

Irv's idea was to hook a program to battle prescription drug abuse with the assistance program. Drug companies, physicians, government regulators, and others would work with and through the public health department to identify practical ways to reduce the abuse. Social marketing would be part of the solution strategies, along with public policy measures that would straddle the conflicting incentives. All would have to be part of the solution, and the solution would have to become real in terms of its impact on local people.

Torrey understood and liked the idea, but he and Irv knew that they were venturing into some dangerous turf. Drug companies were not their most trusted partners, and there were too many politicians in the greater world who were looking to use the underlying issue to their political advantage.

Torrey and Irv led the coalition through a consideration, and the group approved it. Irv implemented the program over a three-month period. There was some resistance from pharmaceutical companies, but no significant revolts. Early results showed that the program was working—deaths and other adverse pharmaceutical incidents were down a third across the county after just three months of program implementation.

So was the use of pharmaceuticals. This became the catalyzing problem that hurt the prescription drug program. Prescription drug abuse was down markedly across the county, but so was the amount of prescribing and the profit margins of pharmaceutical companies within the Pacific Northwest. Local representatives of these national companies came under great scrutiny and criticism from corporate offices and were pressed for solutions. The answer, they said, was to get rid of the county program.

The drug companies unified and hired a national lobbyist to organize a campaign to discredit the public health program. His name was Sam Bridgewater, and he was willing to fight dirty. He recommended they go after it by attacking Torrey, and by attacking the King County executive who had hired him. The County executive position was up for a vote that fall, and Bridgewater organized a campaign raging against the incumbent. The thinking by the pharmaceutical companies was that even if he won reelection, he would need to disavow his public health director or at least the new program along the way.

Instead, in a political surprise, the King County executive was voted out and replaced by a candidate handpicked by Sam Bridgewater. The pharmaceutical companies poured a million dollars into this campaign, some in the form of direct political contributions but also through a secretive political action committee that ran smarmy ads against the incumbent.

The week after the election, the transition team for the new county executive told Torrey that he was being let go as the public health director. The new director would be Phil Welch, a longtime county employee who had ties with a conservative think tank. Welch would undertake a comprehensive retooling of the public health department, employees were told.

Welch met with Irv and told him he was his new boss, and the Healthy Community Coalition and special projects assistant job were over. He said that Irv should find a new job. Welch wanted to fire Irv, but his position was not political and had civil service protections. Irv was concerned about his reputation—he could see the powerful political fingerprints attacking him but also remembered the advice that his next position must show some ability to stay at a job for a while. He told Welch he wouldn't resign.

Welch instead reclassified his position to that of a Public Health Investigator. Welch couldn't cut Irv's pay—not that he made that much as a special assistant—but he could demote him in other ways. His office was moved off the twenty-fourth-floor administrative headquarters and into the bowels of the building. Irv's assignments became mundane investigative matters that few wanted.

Irv was at a loss. Torrey's time in Seattle was at an end, and he moved back to Los Angeles. He told Irv there was a place with him wherever and whenever he wanted, but it would require a move. Johnny was busy in DC and didn't have much time to help Irv navigate this mess. Things had deteriorated at home too. Leaving the Northwest would surely mean the end for him and Mary Beth. Irv went from being at the top of the world to a cellar dungeon, in just a matter of months.

Chapter Eighty-Four

The Dump Site in Mason County

Mary Beth parked her Volvo in an opening behind a patch of cedar and hemlock trees, about a mile down a little used gravel county road just outside of both Union and the Skokomish Indian Reservation, nestled between these political jurisdictions and Route 101, the major drag that ran by the eastern slope of the Olympic Mountains on a sliver of land between the mountains and the water.

When Johnny sent her the coordinates for her GPS, she recognized the road and remembered a sign identifying a county dumpsite just off the main road. She had never been on it and suspected that it was probably used most by teenagers looking for a place to party or gun enthusiasts looking for a place to fire off a few shots.

That was why she was surprised by the busy traffic on the dirt road. First one, then two, three loaded dump trucks barreled down the road at her, forcing her to hug the right side. There was barely enough room for two cars to fit side by side, and a slim margin for error when one vehicle was a wide and heavy truck. They were coming at her pretty fast too—well over the posted speed limit of twenty-five miles per hour.

It was obvious something was up at the end of the road, and it was near if not at her destination. She was headed for the coordinates from the final transmission of the cell phone tucked inside of Jose Rodriguez by Irv in a transport plane. The phone had gone dead after blipping its way across Washington State from the Moses Lake Airport yesterday.

The tracking signal had been lost a few times as it moved across the Cascade Mountains, but had resumed on the western foothills of the snow-capped peaks. It had moved down a state highway toward the town of Enumclaw, somewhat near the cabin where Irv first met up with a body courtesy of the HealthMost corporation. The signal took a hard left onto Interstate 5, the major interstate running north-south through the state, a right at Olympia, and a few miles up the road to where Highway 101 began its northern path to the cities on the edge of the Olympic Peninsula. Then it went fifteen miles to a right onto this county dirt road just after Shelton.

Mary Beth knew the reason for her sleuthing; Johnny had briefed her on the telephone last night and asked if she could do surveillance of the area. He said it carried some risk and she was to abort the mission if she encountered anything out of the ordinary.

She appreciated the concern and knew that the line of dump trucks hurtling down the road qualified. But she was not about to give up so easily in the face of potential danger. Maybe she'd be worried if someone waved a Luger at her, but dump trucks weren't enough of a scare. She would park out of sight along the roadway and walk into the area using a nearby hiking trail that she found on a county map. It was only a hundred yards or so off the roadway and crossed over the road near the county dumpsite. She would be quiet and careful, and take photos of whatever she found.

The road was out of view from the path, though she could first hear and then see two more dump trucks headed toward Route 101. It was about another mile to the county dumpsite, and she stopped short of the crossing when she got there, crouching down behind some trees and ferns before going further.

She used her binoculars to zoom in toward a dust cloud a few hundred yards south of the dumpsite. The winds blew away enough of the cloud for her to get a clearer view, and over a few minutes, she was able to piece together the picture before her. There were a handful of people around the site, mostly middle-aged men standing around and directing a line of dump trucks toward a loading area. There, a large bucket loader was scooping up yards of soil and rocks, pouring them into the backs of the dump trucks. Once full, they would climb the hill from the loading area and set on down the road.

There were five dump trucks waiting for their load when she got there, and in just the first half hour, another two got in line. She could see that hole where the bucket loader was making its drops was a big one, though the dust cloud made it hard to measure in her head.

It was about 4 p.m.—she had chosen to make her trip in the late afternoon should she need the cover of darkness to aid her surveillance. She thought the best thing to do was wait, and she settled into a depression in the forest floor on a bed of ferns, sitting on her small backpack to keep the ground dampness off her clothes. She pulled a thermos and a sandwich from the pack. She had watched enough *Rockford Files* to know she might have a bit of a wait.

At about 5:30 in the afternoon, what seemed to be the last of the dump trucks headed down the road, and the man in the bucket loader got out. He chatted with the group of men overseeing the process, and they moved to several parked cars, got in, and drove down the road. It looked to be quitting time. Using the binoculars, she tried to identify the men as they got in their cars. No luck; she was good with faces, and none struck any chord with her memory. She did note that one of the men looked out of place in a tie and coat. He was tall, with a distinctive mustache, and was talking on a large telephone. It looked more like one of the first portable phones, and that he had a signal at all told her that it was far superior to her cell phone's mobile coverage, which had evaporated a quarter mile into her drive.

They drove away, and she waited another fifteen minutes, just in case someone might return. It also gave time for the dust cloud to settle; the brown particles misted down to the ground, aided by a light drizzle that had begun. They were only about fifty miles from a rainforest, and the wetness was a welcome ally to her investigation.

She got out of her ground hold and slowly crept toward the road and the dirty hole, still listening for any returning vehicles. There was no activity at the county dumpsite yards to the north, nor likely a human being within miles. *Living, that is,* she thought as she remembered the reason for her being here.

Once she got to the hole, and the ramp where the dump trucks had gotten their loads, she could see there was not much left to view. The hole was impressive in scale—at least two football fields across in any direction, and ten feet deep at its shallowest. It was probably closer to fifteen feet deep near the center. Whatever might have been there was gone now, and unlikely to ever be found.

She walked the perimeter of the hole, hoping to find something that might be of use to her. There was nothing but dirt and bits of tree stumps. Puddles were beginning to form from the rain, and they looked like any other puddle in a Pacific Northwest rainstorm.

Mary Beth got out of the hole and walked nearer the dumpsite, hoping that there might be something there. There was one large utility pole, where power lines were hooked, though nothing connected to them at the dumpsite. It was just another hole, this time with old couches, refrigerators, and assorted other junk. She guessed the site was no longer used, in favor of more environmentally conscious dumpsites in the nearby towns. What was thrown into this hole was more likely from those who didn't want to pay the small $8 dump fee at these sites.

She noticed a piece of paper on the pole, nailed to the far side of the post facing the dense forest beyond, making it unlikely that anyone but the most curious of hikers would see it. Walking around the post, she took a closer look.

It was an environmental impact statement, announcing that this site was proposed to be used for the purposes of a data management and repository center. She knew about the EIS process—every project of any size on the Peninsula was required to have one because of the federal lands and endangered species within it. Timber barons had ravaged much of the trees and species, and it was too little too late for most of the objects of concern, but now there were strict requirements in place providing public notice and opportunity to comment on proposed projects within the region that might threaten sensitive habitats.

She took a photo of the notice, which had other information splashed across its contents, protected from the elements by a laminated covering. The numbers linked to the larger filing might prove helpful to finding out more. Though much of that was answered for her by the applicant: HealthMost Corporation.

Mary Beth worked her way back to her car without notice or incident, and drove back to her small home outside of Shelton. She called Johnny to let him know what she had found—or in this case, more what she didn't. Their hope, grisly and revolting as it might be, was that they would find proof of bodies being hidden by HealthMost.

If they were once there, they no longer were.

Chapter Eighty-Five

The Evil Plan

The plan was conceived in a conference room of the Bahama Grand Hotel. Richard Thrust was not surprised when Sam Bridgewater told him that his requested meeting with the Secretary of Health had been scheduled on the island, and that the costs for the trip would be paid for by HealthMost. He understood that there would be an expectation to host the secretary and his family at this island resort. It wasn't the first time, and probably not the last.

Thrust had told Sam to set up a meeting with the secretary so he could explain the problem associated with taking care of illegals and how they might solve it. The record flow of immigrants into the United States was costing HealthMost over $10 million a year, and growing. Most of these immigrants had no health coverage, and many were in great need of medical care. Advocates were telling them that free care was available—all they had to do was go to an emergency room and use the right language to describe their care needs. Hospitals would have to assess them and provide free health care.

The administration had issued an executive order forbidding the use of Medicaid funds to help pay for this care. Their argument was that a confusing clause in an immigration bill gave them the authority to create this restriction. It was in litigation, but likely to be years away from any conclusion. Conservative court appointees were thought to be sympathetic to the administration's arguments.

Thrust thought it reprehensible that he be forced to care for people who didn't have the resources to pay for health care—not just illegals, but anyone. That they were often difficult patients, with complicated diagnoses, only aggravated him more. The truth was that $10 million, while a big number to most hospitals, was little more than budget dust for his mega hospital system. He prided himself on eliminating all waste from his system's bottom line, and regularly cut wages and salaries and laid staff off to maximize earnings for the corporation. He wasn't about to turn his back on a $10 million problem—that would be real money in their pocket.

The rapid growth of HealthMost was also why this problem was so much bigger for him than other hospitals and health systems. The system now stretched across the American West and was prominent in cities across the southern border. The $10 million estimate was projected to grow 10 percent a year over the next decade. Before too long it would become a $20-million-a-year problem.

He came to the meeting with the secretary with a simple and cold plan. They would loosen enforcement of the antidumping rules passed in 1986 by Congress. Then they would defer to health plans as the surveillance mechanism for identifying issues as part of the Republicans' national movement to privatize health care around market theories. If the health plans did not recommend action on any complaint, they would ignore any appeals.

Thrust knew that health plans would mostly ignore the issue, or give it to their staff assigned to deny service. These units had become quite talented in delaying, obfuscating, and saying no to Americans with health insurance who understood perfect English. A language barrier and temporary address were only going to make it easier to dismiss foreign inquiries.

Sam's advice was to first fly the ideas up the flagpole with the secretary's staff. Thrust did not want the usual "we promise to take a look at the issue" response. He wanted the solutions put in law, and soon. Sam had Thrust make a substantial campaign contribution to the president for his reelection campaign, which should have greased the wheels sufficiently to put his solutions on the fast track.

They were a little surprised to arrive at the meeting and find the secretary accompanied not by senior staff from HHS but White House political staff. Security was also unusually tight; perhaps there was a terrorist threat. It seemed odd when the security officers took their phones from them outside of the meeting room door. They were not secret service officers; rather, contract security staff working for some unidentified firm.

The HHS secretary convened the meeting. HealthMost's delegation included Thrust, Bridgewater, and Chief Financial Officer Haynes Dickson. Secretary Olsen was accompanied by two staff from the Office of Management and Budget, one from Homeland Security, and two political operatives on the White House staff. They didn't even offer up their names, and the Homeland Security rep immediately took control of the meeting.

"The secretary has briefed us on your proposal. We appreciate your support of the president and have spent some time reviewing it." Thrust knew this meant that his sizable campaign contribution had been duly noted. "It also matters that Mr. Bridgewater is here with you. We have undertaken other special projects with his participation, and he is a trusted advisor and partner to our administration.

"We are open to your proposal to ease the federal antidumping rules and enforcement. They run counter to our thinking, and you know that one of the many successes of our administration has been administrative simplification."

Thrust nodded his pleasure. They obviously understood the wisdom of his recommendation to them.

"But we think there is a much bigger opportunity to address our national problems."

This statement caught Thrust's attention. He was always the one with the big ideas, and he tensed at the suggestion that someone else was thinking even bigger.

"I am sure you know that we have a major immigration problem in this nation and that this was a big part of the platform that got our president elected. He is intent on fulfilling his campaign promise. You undoubtedly have also seen how our enemies have resisted these efforts, and we are in a battle to make a dent in even illegal immigration. Congress looks to be stymied in its ability to pass anything into law, and we have decided to use our executive authority to solve the problem otherwise."

None of this was news to Thrust or Sam, but they were surprised it was such a prominent feature for this meeting.

"We have been authorized to pursue a special program that would serve our ends and, we believe, yours. My colleagues will present it to you. You may give your assent to it today, if you like. If you choose to take some time to consider it, you will have two weeks to provide a response. However, there will be no written communication about this, and certainly no public announcements. This is a classified communication, and any breach will carry severe penalties. Do you understand? If so, you will sign the confidentiality agreement before you on the table in front of you."

The HealthMost delegation looked at Richard Thrust. He would tell them whether they were okay with these terms and if they should sign the document. Thrust stared at the Homeland Security staffer and the Secretary of Health for about ten seconds. He then pulled the piece of paper in front of him closer, took a fast glance at its contents, and signed it with the pen he pulled from his suit pocket. The rest of the delegation then signed as well.

With that, the two Office of Management and Budget staff presented the proposal. They were quite young and didn't seem to be accountants or people with substantial financial background; they spoke little about financial facts and operational details and far more like political operatives. As they spoke, Thrust saw how superficial they were in terms of program substance or expertise.

The administration shared their antipathy to antidumping laws but was far more concerned with the immigration crisis, including how immigrants were costing the taxpayer money because of their health care needs. They said they were doing all they could to stop the flow of illegal and legal immigration, but that it was now necessary to take extraordinary measures to solve this national crisis. They noted their belief that one-third to half of immigrants crossing over from the southern border had medical needs and were likely to seek medical care once they came to the United States.

With HealthMost one of, if not the largest medical system operating across the southern wall, they were proposing that HealthMost become their partner in a new initiative. HealthMost would contractually commit to taking care of immigrants and their families. This would extend not just to instances presenting at their emergency rooms, but would be supplemented with an outreach program to identify immigrants and families with health needs. This would allow the administration to do media outreach showing their detractors that they were caring of immigrant needs, disarming much of the political flak they had been taking, such as criticism about their family separation policy. HealthMost would participate in the press campaign touting this humane approach.

HealthMost would be paid well for the contractual commitment; they would receive an amount per person to accept the obligation. The funds would move to them as a special insurance payment under a demonstration project authority created by the Affordable Care Act. Obamacare had included a couple of billion dollars for special payment initiatives that inspired bigger change in American health care. The two staffers reveled in the irony that they would now use that money to address the immigration crisis.

They interrupted their briefing at this juncture by noting that this was the general concept and asked for any questions. There was no chance that anyone other than Thrust was going to ask one at this point, and his team looked at him.

He sat back in his chair. "So you are essentially asking us to take a capitation payment to care for the health needs of immigrants and their families, right? That could be pretty expensive—as you said, many of them have great health care needs, and we would be taking on what could be an expensive obligation. Have you run any actuarial projections?"

"No, we haven't," intervened the Homeland Security staffer. "Our thought was that we would negotiate an amount with you to cover what we believe the extent of your theoretical obligation to them would actually be."

Thrust didn't quite understand what he meant. "Are you saying that there would be some limit to what we would have to do for them?"

The aide looked hard at Thrust and chose his words carefully. "I am telling you that once we make our payment to you, we don't care what happens on your end of the deal. Our only desire is that they no longer remain in the United States. If you can commit to this design principle, I believe we will be able to sweeten the deal outside of the capitation payment too."

Richard and Sam both got what the real proposition was and shifted uncomfortably in their seats. Even Secretary Olsen's body posture stiffened with the statement. The other members of the HealthMost delegation could tell that something important had happened but were still getting their heads around what it was.

The proposal was that HealthMost become a surveillance and enforcement mechanism to address the administration's concern with immigration. HealthMost would identify immigrants as they presented, in its emergency rooms or through the outreach program, using the need or attraction of health care as an inducement. Their primary objective would be to get them out of the country, with whatever health care they delivered as a secondary goal.

But how? Thrust carefully chose his words in asking this question.

Again, it was the Homeland Security aide who spoke. "I am telling you that we don't really care. They are not Americans and not our concern. One option is to turn them over to the Border Patrol and let our systems send them back to their country. Our problem has been finding them, not sending them back. You may take whatever extraordinary steps to do so that you must, without interference from us. We won't ask you to tell us how you do this. We just want it done, and quietly."

"But the capitation amount will not be anything that will allow us to provide a great deal of patient care, would it?" Thrust thought it important to get closer to the financial details of the proposal.

"I wouldn't believe so," shared the aide, "but you are the experts in health care. In terms of budget, we are prepared to commit to something in the order of $100 million for these patients. That would make you more than whole. But if you want to do something more with the funds, it will be your call—and responsibility."

His words hung in the air as Thrust and his colleagues worked the implications through their minds. The aide saw this and let the moment stretch by taking a long drink of water from the glass on the table. When he was sure that his audience had processed the proposal, he continued. "The incentives around this deal will be structured separately from the capitation payments. Let us share our idea with you." He looked to the OMB staffers to continue their presentation.

There were more enticements to come. The OMB staffers added one more piece-if HealthMost was able to assure that extraordinary objectives of the contract were achieved, they would also receive an annual grant award of up to $50 million. These funds would not flow through the capitation payment, but through a special Department of Energy award for environmentally sound construction. It was another grant program of Obama's and another chance to take a shot at him.

Thrust pushed back against the back of his chair and stroked his chin as he looked intently at the secretary and his team, spending a couple of minutes rolling the proposal through his mind. This would achieve his bottom line objective for the meeting—eliminating the $10 million cost of caring for immigrants across HealthMost. There was now a lot more money than this on the table. If they were to find a way to minimize the cost of caring for these new patients, it would go right to the bottom line of HealthMost. Thrust figured that the potential profit was at least $50 million, maybe more—*before* the incentive grant from the Department of Energy was factored in. It would be the single biggest profit transaction in his career. It would also be almost immediate, far more immediate and profitable than his usual approach of buying up competitors, cutting their cost structures with layoffs, and ultimately securing a close to monopoly positions within their communities and then leveraging that in the marketplace. All of these took time.

He also liked the notion of exempting HealthMost from the anti-dumping statutes, while his competitors would still have to live with them. He would be reluctant to say so, however, since he had made such a public declaration about the policy wisdom of the statutes being eliminated. But if that was how it played out, he wouldn't publicly object.

There was risk in this proposal. He would need an insurance capacity to take on the obligation. If they structured it right, his insurance partner could be left holding the bag if anything went off the rails. They had been looking for an insurance partner for other corporate strategies, and thought they had found a gullible partner in Associated Life Insurance and its CEO. They would obtain their license so they could receive the capitation payments and use their database to shield this deal from public view. Thrust could probably even convince the ALI CEO to provide the capital to implement the special program.

Nowhere in his thinking was anything about what it meant for patients, or his staff, or his country. This was a business transaction, and caring for people was just like selling cars or computer software or anything else. It was a weakness to get sentimental about your product, and he had used the weakness of others to advance his career and fortune. He would do so again, in an even bigger way.

"We will need a week to review this in greater depth, Mr. Secretary. I can tell you now that we will give it full consideration, and I am inclined to make a favorable recommendation to our board. I suggest we schedule a meeting at the end of next week to continue our conversation."

"Very well," said the secretary.

They met again a week later, this time in Secretary Olsen's Office at HHS Headquarters. It was only Thrust, Olsen, Bridgewater, and the Homeland Security staffer. By then, Thrust and Bridgewater had identified that the staffer was one of the president's longtime confidantes. He was not so well known publicly but he had a direct channel to the president.

Thrust said they were willing to enter into this agreement, with a few changes. Most importantly, he noted that the costs of implementing the program would be extensive. He proposed that some additional incentive grants be included, amounting to another $25 million. It seemed there were grants available in Education and Agriculture and that their staff could identify ways to create companion funding streams to the Department of Energy grant. This was just a negotiation of the price for the deeds; all knew that it was a generous financial proposal to HealthMost, and the supplemental price was agreed to, details to follow.

Thrust also told them that he needed official board approval, but that this was a detail they should not be concerned with. It would be better to do this at a regular board meeting rather than a special telephone meeting so that it would not get too much attention.

The secretary said this would be all right with them. The group brainstormed timelines and public announcements and agreed on a rough schedule. The Homeland Security staffer mentioned that it was time for the president to prepare for his reelection campaign and suggested that Thrust make an even bigger contribution to the SuperPAC formed for his reelection. Sam interjected that he would make sure this request was honored.

They shook hands. Thrust and Bridgewater left the secretary's office and took the elevator to the ground floor of HHS. They spoke not a word until they had left the building and were outside in a private courtyard near Independence Avenue.

Sam looked at Thrust. "Have you done any design of your program yet? Let me know if there is any way I can help with that."

"Yes, we have. We have a conceptual outline and will be meeting daily to put it into operational details and assignments. I will need a few things from you in terms of our relationship with ALI and a few other matters. Maybe with the board at their next meeting. At the end of the day, I think this will be another great success for me and HealthMost. I will be in touch when I need you."

With that, Thrust waved to the limo driver waiting for him on the adjacent street. He got into the car and was whisked away to the airport, where his private jet awaited him for the trip back to Chicago.

Sam watched the car pull away, excited and scared at the same time. This was a big deal and Thrust had not missed a beat when Sam suggested that his annual retainer would need to be doubled to support such an initiative. It was also new and dangerous turf. Sam was counting on Thrust and his health care system to figure out a capable and quiet way to operate the program. They were the best and the brightest—what could go wrong?

Chapter Eighty-Six

What Next in the Investigation?

Irv was as astonished as Johnny and Lance to hear that the dumpsite where Jose was transported was now completely vacant. It had been only a week since they had met in a Colorado hotel, and already the best piece of evidence for their case against HealthMost was gone.

Johnny had texted Irv as soon as Mary Beth reported what she had found to him, saying that they needed to talk ASAP. Irv was seated in his cubicle at work and was ready to respond, optimistic it would be good news. This case was his first priority, and there was almost nothing else going on at work for him anyway. His assignments had dwindled even more since he had first been assigned the case of the body in Kent. If someone was sending him a message about his future at the department, he was starting to consider it received.

Irv announced to his cubicle mates that he was going to get a cup of coffee, and made his way to a coffee shop down the street from his office building. He took his cup of coffee to a small park across the street. It was a favorite spot for the homeless, meaning that anyone following him would really stand out. He called Johnny on his private cell.

Irv was shocked and dismayed to learn the results of Mary Beth's research. Bottom line—Jose and the dump were now gone—lock, stock, and barrel. It had all happened within a week. There was nothing but dust and an environmental assessment notice on a nearby pole.

That HealthMost was the applicant for this environmental permit made it clear who was behind this fast excavation work. It seemed obvious this was not some routine cleanup, but a concerted effort to remove whatever was at the dumpsite. They knew it included Jose, and surmised that there were others there too. Maybe a lot of others.

It was a small mental step to conclude that HealthMost knew someone was on their trail and that a cover-up was now underway. It was impressive in a grotesque kind of way that the corporation could so quickly figure out how to totally eviscerate the dumpsite. Irv should expect this speed and thoroughness around any other trails into the misdeeds.

Lance reviewed the online environmental filing from the photo shared by Mary Beth. There was little information of use, other than it was an application from HealthMost. It had been filed the day after Irv made his escape from the southwestern medical facility. Construction at the site would not begin for another month, but they had been granted an exception to clear the site immediately, and had. There were already a few letters of support in the file, most notably by local and state politicians who effused about the economic development aspects of the proposal—no doubt accompanied by hefty political donations.

Irv and Johnny speculated on the telephone as to why the cover-up had been initiated. They were trying to find some other explanation other than what was obvious—that their investigation had been spotted. HealthMost had figured out someone was digging around and was now getting rid of any evidence of wrongdoing. The only real physical evidence of a crime was now missing.

The bigger question was what it meant for the rest of their investigation. Irv thought it would be hard, maybe impossible, to take another run at spying on HealthMost's special patient disposal program now that the corporation was on high alert. Processes in health care systems could go underground for years and decades, until there was some reason for them to rise to prominence, usually a government investigation or a lawsuit. But covering asses in system headquarters was also a reason to get noticed. Once they were spotted, the attention would mean a fast end to the practices.

Irv also told Johnny about the further decline in his standing in the health department. He wondered whether the powers there would even give him more time off, and he was sure they wouldn't back him up or support any findings of wrongdoing that went up the chain of command. More likely, it would trigger a lecture, suspension, or even firing.

Johnny understood, and shared his own reservations about using the formal command system to report the wrongdoing they had uncovered. This administration had broken new ground in ignoring congressional calls for inquiry, even ignoring reports of inspector generals at the agencies. Johnny had far less standing than these official government auditors, or the committee chairs who were getting bitch-slapped when they reported suspected wrongdoing.

Nor did they believe they had enough to go to the media. Without more and better proof, it would just be another crazy story of what was going on within the current administration. Even if it splashed, the ripples would flatten out days later in the twenty-four-hour news cycle of the times.

It was frustrating. They now knew much of what was going on within HealthMost, and it stunk to high heaven. There was also clearly a direct thread into the federal government, and Irv and Johnny figured that this would prove to be a thick rope if they ever got the chance to pull on it.

It was vital that they find a way to stop this abomination, but they didn't have enough to do so yet. Their best play would be to use the public hearing on patient dumping in Belfair to try to catch HealthMost and the HHS secretary in their misdeeds. There would be press at this event, local and national, and the topic would contain the type of human tragedy that would assure at least a thirty-second spot on the television news. Maybe they could leverage that in some way, along with the proximity of the dumpsite to the public hearing site.

That hearing would be next month, which gave them time to pursue the other research they had initiated on this matter too. They would follow up on that and reassess their best play. They agreed to talk by telephone every Wednesday afternoon between now and then, and meet several days before the hearing in person. Then it would be time to assemble their full team. Mary Beth suggested they do so at the Alderbrook Lodge, about twenty minutes west of Belfair and almost halfway to the county dumpsite.

It was a plan.

Chapter Eighty-Seven

Thrust's Conspiracy Deepens

"What is it?" Richard Thrust barked into the phone. He hated interruptions of any type. Some came with the job, like telephone calls from politicians or board members stopping by the office to say hello. When the interruptions were from employees and contractors, there was no need for any social grace.

Sam Bridgewater was used to Thrust's ways, and he wasn't fazed. He did feel trepidation over sharing information with Thrust that would make him even angrier. It couldn't be avoided, and it wasn't Bridgewater's fault, so it was best to be quick and direct. Ripping off a Band-Aid was generally the best way to deal with Thrust.

"Sorry to interrupt, but there are a couple of pieces of information I need to pass along to you. I am not sure what they fully mean, but you should know of them." Sam waited for some acknowledgment from Thrust that he was ready to receive the reports.

"Go ahead," came the stern retort from the telephone.

"I got a report from our security team that a patient has gone missing today. One of our special cases checked himself out of our facility in New Mexico near the border. We are still not sure how he got out, but our best guess is that he smuggled himself out with a corpse that was on his way for disposal, and still is en route. There has been no report on the whereabouts of our missing patient though. No reports from the Border Patrol or ICE, or other health care facilities. Most likely he has disappeared into the network of illegal immigrants and won't be heard from again until he has another medical episode."

Thrust looked out his window to Lake Michigan. He didn't like speculation, and certainly not when it involved this endeavor. He knew that it involved some risk, but the reward was so high and his ability to manipulate systems so complete that he calculated it was one worth taking. Now there were not one but two recent breaches in the security system he had built.

"Where did he enter our system?"

"Albuquerque. Promise Hospital. Came in on a Sunday night complaining of chest pain and arrived by ambulance. Was flagged for special treatment within an hour and transferred to the holding site overnight. He stayed there for almost two days before disappearing."

"Why do we think he left with a corpse?" There had to be more than speculation. Speculation got people fired, and the culture Thrust had built would not tolerate such sloppiness. He needed a firmer answer.

Sam knew this line of questioning was coming. He was paid to know his clients, and for all of Thrust's harshness, he was wholly predictable. Sam laughed inwardly—*I didn't have to speculate about that!*

"Process of elimination. There was simply no other way for him to have left. Staff found him missing at the start of the day shift, and the only entry and exit to the locked unit other than security rounds was the release of a body. He had to have used that event to get out of the facility."

"And the body? Anything out of the ordinary with that?"

"No. Usual routine. Processed through our facility in Moses Lake."

"Do some more digging. I want to know more about this patient and why he was in our system. And who he was. What was his name?"

"Roberto Hernandez. At least that's the name he gave in the emergency room. Probably dozens with that name in the system."

"You said there were two things. What's the other?"

"It's ALI. Our information system people spotted what looks to be an inquiry into the data set. You might recall that though we were transferring it there for security purposes to keep it hidden, we attached a secret computer instruction to let us know when and if the data was ever accessed."

"Of course I know. I was the one who insisted on this."

Of course, thought Sam. Who else would be so fastidious about corporate fraud and espionage? "Yes. So you know the code doesn't tell us much more than the fact that there had been a data inquiry. The only ones authorized to even make an inquiry are Duncan, ALI's legal counsel, and their chief information officer. We bought off their legal counsel when we made the deal, and this shyster assures us that he did not make an inquiry. He grilled the CIO and is confident that it wasn't him. That leaves Duncan, who we have not approached."

"That little shit." Stupid and unreliable, a damning duet in Thrust's world. He didn't count on loyalty; that was a value for idiots. But any half nitwit in Nelson Duncan's position would understand that Thrust was not to be screwed with. He recalled his private conversation with Nelson—and one of the central points was that any, and he meant any, inquiries into that data system were to be reported immediately by Nelson to Thrust. At best, Nelson had not done that. At worst, he was the one who had made the inquiry.

"What do you want me to do about the ALI situation. Or any of this?" asked Sam.

"Nothing. I will take it from here. But recheck all your traplines. We can't get any of this wrong. And what's new with the public hearing nonsense with Senator Gibson?"

"The hearings are being formed. They are still planning on doing regional forums around the country, with the central hearing happening in Gibson's home state of Washington. Secretary Olsen is committed to testifying at that one. Early signs were it would be in Seattle, but our snooping tells us they are looking into a place called Belfair. It's out in the country about two hours from Seattle, and north of Olympia."

"I know where it is." Thrust was visualizing the map his staff had used to outline the special treatment protocol and systems. His recall was superb and he could see the town of Belfair nestled between inland waterways and a series of low mountains near the Olympic Mountains. He could also visualize the location of their special treatment unit in Union—about fifteen miles due west of Belfair. He didn't believe in coincidence.

"I am sorry to hear that. I told you to stop those hearings. I don't know exactly what Gibson is up to, but we need to be on high alert."

"I understand. I told you that we could not stop those hearings—nobody could. Gibson is a one-off politically. The good news is that nobody will follow him. We just need to contain the event. His staff are still sniffing around the notion of having someone from HealthMost testify. What do you think about that?"

Thrust stared off into the clouds, trying to see what the future held. No man could outthink him—certainly not some political hack. "Yes, it seems like the senator is trying to construct a trap for us." He thought some more, keeping Bridgewater in suspense until his further response. "By all means, let's agree to participate. Tell him that I will be appearing. We will give him some prey that he will never forget. It will bite his hand."

Bridgewater momentarily thought about questioning Thrust about testifying at the Washington State hearing. Just as quickly, he realized that it would be dangerous to do so. It mattered little that he knew more than Thrust about such things. "Roger that. Anything you want to tell me about it now?"

"No, not yet. I will get back to you. And Bridgewater—no more screw-ups. If you want to keep this contract."

With that, Thrust hung up the telephone. No, too many coincidences. Something was afoot. They would regret screwing with him—starting with Nelson. He picked up the phone. "Marjorie, get me the board chair for ALI on the line." He put it down. There was about to be a regime change at ALI. It was a lucky break for their legal counsel, who was about to be promoted. If he continued to play ball with Thrust, that is.

Chapter Eighty-Eight

Johnny's Senate Career Threatened

Johnny's internal warning systems were on red alert as he walked down the marble corridor toward the Senate majority leader's office. He had arrived for his meeting with Senator Thomas Bell an hour early, as he was coming from a meeting in the Capitol Building that had been unexpectedly cancelled. It wasn't worth the bother to head all the way back to his office and then turn around and come back just a few minutes later. Besides, he could have some coffee with Senator Bell's scheduling secretary—she was an interesting woman of past interest and pretty as spring flowers. He would surprise her by coming in the back entrance to the office.

By going the back way, he was now observing Sam Bridgewater leaving the majority leader's office and turning left down a hall to return to the public hallways. Bridgewater didn't see him, as he was looking at his cell phone, but it was out of the ordinary. Bridgewater was known for his Republican connections, not those to Democratic politicians and certainly not the majority leader.

Johnny knew that politics made strange bedfellows and ordinarily might not have thought much of this sighting. It was just too coincidental though. He had seen Bridgewater three times over the past several months after not having seen him at all since the days when they overlapped in the House of Representatives. All three were testy interactions about matters in which Bridgewater's clients—and major political forces—disagreed with Johnny's aims.

This, plus the fact that the senate majority leader had asked him to come by, got Johnny wondering about what was really going on. Maybe it was not about the matter of the meeting—his request for support for a vote on a bill to strengthen hospital patient antidumping laws. He had asked the majority leader what it would take to get a bill on this topic to the Senate floor, and he would get some answer in this meeting, he expected. But the question now was whether there was something going on behind the curtain.

Johnny stopped and leaned against a marble column near a stairwell, out of sight from the office. There was little other traffic in the hallway, as it was a little used back entrance where access was granted only through a special security badge. He thought about the meeting, processing anew what his approach would be with Senator Bell.

He had been in the Senate for almost a year now, and this would be his first meeting with Senator Bell. Bell was the long-term senior senator from Colorado and had been elected majority leader after the Democrats took control of the Senate in 2018. He had introduced himself to Johnny at an orientation session for new senators and was cordial enough. Even then, Johnny sensed an uneasiness in Senator Bell's reaction to him. Since, there had been few times for any meaningful exchanges. Johnny had, he thought, begun this one by stopping the majority leader on the floor and asking him to support his patient dumping legislative effort.

This coldness was something that Johnny was adapting to in the Senate. His relations in the House were generally warmer and more open. The Republicans and Democrats fought like cats and dogs, and there was even intense personal dislike as ideology and party identity had become prevalent in the nation's capital. When he had first gone to the House, there were lots of friendships across party lines, even regular card games and social outings. There was little of this now—you were expected to hang out with your own. Being an independent, he could play with both teams, at least socially, and did.

Not so in the Senate. It was, to be sure, a snootier environment than the House. Senators thought themselves superior to House members and pretty much everyone else they met, something built by the great advantages the Constitution afforded Senate members, starting with six-year terms and the power to confirm appointees. This environment drew a certain type of politician, usually those with even greater egos than the strong ones in the House.

Johnny was an expert at meeting and relating to people though, and he figured it would just take a little more time to break through with his Senate colleagues. Over a year in, it still wasn't happening, and he had begun to wonder why. Instincts told him that it had something to do with how he had snatched this seat away from the Democrats, and that they and the Republicans planned on snatching it away from him next year.

After gathering his thoughts, Johnny hit restart on his stroll to the majority leader's office and walked into a massive reception area. Large pictures of presidents and battlefields were on the wall, barely filling the forty-foot-high walls. There were two sitting areas with luxurious couches and one with a walnut conference table. Doors to the other offices and conference rooms were all about the large space. Unlike his Senate office, there was no one working at desks in the waiting area. Everybody in the senate majority leader's office had a private office, except for a receptionist seated at the front of the room.

He approached her from the backside entrance, taking note of the nameplate on the desk. "Good morning, Jane." He smiled at the pretty woman behind the desk. She smiled back. "I am Senator John Gibson, here a bit early for an appointment with Senator Bell. I thought that Penny might be available so I can say hello. She was the one who set up the appointment."

"Yes, Senator Gibson. It is good to meet you. The majority leader is running behind a bit today, so it might be a bit of a wait. But I will see if Penny is available. I saw her come in a few minutes ago." She picked up her phone and hit the four-digit extension for Penny, and then exchanged some words into the telephone. "She is available and will be out in just a couple of minutes. Could I get you a cup of coffee while you wait?"

"Yes, please. I was counting on that—don't you have an espresso machine? Double shot latte, please." Johnny sat down on the couch nearest the reception desk awaiting Penny's arrival.

Five caffeinated minutes later, Penny Atwater arrived. She was a tall, full-bodied brunette, with narrow hips and ample bosom. She was nearing forty, but the wrinkles of time had not overtaken her face. A natural beauty, she wore her fashionable business suit well. She smiled broadly at Senator Gibson as she approached him.

"Senator Gibson, it is so good to see you." She extended a hand in greeting.

"The pleasure is mine, Miss Atwater," Johnny replied as he, too, extended his hand.

They both burst out laughing, and then hugged.

"How long has it been?" asked Penny. "It seems like only a few weeks ago that we were organizing parades and parties."

"Those weeks would be about thirteen years ago, Penny. Not that you look it."

The two were old friends from Johnny's time in the House. Penny was then a secretary for the House Capitol Office Commission, which coordinated events at the Capitol for House members and oversaw any major building projects on behalf of all House members. The commission needed some representatives to sit on a legislative committee to make its work official, and Johnny volunteered. He was having a hard time getting any plum committee assignments because of his independence and thought he might as well sign up for the party committee.

No one else wanted the job. In addition to the parties, he had met Penny, and they even dated for a few months, during Johnny's brief separation from his wife. That had ended long ago, amicably, and they had not seen each other for several years. Penny had taken a new job with the Senate majority leader five years ago.

They caught up, as old friends and lovers would.

"You are here a bit early, Senator," Penny finally interjected. She was wondering if this was just a social check-in, or if Johnny was fishing for more than that. She had gotten to know his laid-back way of relating to people, and advancing his agenda through it.

"Penny, I was so happy to see your name on the appointment message I got from my staff. I guess I knew this was where you were at, but you know how things go around here. Just too busy with other things to come and find you. But if you have a few minutes, I would like to catch up." He winked at her, out of sight of the receptionist.

Penny knew that Johnny did have something on his mind beyond just seeing her again. "Come on over here, let's do that." She motioned to a leather couch and chair at the far end of the room, set well away from the receptionist and any office doors. It was a good place for a private conversation.

They sat down. "So tell me, what's on your mind, Johnny?"

"I really was coming early just to see you. But on the way in, I saw Sam Bridgewater leaving through the back door. That surprised me. You know his politics and reputation. He and I have been going at it a bit, and I couldn't help but imagine that his being here wasn't a coincidence from my point of view."

She put her hand on his knee as she leaned in so she could be sure her words were not overheard by others. "No, I don't think it was a coincidence. I want to be careful here, Johnny. Confidentiality is the first requirement of my job as appointment secretary for the majority leader. But I like you and believe in you. So, listen closely. Watch your back. When Senator Bell asked me to schedule a meeting with you, he put down a report titled 'Elections Prospects for the Senate Seat in Washington,' and I saw a picture of you in the report as he laid it on the desk. What's more, right after that, he asked that I make sure he met with Bridgewater, and the minority leader, before you came in."

Johnny looked back into her green eyes. "Thank you for that. I won't tell anyone about this. Good to know my instincts are still working, though. I have never felt comfortable over here in the Senate since the day I walked in. Thought I might be developing some paranoia in my old age. Apparently not, though. Any clues what it is about?"

"No. And those are the types of questions that get you fired around here. I will see what else I can learn though, and let you know if I find something. Still have the same old cell phone number?"

"Yes, I do." He fondly remembered texting her double entendre messages the mornings after their dates. Back then, you could get away with things like that. Now, no more. "You better get out of here now. We shouldn't be seen together any more than this. And," he glanced at the receptionist, "the wall might have ears."

Penny and he stood up, shook hands, and said their goodbyes. Johnny walked toward his former seat near the receptionist's desk, stopping at the desk. "It was great to see Penny. We worked together for a bit over on the House side. But tell me about you, Jane. What brought you to Capitol Hill?"

This was Johnny's modus operandi—to be open, interested, and inquisitive of all he met on Capitol Hill. Genuinely. And now he had the experience to know that this often led to positive things for his aims too.

No reason to change now, he thought. *It was what brought me here, and if it takes me out the same way, so be it.* They talked for about fifteen minutes, in between Jane taking phone calls. Then he was called into the majority leader's office.

"Senator Gibson, welcome." Senate Majority Leader Thomas Bell shook hands with Johnny, and then pointed at a seat for Johnny to take. His office was almost as big as the receptionist's office and looked more like a library, with books and paintings surrounding ornate antique furniture around the room. "I am sorry we are a few minutes late. Duty calls, and there was a national security matter that needed attending to."

Senator Bell was seventy years old, a little more than six foot two, and looked the part of a senator in a Jimmy Stewart movie. He had a paunchy midsection, a fine suit that still didn't hang quite right on his out-of-shape body, and a small tuft of gray hair sitting on the front temple of an otherwise bald head. He was a hotel operator before he went into politics, and many wondered about his political connections. The days when the mob strutted around openly were over, but most suspected that they had much to do with his success at the ballot box, along with the support from organized labor that got him votes and key strings within Democratic political circles.

"No worries, Senator. I know you are a busy man. I am sorry we haven't had time to get to know each other since I became a senator. I would be interested in learning more about you and what got you to this place." Johnny was relentless in his way of doing business. He would fish off the relationship pier with Senator Bell, though he wasn't sure that the fish were biting.

They weren't. "Yes, we should do that sometime." Johnny understood that time would not be now, and likely would be never. The majority leader showed little interest in him and moved to the reason for the meeting. Or at least what he would admit to Johnny. "You said that you were interested in bringing up a bill related to hospital dumping? Tell me more about that. What are you trying to do?"

Johnny skipped straight to the matter at hand, knowing that people like Senator Bell were the exceptions to his usual strategy. They would put on the charm when they saw it was in their interest to do so, and Johnny clearly did not command such interest. Johnny shared the highlights of his questioning of Secretary Olsen and told the majority leader that he was in the process of scheduling field hearings on the matter across the country.

"Already we are getting some very troubling reports about hospital practices in this regard," shared Johnny. "I have been talking with committee staff about what we might do to tighten laws on this matter, and they are drafting a set of amendments that would do that. I plan on dropping a bill later this year and have been lobbying our colleagues to vote for them if we can get them out of committee."

"What have they been saying?" asked Bell.

"Mostly that they wanted to know that it would be cleared for a vote by you. They seem supportive of the notion but don't want to go on the record with their support unless they are sure it's a live proposal. I was hoping you would give that commitment so I can build a strategy to get this over the hump."

"And tell me, why should I do that?" It was a cold question, as icy as a popsicle in the North Pole.

"Senator, it would be a natural next step to implement the Affordable Care Act properly. We have been on the defense around that law since it passed. More accurately, I would say that you and your caucus have been—it was and remains a volatile issue for Democrats. The Republicans, on the other hand, have lots of criticisms and no answers. But they sure are raising a lot of money and using it in their campaign talking points. My hope, as an independent, is to bridge these divides and pass some meaningful amendments to the ACA—amendments that would really make a difference to the American people. I believe I am uniquely situated to do that. And the starting point would be a bill that addresses some of the horrible health plan and hospital practices of denying care to sick Americans."

"You don't need to lecture me about the ACA, son. I was here when it passed too."

"Surely you don't think it is really working, do you? I mean fully, as it was intended to and with respect to the great problems of cost and access faced by Americans across the nation. I've got these problems all across my home state, and Washington State government is probably light-years ahead of other places in trying to add home state solutions so it might work better. I don't know how things look in Colorado, but they can't be good." Johnny knew that Coloradans generally supported the law and the notion of going further with its protections; Senator Bell had some vulnerabilities back home on the health care issue.

"I am sure there are ways to make it better. But that isn't really the issue here, is it, Senator?"

"You tell me—what is the issue?" Johnny asked.

"To be direct, you being here. I mean, as a senator. That was some cheap stunt you pulled to get elected. Senator Johansen was a good friend of mine, and I didn't appreciate what you did to him."

Johnny was having none of this attack. "I didn't do anything to him—and you know that I had no part in his decision to resign. He was a friend to me, old school for sure, and we might not have looked at the world the same way. But he was a good man and I don't play the game that way. If you mean I ran for an open seat, I plead guilty as charged. There is nothing wrong with that. I won fair and square."

Senator Bell chuckled. "You think that your little victory is enough to get you standing to actually legislate in the United States Senate, son? Tell me what you want after a few terms, and I will consider scheduling a vote."

"Senator, I didn't come here to fight with you. I am willing to go along with a lot of the demands of your caucus, and I have been a friendly vote on almost all your big ticket votes in the Senate so far. I could change my mind on some of these—and then you would have some ties on your hand. I doubt that the vice president is going to see these matters your way, do you?" Johnny had not expected this to get to the nuclear option so quickly, but here it was—he wanted a commitment or would threaten to vote with the Republicans. The vice president would break the resulting tie for the Republicans.

"Okay, let's not get too far out ahead of things, Senator." Senator Bell was backtracking, realizing that he might have cut to the chase too quickly and too directly. Senator Gibson was not the pushover he thought. "Why don't you get me a summary of the amendments? We've got some issues we would need to work through on just those—the hospitals are a big political donor, and we can't afford to lose their money as we head to next year's election. Maybe we can make a trade."

Johnny sat back in his plush leather chair. "What do you mean?"

"I mean you are done here, Senator. There is no way that you will win another term. Us or the Republicans will take you out. This isn't some insignificant House seat—this is a controlling vote in the United States Senate. And let me give you a little friendly advice. You know those attack ads that have been airing about you? I am here to tell you, boy, that this is the tip of the iceberg. My people tell me there are some much harder-hitting ones getting ready for distribution. Not that I have anything to do with those. I would hate to see such things go public."

Johnny got the threat. He wasn't sure what he wanted to do, but figured he should at least begin to understand the particulars of his choices. "What do you want?" he asked.

"I want you to commit to not running again, and to working with me and our political operatives on how you pull out of the reelection campaign. If we do it right, we can ace the Republicans out of any chance of winning the seat. If you do that, I will commit to getting you a floor vote on your bill, and whatever you want to put in it."

Johnny continued to stare back at the majority leader. He didn't know what to say. That his reelection was going to be a difficult proposition was something he had realized. Hearing the vitriol from a party leader so directly helped him see just how hard it would be. That conclusion was coming at him too severely and quickly to respond.

"I can see you thought you had a chance. Sorry about that, but someone had to tell you. Who knows, you might even get your bill passed. But remember, I am not making any assurances that the president will sign it. I don't think you would find enough votes to override a veto. My advice to you is to take my deal—and structure a very narrow bill that you might be able to squeak by the Congress and the president in a run up to an election. That is your best chance. Think it over, if you need some time. I've got a lunch meeting right now, so go ahead and let yourself out when you are ready."

With that, the majority leader rose and strode out. Moments later, Jane came in to escort Johnny out of the office. She looked at him sitting in the chair and sat down beside him, in the same seat that Senator Bell was in moments ago.

"What's wrong?" she asked. "You look like you've lost your best friend."

"No, nothing like that, Jane. Nothing like that. But I have been told most of my life that I had to grow up if I wanted to really make a difference. Maybe they were right."

Chapter Eighty-Nine

HealthMost's Cover-Up Expands

Richard Thrust strode confidently into the Executive Conference Room at HealthMost Chicago Headquarters. The door closed automatically behind him as he moved to the head of the V-shaped table. It was a smaller room and far less ornate than the boardroom and most of the other conference rooms. There was no view outside; it was an internal office, where security and focus on work were paramount. Two of the four walls had large grease boards, a third a map of the United States with color-coded stick pins denoting HealthMost health care facilities. The fourth wall held a large video screen, and the controls for its state-of-the-art video conferencing were on top of a small credenza in the far corner of the room. It was more advanced than the system's capabilities for online medical evaluations and treatments—cutting corners to save money on telehealth was okay, but not scrimping on the administrative trappings of the Thrust medical empire.

Five men and one woman—all white—were seated around the table on the two wings of the V—Sam Bridgewater; corporate Chief Financial Officer Haynes Dickson, legal counsel Michael Cadmeyer; Chief Operating Officer Lane Stevens; Chief Information Officer Steven Drury; and Barbara Baines, vice president for public affairs. This was the HealthMost executive team, with the addition of its lead lobbyist. All had arrived at the meeting five minutes before its start time of 10 a.m. They knew that Thrust would not enter until just after the hour. His command was reinforced by the design of this room—all attention was to be focused on him at the top of the V when he sat down. When there was an executive staff meeting held without him, no one dared sit in his lead chair—one of many of what were called CLAs in HealthMost—career-limiting acts.

"Let's get this meeting underway, people," barked Thrust, interrupting no one. All conversations had stopped the second he moved into the room. "We are here to consider our next steps to optimize our contract with HHS. Over the last month, there have been some unsettling developments, the product of incompetency to my eyes, though not all of the particulars have been uncovered. You are all aware of the incident in Washington State, which forced us to implement our public health protocol to recover the body and control the situation. Our belief then was that we had contained the situation. A couple of recent developments tell us we should no longer just assume that was the case. Bridgewater, let's start by having you brief the team members about the two additional issues that have complicated our understanding."

"Certainly, Mr. Thrust." With that, Sam Bridgewater provided a slightly longer report to the team than he had provided to Thrust last week by telephone. He had uncovered a few more pieces of information since the call, and inserted these new facts into the storyline.

For one, they had confirmed that it was Nelson Duncan III who had made an inquiry into the secret database in ALI for the project. He had at first denied doing so, and then tried to put it off as just a standard security test that he would occasionally do as CEO. Under threat of a public firing for cause, and the risk of a loss of his pension and other benefits, Nelson relented and admitted that he had provided several files to a staff member of Senator Gibson's. He then resigned his position with ALI, claiming health issues—provided he did not disclose anything else on the matter to the senator or anyone else.

Bridgewater had only a little more information on the mysteriously lost patient in New Mexico. In this case, it was HealthMost's own practices that made it difficult to find out more. Once patients like Roberto Hernandez were flagged, the established systems emphasized limited record keeping. Personnel who had seen him were slim on recollections, though one emergency room worker thought he seemed a little different than the typical immigrant patient. At the holding facility, all they could add was that the patient's mattress was stained with IV solution. They surmised he had somehow managed to avoid the medications that would have put him in a semi-catatonic state through his stay on the ward. That would explain how he could have been alert enough to execute an escape plan—but nothing about why, or where he had gone next.

When Bridgewater was finished with his briefing, Thrust reclaimed control of the meeting. "I believe that we should look at none of this as coincidence or unconnected. Rather, we should look at this as a hostile plot against us and our interests—and we must respond accordingly." He scanned the room and the faces of his underlings; he wasn't expecting opposition, but wanted to take stock of any hesitations.

Surprisingly, Michael Cadmeyer spoke up. "I can see where these events are deeply troubling. But doesn't responding raise the odds that the underlying program will become public, with all of its potential negative consequences? It will make it harder for us to assert our defenses if this somehow moves into civil or criminal proceedings—as legal counsel I am obligated to bring up these possible downsides."

Cadmeyer was trying to walk a fine line with Thrust. The reality was that he and the entire executive team were deeply troubled by the arrangement they had made with the federal government to help deport illegal immigrants in exchange for secret government grants. Its moral ambiguities troubled them, but it was the chance they might get caught that made them nervous.

For professionals like Cadmeyer, discovery would mean not just public shame but likely loss of his license to practice law. When the additional system protocols were added on to the scheme, his concerns had risen exponentially. Where before he could see the risk of moral failings being prosecuted in the court of public opinion, the special treatment program now carried with it clear labels in American criminal law—kidnapping, assault, homicide, bribery, and extortion. A lost license would be a small matter compared to spending several years in a federal penitentiary.

But he, like the rest of the executive team, was too far engulfed in this—and the entirety of HealthMost's corporate approach to business under Thrust. They were feeling more and more like Nazi prison guards—wondering whether their involvement in the scheme, and enthusiasm for the greater cause, would protect them if things turned sour. Knowing that desertion from duty would carry severe penalties for them and their families, they were still willing to double down further and engage in additional questionable conduct.

"What are you suggesting, Cadmeyer? That we shouldn't have done this? That we should fold our hand because some politicians and bureaucrats are complicating our business practices with their meddling?"

"Uh, no, sir. I just wanted to express for the record that we have considered other options in light of these circumstances. It will be important, should the worst happen. Again, as your legal counsel, I am just trying to provide you all the protections we can." He was now making legal shit up. Thrust had called his bluff and made it clear that it would be full steam ahead. Cadmeyer also knew that meant that any deserters or even malingerers would be shot without question, at least metaphorically.

"Damn lawyers. Always speaking out of both sides of your mouth. Your advice is duly noted, and you can also note that we are rejecting these other options. Instead, what we are going to do is make sure our investments and strategies are protected. In any way we need to. Understood?"

All of the persons around the table nodded and mumbled assent. Unanimity was in place—a common outcome from meetings in the Executive Briefing Room.

Chief Operating Officer Lane Stevens went further; he had no misgivings about the project and saw himself as Thrust's eventual successor. He regularly looked for opportunities to position himself with Thrust for his favor and possible anointment down the road. This seemed to be one of those occasions. "Yes, I agree completely, Mr. Thrust. This is an extraordinary program that you have conceived. It is achieving a vital national interest and bringing hundreds of millions of dollars in income to HealthMost. Anyone interfering with it should be viewed as a traitor and a thief, and we should do all we can to uncover and punish them. Chief, what do you see as our next steps?" He liked to call Thrust "Chief" so as to feel special—and for others to perceive some intimacy with the boss that they did not have.

Thrust smiled. He liked the special handle. Not because he needed the affirmation, but because it proved him the subserviency he demanded. It would help bring others in line too. Not that he had any inclination to do anything for Stevens if he ever did decide to leave HealthMost. He wasn't smart enough to do the job. But then, who was?

"Two things. First, we immediately shut down our special treatment facilities in Washington State. Wiped any trace of them off the map. That way, if anything ever does break because of these security breaches, we will have plausible deniability that any of what will seem to be wild assertions are true."

"Second, we need to scare off or preferably take out those who are attacking us," Thrust continued. "While it is possible he may have some helpers, what we know is that this starts with, and maybe ends with, Senator Gibson. Bridgewater has told me that Gibson has virtually no chance of retaining his Senate seat; the Ds and the Rs are after him, and we will also be putting money into a private campaign to make sure the voters of Washington know who he is. Bridgewater, I want you to take the lead on this."

"Will do," replied Bridgewater. "This has largely been our plan anyway, and we will give it even greater priority now. It might cost a bit more to pay for our campaign, but we are already in league with some others to uncover the senator's dirty little secrets. Soon, the world will know about them."

"I look forward to that." Gibson's insolence toward Thrust would not be forgotten quickly. "But it's not enough."

"What do you mean—uh, what more do you want to do?" Bridgewater was, for once, surprised out loud by a statement by Thrust. Gibson was already a very short-term problem, and one with somewhat of a political muzzle for the few months now left in his public office career. Outcomes were what mattered in his world, and those that got emotional or spiteful usually lost.

"I want to expose him for what he is. It isn't enough that he loses his Senate seat; I want to show the world that he is a sanctimonious ass."

"Yes, and we will try to do much of this through the private campaign. We've already got the Swiftboat people locked up and ready to transmit our message when we've got it fully cooked."

"Well, I want to put a little contemporary incompetence out there for voters and the public to see. The problem with things like the Swiftboat ads and other voices of the past are just that. Past transgressions brought to public reckoning decades after they have happened. Just about everyone has something in their closet—or enough to put something in their closet. I want something more immediate that will make his shame obvious in real time," said Thrust.

"Okay," headed Bridgewater. "My general rule is to let sleeping dogs lie, especially if they are already in the process of being put down. But if this is what you want, we will put something together. Do you have some idea in particular?"

"It seems to me this nonsense about the public hearing in Washington State is intended to be some type of a trap for the secretary and us; that much seems obvious already. But I don't think we should see it as a coincidence that the location is so close to our disposal facility in western Washington. I think that is what the record keeping espionage with ALI was all about, and that he is angling to make some special revelation with the cameras rolling."

"How much could they know?" interjected Cadmeyer. He was getting nervous again.

"We don't know, but we should assume a lot," Thrust replied. "Which makes it a perfect opportunity to also prove the accuser to be an incompetent fool. I say we agree to testify at this hearing, and I will do it. Bridgewater, we will need you to figure out what their plan is. Bring Secretary Olsen into this if you like—the more he is on the hot seat, the more we will be protected. But ultimately, let's get Gibson to set his trap and then show the world there is nothing in it."

"Yes sir." Bridgewater knew there would be no further debate. "It helps that the disposal facilities in Washington State are now gone and erased."

Thrust confidently nodded his agreement. "Now you are starting to see the big picture. You've got your assignments. Barbara, I want you to work with Bridgewater on our media plan around the public hearing." Thrust liked to call his female staff by their first name, suggesting an intimacy with the other sex that male counterparts would respect. "There will be an executive team meeting on this every week until we get to the hearing. Everybody is to be here for those meetings. Wipe your calendars clear, including vacations, weddings, or funerals. This is now our top priority operation."

Thrust got out of his seat, picked up the files and pad of paper from the desk, and quickly left the room. The others stood as he did, but waited to pick up their materials until the door had closed behind him. They quietly gathered their belongings and left the room too. All might have been uncomfortable with where they were going, but there was nothing to be gained by sharing this with others. They all knew they would need to build their own path through, around, or into this, just like Nazi prison guards.

Chapter Ninety

Johnny and Nancy Meet

Johnny strode into Nancy Jones's Seattle office, surprising her with his sudden and fast entrance. He kept walking toward her, and then detoured around the desk separating them, giving her a big hug as she got to her feet.

"No time for anyone else now, Nancy—Johnny is here!" exclaimed the senator.

She closed the laptop computer on her desk and motioned to a small conference table on the other side of the room. It offered a good view of downtown Seattle and the waterfront. "Johnny, you know there is never any time for anyone else but you. How is my favorite client?"

"Oh, we'll get to that soon enough. Tell me about you. Have you sold out to the man yet? Or are you finding more provocative ways to make a living?"

"Come on, Johnny. From the day I started working with you, the man hasn't had much interest in me. Oh, they might humor me, but really, you have made me a suspect in my own friendship circles. Maybe not with candidates, but with the party bosses. If I want to make a living, I have to reach out to lost and difficult causes." She laughed. "But that is my thing, isn't it?"

She pointed to the table. "Let's sit here. I got us a couple of box lunches. Still off of meat, right?"

"Too late for me to turn back. Haven't had a taste since 1980."

"Here, you take the falafel." She handed over one of the box lunches. They opened their lunches, ate, and caught up on old times and acquaintances. There was plenty of time to get to the new business at hand; both knew it was going to be less fun than reminiscing.

When they were done with their lunches, it was time to consider the current state of affairs. Nancy kicked it off. "All right, tell me, Johnny. Who have you pissed off now and what do you want me to do about it?" She already knew, but it would help her to understand how much he knew of the bad space he was now in.

"Same people as before, Nancy. They just seem a lot more intense than before. Things really have been different since I moved over to the Senate. No regrets, but they are a sordid bunch." He gave his account of his meeting with the Senate majority leader. Nancy was attentive to his every word.

She stroked her chin, contemplating how much to tell him, and how quickly. "Unfortunately, Johnny, this matches up with what I was hearing. Your version was a lot more direct about how the Democratic Party apparatus is now seeing you than what I got from my sources. But it was the same point—they want you gone and out of the way and don't intend to let anyone or thing get in their way. They were even telling me that I would not get any other Democratic clients until I dropped you."

"So, you going to do that?"

She laughed, as did he. "Yeah, right. A little late for that, buddy. You and I are joined at the hip for better or worse. No, I am still your political consultant if you want me. Besides, they were just blowing a lot of smoke up my ass anyway. There are a number of democratic women candidates who have told me that they want me to work with them, and they won't give a shit what the party office has to say about that."

"Do you think I should even give it a try?" asked Johnny. "I was thinking of taking the majority leader up on his offer."

"That would be your call, Johnny. My advice to you, as your political consultant and friend, is to wait before you make a decision. It might be that you want to make a deal now. But the terms are up for negotiation if that is the case. And what you want is more leverage. If you decide now not to run, you have none. Waiting, and better yet announcing you are running will give you something to work with. And if you decide to run again, you will be well on your way."

"You always make these political choices seem so much clearer. Thanks, Nancy. I was kind of getting lost in the fight. These things usually don't get to me, but this one got me mad."

"Understandably. There is a lot at stake and they are being particularly nasty. And you've always had good instincts, so what you may be feeling is some sense that this is bigger and nastier than you think. If so, I am here to tell you that this would be true."

"What do you mean?"

"I laid my political traplines out across the state to see what is out there about you. The hostility of the Democratic Party to you was part of what came back. It is what you described—they think you stole their seat and they are out to get you. They might even silently admire your political moxie, but this is about control of the Senate, and they are not going to play around with you. This we knew—and so do you. What is also troubling is that I got some of this from my Republican Party contacts. They have their own take on this, and also think you stole the seat from them. So, they want you out too."

"I would have guessed that too. But they didn't reach out with any direct threats like the Ds did. Are you saying that I should be watching out for that?"

"Honey, you should always be watching out for that—and you know it. What troubles me is that I got a report that the two parties might even be working together to get you out of the way."

"What?"

"Yup. It came from someone high up, an old friend that I really trust. He wanted to make sure I didn't get hit in the crossfire to come. I won't betray his confidence in who I got this from, but what he told me was kind of chilling. Seems like you are about the only thing that has brought our two political parties together in America. They are working on a joint campaign to get you out of the Senate and putting money into a special fund to buy up ad space to keep your ads off of television and to run theirs. A special committee has been formed to do negative ads about you. They are already running a few test ads and are also organizing a digital media campaign to discredit you. They have contracted the Swiftboat people to put together some smears to really hit you where it hurts. Their goal is to make it impossible for you to resurrect your candidacy using your past campaign tools. It was why my friend was concerned for me. Once they jointly conclude you are toast, they will end the joint attack and go back to their usual party-to-party dirty politicking. But for now, they have both agreed that getting you out once and for all time is the first and common objective."

Johnny sat there absorbing this news. He did find it shocking. Maybe his instincts had picked up on this but his brain certainly hadn't. "Geez, Nancy. Other than that, how was the play, Mrs. Lincoln? Anything more?"

"I sent my political detectives to do some sleuthing in the smarmy underbelly of PACs and issue committees and the like to see if they could find out more about this joint campaign. They found enough to confirm that it was happening and that it was being led by Sam Bridgewater, from the firm of Bridgewater, Atkins and Lacey. Know this guy?"

"Not well, but we've had some jousts in the last year. I used to serve in the House with him way back when. He sold out a long time ago, and has some seedy corporate clients as well as a strong link to party leadership for the Rs. Wouldn't trust him as far as I can throw him before you shared this with me." Johnny stood up and walked over to the window, looking down below at the Seattle waterfront. "So, tell me, my friend, what do we do?"

"I've got to be honest with you. I believe they have your number this time. If it was just a House race, we could do some things. But statewide, with the firepower they plan on coming at you with, it will be really hard. The only possible way to counter it is with a counter version of their playbook. And, my friend, your attraction to voters has always been that this is exactly what you are not."

Johnny kept looking out the window.

"If you want to fight this, count me in," said Nancy. "I will always be in your corner, to the end of time. But it might be time for another play. That is your decision. I've got some ideas if you want to go that way, but you have to let me know what you want to do. And for now, I suggest we get you some more leverage by announcing your candidacy for reelection. Maybe we can roll something out this week, while you are in town."

Johnny turned from the window and looked at Nancy. The usual grin was gone from his long face. "Let's do it. Just tell me when and where you want me and what I should say. I've got some thinking to do. You know I can't do this without checking in with Irv and Mary Beth first. But I can tell you that I also have some ideas if we go in this direction."

"It's been quite a ride, Nancy," he continued. "If this is the end of it, let's make it a good death. A death that can give life to others."

"I would expect nothing less than that from you, my friend."

Johnny and Nancy hugged again, squeezing out the bad mojo of the current times and replacing it with new possibilities for the future.

Chapter Ninety-One

Irv Crashes

Irv accepted his demotion to public health investigator as best he could. It was a bitter pill to swallow.

Only months ago, he was leading innovative projects that were fundamentally changing the health care system for the better. Now, he was a low-level investigator who got the assignments no one else wanted, which usually consisted of inspecting restaurants or septic field problems. Once in a while, he gave a guided tour to a high school class.

He hoped that he might eventually come across some more important projects that might help him make it through this bad phase for his career. He quickly learned that most of his projects were being assigned personally via the office of Director Welch and he should not expect any change in his situation.

He did figure out that he was eligible to be part of the "on call pool." When it was your turn for the hot lead—on nights, weekends, and holidays—an investigator would not only respond but get the case assignment. Director Welch couldn't intervene in that. Being on the list came with extra pay, and Irv was saving as much money as he could so he could soon move on to a better situation without money as a limitation.

It was common to get a call, but far less likely for it to become an interesting longer term assignment. But Irv did get one in his first year in his new demoted capacity—an E. coli outbreak in the international community. Business people affected, including some wealthy donors to the new county executive, were looking to quietly bury the real problem Irv had uncovered. Irv had defied these efforts by slipping the story to reporters, which made his relations with Director Welch worse.

Still, he was going to hang on as long as he could. His aim was to get close to five years with Public Health; this was the general time frame for staying in his next position offered by advisors during his last job search. He figured that he could shave some of that time off under these circumstances. The issue now was that he didn't have any idea or interest in finding this next job.

He was depressed, partly from the job problem, but also because of the growing distance between him and Mary Beth. A couple of years ago, she had moved to southwest Washington to take an executive director job. It was a direct consequence of her losing her former job at the bakery, but was also related to their struggles as a couple. Cancer had triggered this, but Irv knew that he was also the problem.

They never technically broke up. Rather, they were just living apart and would get together on weekends and holidays, as best they could. She was busy with her new job and didn't have time to come to Seattle often. Not so long ago, Irv was also busy with his important work with Torrey. Irv and Mary Beth's get-togethers became more and more infrequent as time passed.

Now he had the time but no idea how or even if he could resurrect their former magic. He visited Mary Beth a couple of times after his demotion, but she was incredibly busy with work and unable to devote her time to him. Nor was he putting his best foot forward when he did spend time with her in his current state. An idle and depressed Irv was not the most fun person to be around.

So, Irv spent most of his time after his demotion in Seattle alone, trudging through the day at work as best he could. Then he spent his time in the Wallingford home, surfing television shows and the Internet and otherwise watching time pass. He was trying to find a better spot, but failing—slipping deeper into his dour state of mind. Most of a year passed, and nothing had gotten better. Time was marching ahead, but not Irv.

He was considering drastic action. He didn't know what, just that he had to do something and soon. He would keep saving up as much money as he could and leave by the end of the year. Where he might go, he did not know. It would require a lot of energy to figure out what to do, and he was hoping to find some resolve to explore this in the fall. Then, one early spring night, his beeper went off in the middle of the night.

There was a dead body in a house in Kent.

Chapter Ninety-Two

Mason Health Foundation Threatened

The Mason Health Foundation's plan to become a not-for-profit health insurance broker was working. It took three months to launch the patient navigator and insurance broker service and, while complicated and time-consuming to develop, the necessary changes were not all that difficult. The foundation needed a more thorough organizational infrastructure and several state and federal licenses. It needed to get certified by health plans operating in Mason County. Staff needed to review their navigation service to make sure it was thorough enough to take on this new challenge, and brainstorm what new pieces they might add to make it better.

There would be more to do as they learned about the business, for sure. But they had enough to start up. Mary Beth also wanted to make sure that they tested their new activity regularly and grow it organically, rather than presume they knew everything about it from the start. It was especially important since the foundation was committed to build something in full relationship to their social mission, not just operate a business using their not-for-profit status as a tax dodge.

The foundation was able to get the service officially up by the time of open enrollment period for Medicare in November. This was also a time when many companies made their health coverage decisions for the next year. Mary Beth and their two caseworkers networked across the county, one person and organization at a time, starting with the list of partner organizations of the foundation. A small but growing number of small businesses and individuals decided to sign up as clients of MHF. By the end of the year, they had 238 clients.

It was, as expected, only a small stretch to reconfigure their personal health navigation service to include health coverage broker services. Staff had to learn more about the specifics of health coverage and different health plan offerings, but they did already know far more about health coverage than general insurance agents. Their challenge was learning how to customize personal health needs with these standard insurance offerings, observing that it was not something other brokers did.

By the end of the first quarter of the next year, commissions were rolling in—over $3,000 per month—and the business was growing incrementally, about twenty clients a month. They were in discussions with several small employers about being the broker for their employees. Planning was underway for the fall open enrollment period, and Mary Beth and staff had new ideas on how to market the service. Their conservative projections were that they would have about a thousand clients by the end of the year and monthly commission revenue of over $10,000.

Nor was there any reason to believe that growth would not continue into the future. MHF had been approached by individuals and small businesses in adjacent counties about serving them, and Mary Beth could not find any legal or practical reason why they could not do so. The board was reviewing how they might expand the geographic scope of their mission to include these outlying areas. This alone would grow revenue by another 25 percent.

Property tax receipts for the next year had taken the expected hit—$23,000 less on top of the $50,000 loss from last year. They would more than make up for this loss with business already signed up, and by next year, they would be approaching the possibility of matching their property tax revenues with just commission revenues. Even with the added expenses of establishing and running a broker business, the foundation would be operating at better than breakeven.

Just as exciting to Mary Beth, the staff and the board were seeing the great potential to impact health across the county, maybe even the region, more profoundly. The personal service they were providing was improving regularly, especially in how it advanced people's health. Staff learned how to customize health coverage decisions to personal circumstances and health needs, and identified tools that would help them and their clients do even better. They now had sufficient revenue to add another two staff to help grow their idea, and several new program ideas to enhance the services under development.

It was with this backdrop that Mary Beth was now driving to Olympia for a meeting in the insurance commissioner's office. She had received a phone call asking her to come to their offices, and it was troubling at the time that they suggested she bring along her legal counsel. They wouldn't say more about why, and Mary Beth invited Jim Reynolds to come along. He was a member of their board and occasionally provided pro bono legal counsel to the foundation. His day job was as a general practice attorney in Shelton, and he had done so for thirty years after having taken over the practice from his dad.

The insurance commissioner's office was located in the Capitol Building on the grounds of the state capitol near a small inlet at the base of Puget Sound. The campus was one of the more beautiful capitols in the nation, especially when the sun was out. This was a wet summer day, but still pretty as the rain bounced off the many shades of green across the campus.

They parked their car in a commuter lot and walked the half mile to the capitol, and then up the marble stairs into the Capitol Building. Looking up, they were impressed by the massive rotunda and the white marble columns rising up to it. To the right of the first hallway was a high portico and massive door with the words "Office of the Insurance Commissioner" etched in stained glass over the doorway. They opened the door, stepped into a reception area, and announced themselves.

The receptionist told them that the others had already arrived, and she walked them down a short hallway to a large conference room. Who were these others? The person who called for the meeting had made no mention of them.

There were four people sitting at the rectangular table filling the room, on the long side across the other side of the room. They filled half of the length of the twenty-foot table. Seated at the shorter head of the table to their left was a man in a dark three-piece suit. Next to him was a woman with what looked to be recording equipment in front of her. The only two chairs available were at the other long side of the table in front of them.

"Please, have a seat," said the man at the head. He motioned to the two seats in front of them. As they sat, the man went on. "I would like to call this hearing to order."

"Excuse me," interrupted Mary Beth. "What hearing is that? I was asked to come to a meeting, without much of an explanation."

"Well, perhaps you misunderstood. My name is Alex Cross and I am an assistant insurance commissioner. You have been asked to appear because of your apparent violations of insurance law in our state. With me today are two investigative staff from our office. We also invited two staff members from the State Department of Health since some of your alleged violations relate to the state's role with health improvement."

Mary Beth's legal counsel stepped into the breach. "Mr. Cross. My name is Jim Reynolds. I am a member of the board of the Mason Health Foundation and I also provide pro bono legal services to the organization. My understanding is that if there is some complaint, you need to provide us notice in writing. We have no such notice, and really no idea of whatever it is that has been alleged. We believe that our organization is operating in full compliance with all operable state and federal laws, and your investigation takes us completely by surprise."

"Let me be a little clearer then. We are convening this under our emergency enforcement powers, which authorize us to convene an investigation with reasonable suspicion of an activity that violates our laws and might endanger the well-being of the public. That is indeed why we have the Department of Health staff here as well. Perhaps we could have been a little clearer in our scheduling of this meeting, but know that we don't have a legal obligation to do more than we have done in bringing you here. In the interest of fairness, if you would like to reschedule this meeting for a day later this week, I would allow that. Or we can proceed now."

Mary Beth and Jim huddled to figure out their next steps. "I have no idea what they are talking about," she noted.

"Nor do I. But we talked about this on the drive here." They had wondered with concern as to what they were walking into. Jim had followed up Mary Beth's invite to him with a telephone call to the insurance commissioner, a personal friend, who was not willing to share anything he knew about the meeting, but did tell Jim that there were people out to "get," in his words, the Mason Health Foundation.

Jim offered his legal advice. "I say we go ahead and hear what they have to say. We have no obligation to respond in any way, and will have time under the statute they are relying on to develop our response. Our aim should be to draw out as much information as we can so we can understand what we are up against."

Jim turned to the assistant commissioner. "We will, under duress, agree to the convening of this hearing. I do want to state for the record that the Office did not provide any notice to us of any charges or complaints, and that we are voluntarily agreeing to remain only for the purpose of understanding what the nature of your investigation is."

"Very well," said Mr. Cross. "Shall we proceed?"

"We shall as soon as your stenographer actually enters what I just said—I want it on the record." Jim could see that the assistant commissioner was preparing to cut every legal corner he could. Jim was ready for a legal fight, if need be.

Cross nodded to the stenographer, who made an entry. "Thank you all for being here today. We are convening to investigate a series of complaints made against the Mason Health Foundation. It has come to our attention that the foundation has opened an insurance broker business and is now providing insurance advice to clients in Mason County. We have received several complaints about this business, alleging that it is fraudulently representing itself to the general public in violation of Washington insurance laws. We have also received complaints that it is endangering the health of the public by otherwise offering medical advice outside of the expertise of the organization or the people working at it. These allegations are detailed in the report that we are sharing with you now." One of the staff members across the table got up and walked over two copies of a bulky report and handed them to Mary Beth and Jim.

They both quickly flipped through the report. It was over fifty pages long and included a series of allegations and recitations of Washington law. It would take time to digest exactly what they were alleging. "It will, of course, take us some time to review these materials. Perhaps you could provide us with an overview of what is contained so that we might ask some clarifying questions?" asked Jim.

"All right," Cross replied. "There are two general allegations against the Mason Health Foundation, and both are substantiated by extensive documentary evidence. First, that the foundation has provided misleading information on its broker services to prospective clients. Second, that the foundation is endangering public health by providing advice that it is not licensed and qualified to provide."

"Let's take these one at a time," Jim asserted. Mary Beth was busy speed-reading the report—a skill she had learned years ago that served her well now.

"Fine. The first allegation arises from the broker service that the foundation opened late last year. We have received a series of complaints that the foundation has misrepresented itself in its service offering. That is in violation of Insurance Commissioner regulations, and we are considering a cease and desist order upon the foundation because of these violations." Cross paused.

Mary Beth jumped in. "My fast read of this report is that the allegations are all the same—and repeated a number of times by different people." She opened the report and looked for the key words she had found. "It seems that they are all about our using the word 'free' in our written materials offering our broker services. Is that right?"

"Yes," said Mr. Cross, "though with the number of complaints, we see that there is a pattern of potential deception at play here."

"What pattern? They are all in reference to the same statement on our website that we are offering to provide free advice to the people using our service. Just because a number of people complain about the same language doesn't make it repetitive?"

"But it is not technically free—that is the complaint. And by suggesting that it is, you are misrepresenting yourself to the people of Mason County."

"What do you mean it is not free? Of course it is. Any funds that we receive for providing advice comes from commissions paid by the health plans they might select. We don't charge a penny to anyone using our service. In fact, if some health plans don't agree to pay us commissions, we will still provide the service—without any difference in what we do—to anyone. That is free, isn't it?"

"No, not to us. The reference manual to insurance broker materials labels commissions as 'no cost,' not 'free.' We contend that it is not free, but without cost. What's more, no other broker in Washington State refers to these as free services."

Jim took up Mary's cause. "That sounds like a distinction without a difference. And why is it important what other broker agencies say?"

"It sets a standard of appropriate behavior and point of view, and is something that our office relies on in interpreting Washington enforcement statutes," countered Cross.

"Are any other brokers operated by not-for-profit organizations, like ours," asked Jim. "That might be one big reason that they don't use the same language. They are in it for the money, not the cause."

Cross looked back at Jim. "You can see the allegations, and I believe we are on solid ground to enforce what we view as significant misrepresentations."

"Can you tell us who made these complaints? Looking at them, there is no indication of who made them. Or if one person made them over and over again, for that matter."

"No. That is privileged information. We have, we believe, verified that the complaint is accurate. The only question we have considered is whether it violates our statutes, and you are now hearing our view that it does."

Mary Beth was about to ask another question but Jim nodded at her. It was time to stop digging on this allegation. Their objective was to get as much information as they could about the complaint, without somehow creating a legal trail that could make their next legal steps more difficult. It was obvious that the assistant commissioner was hostile to them, though neither Mary Beth or Jim had any answer as to why.

Instead, Jim moved the conversation toward another line of questioning. "You said there was a second set of allegations. And that these were what made this an emergency enforcement? I think we need to understand a lot more about any such allegations." Mary Beth was now busily speed reading this section of the report.

Mr. Cross flipped through the notes in front of him. "Very well. The second set of allegations pertains to the foundation not limiting their advice to clients to decisions regarding the purchase of health coverage. The foundation is going beyond the traditional role of an insurance broker by doing so, and we have received several complaints about that. In reviewing these allegations with our colleagues at the State Department of Health" —he pointed to the two staffers seated across the room—"we believe that this advice is endangering health for the public by providing physician-like advice without a license. This threat is why we are convening this hearing as an emergency petition."

Mary Beth again took first crack at uncovering what was at play in this second set of allegations. "In looking at the materials in this report, you seem to be referencing the personal health navigation service that we have provided over the last two years to the residents of Mason County. We've never heard any complaints or criticisms about this. Nor are we providing anything like physician services, or those provided by any other licensed health care practitioner. Our role is limited to helping people navigate their way through the medical care system. Especially when they are confused by it—which, by the way, is almost all of the time. It also seems worth noting that at times this is because of or worsened by confusing materials and answers provided to them by the state."

"That doesn't mean we haven't been questioning what you were doing," interjected one of the two Department of Health staff. "If someone was going to do this, it should have been the local public health department."

"Sally, there is no need for you to respond to their statements." Cross tried to silence his public health colleague. "We will have ample time to respond to their defense of the allegations."

Mary Beth was loaded and now ready to take up the fight, here and now. "But public health in Mason County wasn't doing this, were they? In fact, public health isn't doing this in any county in the state, are they? Nor is the state department of health doing it. We are doing it precisely because no one else was doing it—and it is so needed by people."

"Yes, but now you are making money doing it. That's not right," Sally, a self-appointed defender of state public health, registered.

"Oh, so this is the issue. Now that we are able to do this with a revenue source, it is wrong? And let's be clear—we are not providing anything close to medical advice like that of a doctor."

"We weren't happy about it before you were making money, just to make that clear. You were getting a lot of strokes for doing something that is more appropriately a role of government. Because we are the government we can provide the type of advice you do, but you can't."

"Like what?" asked Mary Beth.

"Immunizations, for example. We know you get calls about that and advise people what to do—that is like practicing medicine."

"That's ridiculous. First of all, we tell anyone who calls about immunizations that they should talk to their doctor in making that decision. If they have one. And we provide them what is publicly available about this personal decision and some tools for making a decision, especially if they don't have a doctor. We actually provide them with the State Department of Health's materials when we do this. We also provide them references or copies of studies about immunizations, always making it clear that it is their decision—and that we are not doctors."

"I am going to cut this off," interrupted Cross. "The purpose is not for us to argue with you about our allegations, but to provide you a chance to respond before we take official action. Do you have any defense to offer?"

Jim took the lead again—it was time to call this charade to a halt. "Mr. Cross, as I said at the beginning, we are not prepared to offer a defense to any of these allegations. They seem misguided, but we only agreed to hear and better understand your allegations, which have gone unreported to us until now. We will not be making any further statements about these at this time, other than to assert that they are baseless and frivolous allegations. I will follow up with you with our official response at a later time."

"Very well, that is your right. I will then close this hearing, for the record."

Mary Beth and Jim stood up and immediately left the room; there was no reason for social niceties. There was no mistaking that this was a deliberate and calculated attack on them and the foundation. They debriefed on the car ride back to Shelton, while trying to chill their anger.

"They can't seriously believe these charges will stick, can they," asked Mary Beth.

"No, I don't think so. They may have hoped that we would roll over and play dead, but they really are pretty flimsy charges. I am confident that I can draft a response that will blow their allegations out of the water. I have to believe they know that, and this little stunt is more about something else. We need to understand the bigger picture of what might be going on here. I suspect it will be coming at us, and soon."

"So who do you think is behind it?"

"I was hoping you might know." Jim thought about this for a minute or two, looking out the side window at the water in the distance. Mary Beth was driving. "The most likely starting point is some insurance brokers, or their association. I've heard that they weren't happy with what we are doing."

"But there aren't any brokers offering advice on health care coverage to individuals and small businesses in Mason County. The few that are in town do this only for bigger businesses and don't even offer the added-on support we provide. It is a whole different thing."

"That is their objection. You are doing something that they don't want to, but they might change their mind at some point and want to preserve it for themselves. And that you are providing a ton more service than what brokers usually do for their commissions makes it far worse. They've been riding a pretty sweet money train for a long time."

Mary Beth recalled what a national consultant shared with her at the outset of her research. He referenced insurance commissions as largely a scam in search of a better purpose. Brokers would do minimal work to enroll clients, and then get ongoing commissions for long periods of time. Their fees would go up with health cost inflation, as this got added on to higher insurance rates every year.

Nor did they have any reason to recommend cheaper plans to their clients—they got paid more for more expensive products. The consultant had suggested that even if the foundation wasn't successful in what it was trying to do, it would be a worthy endeavor if their effort to provide real value forced changes in the broker business model. Change was hard, she thought, and cheap shot defenses like this easier than creating real value.

Jim continued. "They've also owned the Insurance Commissioner's Office for a long time, just like the health plans. These offices are historically a great example of industry-capturing regulators, all across the country. Just like when the railroads essentially took over the old railroad commissions and the airlines the old Civil Aeronautics board. Washington State probably has a lot more gumption in trying to actually regulate insurance than other states, but it doesn't change the reality that power and data and lobbyists put greater control in the hands of the industries they are supposed to regulate than public needs."

Mary Beth agreed that this was likely a source of the allegations today, but also knew there were some jealousies at play through the Department of Health. Jim went on. "Cross and the other low-level staff there might have been silly enough to think that these charges could actually stick. The real power brokers are too sophisticated to believe that would be the case. I am wondering more what their next play might be."

"Any guesses?"

"The obvious one. That this emergency hearing was mostly about making sure it happened so it could get reported. I would expect that we will see some newspaper articles about it soon, and maybe some other media reports. In our new media culture, the investigation and dirt are what opportunists are after."

Mary Beth understood what he was describing—it was a tool she had observed used for good by Johnny in his political campaigns—spreading information that more people should know outside of the standard media circles. But his was truthful information. "Some are just making things up completely and then paying messengers to spread them. The Internet is now rife with such garbage—and Facebook makes a pretty penny off of them. That is the real fake news."

"Exactly. That is my real concern, Mary Beth. I believe my friend, the insurance commissioner, was telling me that someone who matters politically is coming after us. This investigation might be part of this attack, but I think we want to be on alert for something more. Someone doesn't want us to succeed—hard as that is to believe."

"What's that old saying—if all the rational explanations for something don't prove accurate, then whatever is left, even if it isn't rational, must be what is going on."

Just last week, Mary Beth was beaming with pride over the foundation's clever and purposeful idea for sustainability and its progress. Now, it and they were under attack. *Does this ever get easy?* she wondered.

Chapter Ninety-Three

Nancy Confirms Johnny's Political Problem

"Nancy. Good to hear your voice." Senator Johnny Gibson was speaking loudly into his cell phone as he walked across the street toward the Capitol. There would be a vote on a budget matter in about ten minutes, and he needed to cast his vote against the proposal. The fine day brought him outside for a walk, rather than the usual bramble through the underground tunnels connecting his Senate office building to the Capitol Building. For summer in DC, it was unseasonably cool, meaning eighty degrees and low humidity. Normally, August in the nation's capital was like serving a sentence on a prison farm near the equator.

"Right back at you, Mr. Senator. What's all that huffing and puffing?" Nancy Jones was surprised to hear the normally fit Johnny Gibson gasping for air as he spoke on the phone.

"Nothing to be concerned about. Just out for a walk before a vote. Must admit that the four sets of stairs down to the ground floor winded me a bit."

"Going to get out of there anytime soon? Sounds like the majority leader is intent on keeping his opposition busy all summer." Normally, Congress would be off on a summer recess, but the Senate majority leader was doing all he could to preserve his party's majority by making it difficult for Republican candidates running for reelection to be home pressing the flesh for votes.

"I think we will at least get off around Labor Day—or he is going to have a revolution on his hands within his own party. Either way, I plan on getting home around then and staying through till our field hearing in early September in Belfair. What's on your mind? I got your message that you wanted me to give you a call."

"Are you by yourself? This conversation should be for your ears only." Nancy had the ability to make any situation seem more dramatic than it really was, but her tone suggested this was no drill.

Johnny sensed that this telephone call would be different. "Hold on for one second." He moved away from a crowd of tourists and toward a park bench at the far end of the lawn, where he sat down; the bench overlooked the Library of Congress and the Supreme Court buildings. "Now I am."

"Johnny, this is a follow-up on our conversation about your reelection prospects. I know you've been thinking about that since we met and sent out the announcement that you would be running. We've done some more research on your prospects and had a few things thrown our way, too, that I need to catch you up on. None of what I have to tell you is good news. I would be surprised if you don't know some of what I have to share with you."

"I can't imagine you have any good news, Nancy. You didn't then and if anything, I've sensed even more hostility since my reelection announcement. If cold stares translate to leverage, mission accomplished. The majority leader glared at me on the floor the other day. Are you saying that we have to make a final decision soon?"

"More than that. I am telling you we have to decide by the end of September. And if you do decide to run, a political action committee is about to unleash the fury of the titans on you."

"I thought that was generally the timeline, and you thought they would get ugly if I didn't get out of the way. What's different?"

"What's different is that I now know this is not just speculation. They reached out to me as your campaign consultant. That guy Bridgewater came by with a couple of other operatives and showed me some video clips that they plan to go viral with if you don't step away. It was some real nasty shit—suggesting everything from marital infidelity to meeting with terrorist groups. He let me know that there was even worse stuff to come. Fifteen minutes after he left, the majority leader called me up and asked if I had a good meeting. He said he hoped that this information might help change your mind about running and that if it didn't, it was only the tip of the iceberg of your problems. It is not often the two parties get together on something. Congratulations."

"Any idea what bullshit they are coming up with?" asked Johnny.

"I asked, as delicately as I could. Let's just say he artfully made allusions to IRS audits, federal election commission complaints, and even people in your office who would testify that you had molested them during their internships."

Johnny fumed on the park bench as he listened to these secondhand charges. None of them had a shred of truth attached to them, but he knew that would not matter in the immediate media reaction from such attacks. He gathered himself, trying to refocus his energy to something more productive. "So, are you saying that it is the end for me?"

Nancy also needed to collect herself. This was the message she was calling to tell him, and there were few ways to make it less harsh. "Yes. You can fight these charges, and to some extent they will blow away. But what I also have to tell you is that we have done some statewide polling on your election prospects. The underground rumor mills that the opposition PAC has been generating over the last three months have really undercut your support. You are still strong with independents, but registered Democrats and Republicans are both saying that they will vote for the party candidate, not you, in the upcoming election. You are twenty points down even before the real smears start happening. I am sure that Bridgewater and the majority leader have done their own polling and know this too. It wasn't an accident that they chose now to come talk to me about you."

Johnny breathed deeply into the cell phone. It was as if ghosts were blowing out the candles of his birthday cake of a political career into the receiver. He watched a squirrel run up a tree trunk, taking an acorn up to his nest for later munching. Probably the only option left for him too, he thought.

A couple of minutes passed; it seemed like an hour but Nancy wanted to let her friend and client process the bad news on his time frame. "Talk to me, honey. What are you thinking?"

Johnny smiled, to himself and the squirrel, who was now sitting on a branch looking down at him. "I am thinking this has been quite a run. But all good things must come to an end—so we can find new good things. Seems like that is what I have to do." He and Nancy shared a couple more minutes of silence.

Johnny continued, "But before I go, I want to do one more thing. You know, I would be willing to fight this a bit longer, but the bad press about me will minimize the news I want to make at this hearing in Belfast. And that is far more important to me. So, let's just tell them that I will likely be stepping aside, but they will have to wait for the decision and announcement until after that hearing."

"Got it. I suspect that this may temporarily call off some of the dogs. After all, their alliance is a fleeting one—they are itching to begin trashing each other's party candidates, so they will be content to just let you fade away. As long as you are officially out before October comes along."

"One more thing. The majority leader promised me a vote on my bill if I stepped aside. Tell him I want that commitment as part of our deal if I do step aside. Tell him that I will be coming to see him in early October and I expect him to honor our deal."

"He will know what I am talking about?" Nancy asked.

"Sure. An old warhorse like him never forgets a political trade. He might have hoped I forgot, and your job is to make it clear that I haven't."

"Why do I think this has something to do with your hearing . . . " mused Nancy. "Did he make any commitment to vote for it?"

"It does, and no, that wasn't part of his offer. Nor am I asking for it. Just tell him I want what he promised when we met in his office."

"There's more to this than meets the eye, isn't there, my friend?"

"You could say that. How about I tell you more about this in person when I am out there around Labor Day. Think you can clear your weekend around the holiday? Irv and Mary Beth and I have a call tomorrow, and our tentative plan is to get together to prep for the hearing somewhere in Mary Beth's neck of the woods. It would be great if you could be with us too."

"Deal, Johnny. Wouldn't miss it. I must say, dear, you take rejection better than most of my clients."

"Rejection, what rejection? Your news caught me a little off guard, but really, I think you and I both knew we were already at this point even before this conversation. Every new beginning has to have an ending of what was before first, and you have helped me understand that this is where I am now. Thank you. To tell you the truth, it is liberating."

"You always surprise me, Johnny. Now go get your vote in."

"Oh screw that. It was just a showboat vote for the cameras. Nothing I need to worry about now. Think I will see a man about a squirrel." He stuck his tongue out at his furry little friend still gazing down upon him from the branch.

Chapter Ninety-Four

A Campaign Against Mary Beth

Jim Reynolds' words proved prescient. It was the next week when a shitstorm started to flow toward Mary Beth and the foundation. The first new attack was something she discovered while shopping for groceries at the local supermarket, where a group of women were whispering in the corner of the store. One was pointing at her.

A shopper who was near the group walked by, swinging her cart in Mary Beth's general direction. She seemed to mostly be interested in shopping, but Mary Beth stopped her. "You know what's going on there?" she asked.

The shopper turned her head and understood that Mary Beth was talking about the impromptu bitch circle at the other end of the store. "Oh, those biddies. They are always messing around in other people's business. I give them a wide berth. I did hear them say something like 'She is the one who had the abortion.' Sorry, that's all I know."

As soon as Mary Beth got home, she made a call to a local friend. While putting her groceries away, she asked whether she had heard anything about her around town. "I was about to give you a call, Mary Beth. But I wasn't quite sure what to say. It really isn't any of my business."

"What isn't any of your business?"

"Oh, so you haven't seen it."

"Seen what?"

"You know about the Daily Fire blog?"

"I've heard of it but have never looked at it." The Daily Fire was a local blog that carried a cross between real news, opinions about the issues of the day, and some questionable stories that regular news sources would not give air time to. Mary Beth hated sources like this—they were just forums for anonymous criticisms and conspiracy theories.

"Yesterday, they ran a story about you. It was about how you got an abortion years ago. I don't spend any time on that piece of shit blog myself, but I took a look when I heard about it. It is scandalous and mean-spirited. But what was also notable about it was that it actually had some of your medical records attached—showing that you had the procedure."

Mary Beth was shocked by the news. She ended her call with her friend and stopped unpacking the groceries. The ice cream on the counter slowly melted as she opened her laptop computer and searched for the Daily Fire blog. There was the story, there were the nasty anonymous comments, and, most surprising of all, there was her medical record for the procedure.

She didn't know what to say or do. This was such a personal thing; no one had any business even knowing about it, let alone publishing it and her medical records. It was a difficult time in her life, when she had learned of her pregnancy a month into cancer treatment. Irv and she had discussed it, and they were at first surprised and then excited to have a baby in their immediate future. It was one of the testiest moments of their relationship when they learned of her oncologist's concern over the types of chemotherapy being used for her treatment, which carried warnings about birth defects—severe ones.

Reluctantly, she chose to terminate the pregnancy. Irv was outwardly supportive, but she wasn't sure he agreed with her decision. It was another chip at the foundation of their relationship; a foundation that they were still trying, sort of from a distance, to rebuild. But all that was beside this point. It was nobody's business but hers. Who would print such a thing? Who would provide the records?

She immediately thought of Jim Reynolds and his words. She called him up on her cell phone. "So, you've seen the blog," he asked immediately.

"Yes, I have. It's nobody's business, Jim. It must be illegal for my records to be used in that way. Can I sue them for publishing them?" Mary Beth was pissed, a ground hornets' nest that had been stepped on by a big and heavy boot.

"Mary Beth, this is not anyone's business, including mine. I can understand why you are so pissed off. We can talk more about it if you like—as a friend, or even as your attorney if you really want to. My free advice to you is that taking action against the blog is only going to give the story more of a shelf life. It will end up not just in this piece of shit blog but the *Shelton Herald*. I don't think you want that."

"Well, what should I do," she asked.

"Be pissed off, to start. Scream to the high heavens, beat up your old car with a tire iron. Do whatever it is that helps you blow off steam."

"How are people around here going to react to this? It has only been over the last six months or so that I've started to feel like this community was a home for me, not just a place to work."

"To anyone you care about, really, it won't matter, at all. Sure, there are some who might disagree with your choice, but I think they would respect that it was yours to make. And they don't know anything about your choice."

Mary Beth thought about sharing the full story with Jim but chose not to—it didn't really matter to him or this situation.

"Yes," Jim continued, "this is a pretty conservative county, and there is an active pro-life group in town. But I don't think it will do any terrible damage to you."

"But you do think it will do some damage, don't you?" she asked.

Jim hesitated in his response, trying to find the right words. "The harsh answer to that is, yes. It will damage your reputation around your work for Mason Health Foundation, by those who don't know you. You have been somewhat of a mystery and an icon for people in this county, having moved out and revolutionized our local health care relationships. You've touched hundreds of people directly and have an outstanding reputation with them. I don't think that will change. It is the thousands who have heard about you in glowing terms from your general and lofty reputation. They didn't have a lot of information in making this conclusion, and unfortunately, some of them will reprocess that with this news."

"Just a girl's lot in life, huh." She felt a little bad bitching at Jim. He was only trying to be helpful, but who else was there right now to vent at about this nonsense?

"Yup. You and I both know that it would go down a whole lot easier if you were a man and this was some other story. I can't change that, and neither can you—at least now. Buck up and get over it. It is one of the qualities that draws so many people to your leadership—you are so courageous and calm in the midst of storms and crisis. Be yourself, and find the high road, even on this. That is who you are."

She greatly appreciated the kind words from Jim. When some of the foundation board members once shared with her that they also thought she was "courageous," it took her by surprise. She didn't even understand what they meant. Over time, she realized that was how many saw her optimism and belief and stick-to-itiveness in the face of big challenges. To her, it was just what one did.

"I will do my best with this, Jim. Thanks for that. I appreciate you hearing me out. I didn't call just for that though. Last week, you suggested we be on the lookout for the next shoe to drop. This is it, isn't it?"

"I've got to believe so, Mary Beth. Too much of a coincidence for it not to be. I also just got a call from the local publisher of the *Herald*. Not about this, but about a call he got pushing a story about the Mason Health Foundation. The source was telling him that there would soon be an announcement about an investigation of the foundation and that it would involve some very serious charges. The source was making the case that the *Herald* should be ready to run a major story about this; maybe even do its own local research to expose the corruption at play."

"Lots of shoes dropping," noted Mary Beth. "Is he going to bite on it?"

"I doubt it. Sure, he will have to run a story if a press release gets issued or the major papers in the region run a story about it. He would at least have to pick up the wire service story and put it in the paper. The good news is that he is suspicious of his source and a big fan of the foundation. He is actually one of our clients, and your team did a fabulous job of making sure his son got the treatment that he needs for PTSD."

"Was he in our special program for veterans?" She was thinking of a special program they had put together in the patient navigator service for returning servicemen—and their families—from the Middle East wars. Many were suffering from serious post-traumatic problems, and the Veteran's Administration had turned a blind eye toward them.

"Yup."

"Great to hear we were of help to him. Anything I should be doing on that front? If I can't bitch to the world about this piece of shit story about my abortion, maybe I can on this?"

"Let's think about that. I don't think we want to respond without putting some serious thought into what we should say. The advantage we have is knowing what is going on here. It is clear that there is an organized campaign. And unless you have some major ghosts in the closet, which are also none of my business, we can probably conclude that this is an attack on the foundation. Not to get you, but to get it, and what it is doing. Whoever it is might see you as a combatant and maybe a casualty in this, but it is important for us to remember that you are not the real objective."

"Good advice, Jim. Let's noodle on this. Maybe call an executive committee meeting after we've got some better ideas on a response. Oh—and I can assure you that you have now seen most of what I have in my closet."

"Good to know, Mary Beth. Sorry for this nonsense. It can be a harsh world out there. As an attorney, I regularly get to see the worst of people. It is one of the reasons I love the foundation and its work so much—it is all about the good that is out there, a good that we are trying to find even while the people it serves are getting served major doses of crap in their lives. We've got to keep it going—and grow it some more. There are so many more people who need it."

Mary Beth shut off her phone with a smile on her face. Calling Jim was the right thing to do. Sure, he had his usual common sense advice. What she appreciated even more was hearing his view of the work that they were doing through the Mason Health Foundation. It was how she felt about it, but another thing to hear someone she so respected spontaneously gush its praises. She needed to introduce Jim to Irv and Johnny—he would fit right in.

The personal meddling in her business was already getting pushed to the side, though even a glancing thought about it got her blood boiling again. It might take a day or two to cool down and respond tactically. This blog was not going to define her. The regulatory conspiracy was not going to end their service. None of this was going to stop her, or the Mason Health foundation. *They don't know who they are screwing with. Whoever they are.*

Chapter Ninety-Five

Irv Resigns, Under Pressure

Irv sat in the guest chair outside of Director Phil Welch's office for the second time in the last six months. Like before, he was called to the office with a note of urgency as he arrived for work in the morning. He quickly made his way up to the director's office and found Rose typing away at her desk just outside the office.

The director was in his office this time, with the door closed. Rose called in and let him know that Irv had arrived. Irv tried a couple of times to engage Rose in playful banter, but she didn't bite. She was either really busy or anticipating a difficult meeting for him. Her demeanor only reinforced his instincts.

He couldn't recall a good meeting with Director Welch, nor had they even talked since the pandemic scare a number of months ago. As far as the director knew, Irv had dropped that case like a hot potato—pun intended. It was possible Welch had uncovered that Irv was still on the case. But how? Irv had been exceptionally careful with every step and had used his vacation time for his absence from the office.

Could it be another case? Unlikely. He had been mysteriously removed from the investigator-on-call list after the flu incident. It seemed someone was trying to get him even further out of the way. That was fine with Irv, as he had other things to do with his time. The case had gotten him out of his doldrums, and he was now ready to figure out not only this case but his next career move. Still, the obvious shift for the worse in the public health department had him wondering.

The phone rang on Rose's desk and she picked it up. "You can go in now," she told Irv. No smiles, or winks. Yes, something was afoot.

Irv opened the door and walked into the office. Director Welch motioned for him to sit in a chair at his small conference table. "Close the door behind you," he stated. Not even a good morning.

Irv sat down and watched as Welch took a brown file from the middle of his desk and walked over to the conference table. He sat down across from Irv, palms down. There was a bead of sweat on his forehead, even though the office was very cool. Irv told himself that he would welcome the chance to play poker with the director.

"As you know, we have been making a number of changes across the department since my arrival. We are following the directive of the new county executive to reduce the size of government and the number of county employees. I am meeting with employees who are on our list for dismissal or reassignment. You are on that list and why I wanted to talk to you this morning." Welch had said all of this with the flat tone of a recorded computer message, while staring at Irv's second shirt button from the top.

So that was it. They were coming after him. Irv still had a residue of wonder whether this was just their general dislike of him and his background, or if it had something to do with recent actions. He would dig. "So, is this a termination meeting?" he asked, staring directly into the director's eyes.

"No. We are not in that stage yet. But we will be soon. The purpose today is to put you on notice of our evaluation. You, of course, have the opportunity to respond in writing or even to request a personnel meeting. I am also hoping that we might find a way to deal with this matter another way, should you be agreeable."

Irv stared at the director. He stroked his chin for a few seconds, processing his thoughts and next words and letting Welch stew in his own juices for a while. "Maybe," he said. "But before we get into any deal, I want to know why I am on your 'list,' as you referred to it."

"It is our evaluation of your work that it is barely satisfactory, Irv. You have broken protocol a number of times, and there is low confidence by the authorities in the department that you are loyal to this administration."

"Sounds like bureaucratic code words trying to say that I was not your political choice, and that I am willing to push and even fight for the truth in protecting the public's health. Instead of pushing things under the carpet like some people." He raised his eyebrows toward the director, making sure that the accusation that he was on this list was obvious. "You and I both know that I have glowing personnel evaluations and recommendations from the previous director, and that any criticisms started with your time in this office."

Director Welch gazed back at him, not sure what to say next. "All the same, there is an ample record of poor performance now." Irv was pretty sure that this outcome had been in motion for some time, and that the director and the personnel department had been inserting the necessary paperwork in his file to be ready when they thought the time was right. The Labor Day holiday was coming up, and the time seemed to be now.

But he had to be certain. "Did this have anything to do with the last case I worked with you on? You know, the bird flu case. You were pretty insistent that I narrow my role in that case. Did I not do that?"

Welch looked away when Irv asked the question. Yes, this clearly had something to do with them getting to this moment.

But Welch was not going to admit that. "No, this is more about your general performance. The federal contractor was not a fan of yours and asked us to remove you from the case entirely, but we didn't need to do that since we closed it the next week. But it is a good example of where you are lacking—important people aren't impressed by you and think you are a hindrance."

"You mean political hacks representing the current administration, don't you. Like you."

The director's face began to redden. *If only we had a deck of cards here*, thought Irv. *I would play him straight up for the pink slips on our cars.* Welch began to stammer out a defense, but Irv cut him off.

"I don't want to hear it, Welch. You being a political hack and a second-rate director of health is not going to change whether I stay or go. Tell me about this 'deal' of yours."

"Simple. You would be entitled to three weeks' pay if we go ahead and decide you are on our termination list. Or you can voluntarily resign today and get six weeks of pay. You have until this meeting is over to accept this deal."

"That is not very generous. A few more weeks in exchange for getting out of your hair immediately. Why, it will take you the extra three weeks to process my termination."

"All right, make it nine weeks then. And we are ready to move ahead with your termination within the next ten days. If you want to fight it, I can promise you that we will do everything we can to make sure your reference checks make you unemployable into the future."

"And what if I accept the deal?"

"We will acknowledge that you worked here, and that is it."

"All right, I will take it. I assume you have something for me to sign in that folder."

The director opened it and handed Irv two copies of a resignation letter prepared for him. Rose probably had typed this up for him and explained her reservations while he waited. Irv read it. It was pretty straightforward administrative crap, including a nine-week severance payout. That was the deal all along. He took a pen from the director's table and signed both copies of the letter. He put the pen in his front shirt pocket, letting Welch know, *I will take this souvenir too.*

"Date it too," noted Director Welch. He arose from his chair. "There is a security guard outside my door. He will accompany you to your cubicle, and you will have ten minutes to gather your personal belongings. I will take your county identification card and keycard. Your county vehicle will no longer be available, so you will have to find some other transportation home. That will conclude our business."

He certainly had his administrative ducks in a row. Probably took him the weekend to memorize all the steps. Irv reached into his pocket and took his keycard out of his wallet and handed it to the director. He pulled the county identification card from around his neck and threw it on the table.

Welch extended his hand, as if a handshake would remove the stain of his treachery. "Bite me," said Irv and turned and walked toward the door and out of the office. He looked at Rose, who peeked up from her typing assignment. He shrugged and followed the security guard down the corridor.

So this is what unemployment feels like, he thought.

Chapter Ninety-Six

No Confidence Vote

"Let's convene this board meeting of the Mason County Public Hospital District." Ken Sonnberg bellowed the words, trying to bring some order to the mass of people standing around, but not in, the chairs in the auditorium. Normally, their monthly board meetings were barely attended by more than the elected directors and staff. But this was no normal meeting—this was Peyton Place Two.

Sonnberg banged the heavy gavel down on the wooden table in the front of the room, showing the attendees he meant business. The commissioners took their seats at the north side of the table, with him in the middle. It would be strange to not hold a meeting where they sat around the table, but all wanted to be able to look directly at the crowd for this meeting.

It took a couple of minutes for the fifty or so people to take their seats in the metal chairs in the small auditorium. The first couple of rows were empty except for a reporter from the *Shelton Herald*, who was center cut in the first row, pad in hand. Whatever happened next, this was big news in this town.

"I will call us to order. My name is Ken Sonnberg and I am the board chair of the Mason County Public Hospital District. I am joined here today by my fellow board members." He proceeded to name them one by one, and each waved or nodded to help the attendees know who was who. Though none of this was a mystery to most there—they had known each other for much of their lives. Maybe it was just a polite nod to the unknown tall man in the suit in the back row.

"Seated at the end of the table to my left is Mary Beth Collins. She is the staff head of this district, and acts as CEO of our primary concern, the Mason Health Foundation. Behind her in the wings are the staff of the foundation. I would like to welcome them and thank them for their excellent work and service to this community. They normally don't attend our meetings, but they called me up and insisted that they would attend this meeting, given the topic at hand.

"Let's get right to that. Normally, we begin our meetings by approving minutes, reviewing the treasurer's report, and hearing some progress reports from committees and staff. Today we will defer these agenda items until later in the meeting so we can deal with the item that brings most, if not all, of you here today. That is the proposal of a no confidence vote directed at Mary Beth.

"Commissioner Kastner, allow me to call on you. You announced your intention to introduce this resolution in an op-ed in the *Herald* and provided some of your reasoning there. You weren't shy about your criticisms and your call to action for the board. Personally, and as a board member, I must say that I completely disagree with your conclusion and even your recollection of events and facts. But as the board chair of this district, I must provide the forum for you to express these opinions and to propose action."

An audience member shouted, "Let's get rid of her and fast—we don't need to waste time with any storytelling!"

Chair Sonnberg banged his gavel down even harder than before. He was ready for the crowd to get vocal and intent on not letting it devolve into anything akin to the nasty political rallies that were on the nightly news.

"We won't have any of that here," he shouted to the crowd. "Charlie, that sounded like your voice. You better know that I will toss your ass out of here if you do it again. And that will only be the half of it, as I will come to your house afterwards. Maybe Thelma thinks you were at the Rotary meeting last Tuesday, but I know better, don't I?" There were chuckles in the crowd. Ken had, for the moment, tamed the lions with his dry humor and show of authority.

"Thank you, Mr. Chairman." Anne Kastner, a local beautician, stood up to address the attendees. She was a relative newcomer to the board but not to the community—she was born in dreary bogs just outside the mill town of Aberdeen about thirty miles to the southwest, and had moved with her parents to the big city of Shelton as a teenager. She had seen tough times over her fifty years, as the timber industry dried up on the lower peninsula and unemployment and alcoholism engulfed her family.

Up to now, she had been a pretty quiet board member, soaking up knowledge about the district and its health activities. No one really thought of her as a troublemaker or a rabble-rouser, though she was a central piece of the town's gossip mill. She seemed to have a good heart, which made her attack on Mary Beth hard to understand.

She had a yellow legal pad in her hands and proceeded to present a vicious case against Mary Beth. It was a scripted and detailed argument, more like a case presented by an attorney than a hair bun specialist. It suggested she had help with it, as Anne had barely finished high school. Every once in a while, she would cast her gaze at the tall man in the suit in the back row while reciting it; it seemed he had something to do with it. Her delivery was a bit rough, but adequate enough. She had trouble with some of the phrases used, too many adjectives to smoothly roll off her tongue without a full breath. It was a damning story, and it echoed through the now quiet auditorium.

She told of Mary Beth moving to Shelton to try to resume her career after questionable life decisions and the loss of her job in Seattle. She did not say the word "abortion," but all knew the reference to "highly objectionable morals of the big city." She reported that Mary Beth was in need of fast cash to reckon for her sins, and implied an illicit drug habit. She suggested that the county's meth dealers and the opportunity to swindle the foundation out of some money were what brought her to their community.

All eyes were on Mary Beth. She sat stoically, straight in her chair and with her hands folded before her. She was staring at the table, struggling to look as calm as possible. She wasn't that good an actor—her face was flushed, the rage pushing against her cheeks and forehead. Those at the table could make out small teardrops in the corner of her eyes.

Anne Kastner continued. "I suppose that is now all water under the bridge for most of you. After all, we can't prosecute her or the board for past bad decisions. And let me be the first to say that some good has come from her being here. I think she has gotten far too much credit for it, but God does work in mysterious ways. We should not forget about her background as we now look to the future of our community and hospital district though. That is why I am introducing a resolution censuring her for her recent misdeeds and errors and, perhaps, crimes. And why I am asking my fellow board members, who seem unprepared to fire her outright, to adopt a vote of no confidence that will put her on notice that her bad behavior will no longer be tolerated. It will tell our community that some of us care about them and what is at stake, even if those in charge don't."

With that she outlined the abuses perpetrated by the foundation staff and Mary Beth over the last year. Among them, squandering public resources on a lavish lifestyle, violating public employment guidelines by not hiring local applicants for jobs, and misrepresenting themselves as health professionals to patients in need. She waved around a copy of a newspaper, noting a story on how the foundation and Mary Beth were being investigated for defrauding the public through an insurance scam operated by the foundation. By the end of Kastner's rebuke, Mary Beth was thinking that she might have to vote for her own censure—anybody half as bad as what was described would deserve that and more.

When she was done reading through her long script, Kastner put down the pad, looked first at her fellow commissioners and then the audience, and stated, "And that is why I now make a motion of a vote of no confidence against Mary Beth Collins today." There was applause from the audience, and Anne smiled and sat down.

The gavel came crashing down once more. Several board members were beginning to speak up, and members of the crowd began talking to each other. "Order, order. Before we go any further, I must see if there is a second to this motion."

"I second the motion," said Commissioner Jake Olinsky, raising his hand. Olinsky was a retired insurance agent who had served one term on the board. He had been a supporter of Mary Beth and the plans for the foundation for most of time, but had lately become more critical. Suspicion was that the insurance lobby had gotten inside his head, telling him that the not-for-profit broker idea was a bad idea.

"Okay, we have a motion and a second. Is there any discussion—and before you in the audience start shooting your yaks off, I mean by the board members seated here, not you."

With that, twenty minutes of denials, assertions, accusations, reprobations, and occasional personal insults flew across the table like ping pong balls. Chair Sonnberg vehemently defended Mary Beth, and Kastner and Olinsky continued their attack upon her and her defenders. Two commissioners sat mostly silent through the battle, taking notes and shifting uncomfortably in their seats.

One of them, Commissioner Patrick Johnson, the owner of the local tire store, spoke up. He was thirty-five and had taken over the business from his dad, who taught him that he had a responsibility to watch over the greater community because of the company's success. "Does Mary Beth have anything to say about these charges? I would like to hear from her."

"Good call, Pat. Mary Beth, I would like to thank you for your long and devoted service to this organization and the community. I am so sorry that you are being put through this now. What would you like to share with us before we call for a vote?"

Mary Beth looked up from the table she had been staring at for most of the meeting. She looked at the commissioners. She turned and looked at her staff. She gazed across the auditorium at everyone in attendance. Finally, she stood and spoke, to the audience, not the commissioners.

"I would be a liar if I said the talk around town has not hurt. It has. There is so much of the rumors that are so difficult for me. I've made hard decisions through much of my life. Probably no more so than just about everyone in this room. But it is mine that are on public trial. All I can say about those stories is that there is always more to a story than appears on the surface. You all know that in your own lives. And aren't called on in a public meeting to somehow explain why you did what you did. I don't feel like I have any reason to do so either, and won't.

"More troubling to me is the allegations that something is wrong at the Mason Health Foundation. That we are doing things that are illegal or immoral or just plain wrong. You know that is not the case. Many of you in this room have used our personal health advice service. You know from your own experience how professional and caring our staff are in attending to your needs. Does it make sense to you that we aren't that way with everybody who calls?

"And I can assure you that we are doing so legally, and ethically. Yes, we have legal counsel, and we have run all aspects of our operation by them to make sure. But that is not even the crucial point. My approach to being the CEO of this organization is that we live and die by our values. Not the ones that some organizations put up on their walls or websites and make-believe they follow in practice. What we live and breathe and believe in every day. These are about honesty, the importance and centrality of each person who seeks our help, the belief that health care is a right, especially for those of us who are sick or whose loved ones are sick. If we can't make a positive difference living these values, and sticking to these values, then let God strike us down.

"All I can tell you is that this is who we are. That is who these wonderful people who are the staff of our Foundation are. That is who these commissioners are—even those who now have found reason to attack me. That is who this organization and special purpose government is. It is who you in this community are. Abraham Lincoln once told us, faced with his own time of public challenge, that we should speak to the better angels of our nature. That is all I can ask you to do today."

With that, she sat down. For seconds, maybe a minute, nobody said a word in the room. The silence hung like drapes, cloaking the room with deeper thoughts by all within it. Themselves, their families, their very community. Then, slowly, a clap or two came from the audience members. It continued and grew, and soon half of the room had stood to direct their applause at Mary Beth, or the organization, or whatever good they had discovered in her words.

Commissioner Johnson spoke up. "Mr. Chair, I call the question."

With that, the board voted on the no confidence motion. It passed three to two. Ginger Bettis voted along with Kastner and Olinsky to approve a vote of no confidence in Mary Beth. The crowd groaned as the vote was announced. It was no longer a popular decision, but it was now official.

Chair Sonnberg called for a break in the meeting. They all needed to catch their breath, and the audience members were already beginning to leave, noisily. It would be difficult to proceed with the rest of the agenda until they had departed. Board members got up from their chairs and moved about the room, talking with audience members.

Jim Reynolds walked over to Mary Beth, who remained at her seat. He whispered in her ear. "I still don't know why you wanted to go through with this."

She whispered back. "Trust me, Jim. It had to happen that way." She peeked over his shoulder to the back of the room. She could see the tall man in the suit making his way out the door, talking on his cell phone.

"They need to think we are weak and crumbling. We can only hope they call off the dogs so we can get some time for our next move. As I told you, if you can keep the board together, I will take care of the rest."

"When," he asked.

"Soon. We've got to get through the public hearing in Belfair, week after next. We've got the answer under development. It will explain all, including this vote. Eventually."

Jim stood straight up, raising his voice. He didn't care if what he said next was overheard by anyone. "Mary Beth, you have surprised me time and time again. But you have never disappointed. I believe in you, and I say this entire board believes in you, even if we have a vote in hand that says they don't."

Mary Beth stood and gave him a hug. Tears were forming in her eyes again. This time from pride and companionship, not from the pain of personal attacks. "Jim, I won't let you or this community down. Ever." She kept hugging him, and thought about another who she wished was here with her now—the man who had taught her that values mattered, especially when times got tough.

She so wanted to tell Irv that she now understood what he meant. But first she would have to tell him about this whole sordid episode, including the link to her abortion. She couldn't figure out how to start the conversation when they spoke on the phone three nights ago. If there was anything she regretted now, it was this decision, not the rest.

She looked at her phone. *The Lord does work in mysterious ways.* She had a voicemail message from Irv.

Chapter Ninety-Seven

Mary Beth and Irv Hook Up Again

"Lost your job—are you shitting me?" Mary Beth blurted out while rolling off of Irv. Her old bed and mattress creaked with the movement. They had just finished a frolic in the hay, and instead of a snuggle, he had chosen then to let her know he was now among the unemployed.

"Yup. They forced me to resign on Monday. That, or worse to come if I didn't take their deal. You can guess the rest of the story."

"Did you do anything? I mean, did you do something that forced them to do it?"

"Of course not. Or at least not anything they knew about. Now, if they knew, then that would be a different story. But pretty sure it was just them concluding it was time to get rid of me once and for all. I do suspect that prick Bridgewater had something to do with it too. Did you think I had it coming?"

"No. No and no. I am just a little surprised. Actually, a lot surprised. Not so much that it happened, but that you chose this moment to tell me."

"A little too melodramatic," joked Irv.

Mary Beth frowned at him, pulling the cover over her breasts. "Please, you ass. Just not very cuddly. And here I thought you came out on a Tuesday night just 'cause it was killing you to not be with me."

"That part is true." Irv was starting to understand he had bungled his announcement. He thought telling her post coitus would be a cute thing to do, but he had overshot his mark, he thought. A cute pun occurred to him, but he gathered himself and let it float through his mind and not off his tongue.

"Thank God," said Mary Beth, scooting up close to him again. "You know if you want pity sex, all you have to do is ask."

"That's just it, Mary Beth. It wasn't about sex at all. I just wanted to talk to you—and be with you for a change. I was sitting around the house feeling sorry for myself, in between my bouts of anger, and that was when I realized there was an upside to this indignity. Several actually. The first one I thought of, though, was that I could spend more time with you. If you will have me, that is."

"Oh Irv. It's been such a long time since you've talked like that to me. We've been doing this sporadic girlfriend-boyfriend thing for almost three years now. I've kind of gotten used to it even if I still don't understand it. Knowing that I could talk to my best friend on the phone whenever I needed to helped. Maybe it was even easier at times to not mix it in with the drama of other stuff."

"So that's a no?"

"No, you ass. That's a 'you just dropped this bomb on me' and I don't know what the heck to say." She needed to buy some time to give him a better reaction—she knew deep down that she was not rejecting his overture. But it wasn't aligned with her current situation. Nor had she fessed up to him the challenges she had been dealing with over the last week.

"Tell me the whole story, Irv. Let's take it from the top." That would give her some time to process all of this. Just in case he wasn't buying her ruse, she slipped her hand under the covers and rubbed his thigh. It was an old, but effective, trick.

Irv bit like a trout and told Mary Beth the whole story. He had shared most of the tale of his public health sleuthing with her already, maybe not all, but most. It seemed that might have something to do with the rug getting pulled out from under him now, but he knew this was a long time coming. Mary Beth knew the longer saga of his banishment with the change of public health directors and political leadership in King County. His former dream job had turned him into a rogue operator within King County's public health apparatus, far from what he once was—a rising star in the department. Irv took an odd pleasure in sharing his "bite me" farewell to Director Welch.

Mary Beth listened intently, staring into his eyes as her fingers did the walking. She had Irv's full attention. It was giving her valuable time to work through her own confusion and confessions to come. She was also curious about what he might not be telling her. "You said you thought that your investigation maybe had something to do with this?"

"Well, I don't know that. And Welch didn't seem to be making any major connection between the incident and my being asked to go. Though he did mention that the feds didn't like my attitude. That's all it could have been—I really don't think he or they know anything about the rest of my extracurricular activities."

"Or maybe they know more than you think. Or who you hang out with," she commented.

"You mean Johnny? I guess that is possible too. It isn't a secret that he and I are tight, and I know that the campaign operatives have been going after him. But I never really thought our connection mattered that much to the bigger world out there."

"Yeah, well, maybe it's Johnny. Or maybe it's me. You are not the only one under the gun, my love. I've got some current events to catch you up on too." With that she outlined the past couple of weeks of attacks—on the Mason Health Foundation, on her professionally, and on her personally. She finished her story with the vote of no confidence that had happened on Monday evening. Irv surmised this had happened about the same time he was wallowing in his bourbon about losing his job. "It hurt, for sure, and I was really surprised. I just never thought anyone would go to so much trouble to get a political or business advantage. So maybe it is not crazy to wonder whether your troubles were linked to mine."

Irv was absorbed by her story. She had recently made offhand comments about work issues during their recent telephone chats, but never offered up many details. Nor had he, or Johnny, when he was on calls with her, asked much about her world, obsessed as they were with the investigation. He now felt bad about it. When she shared that public criticism of her abortion was part of the tale, he felt miserable. That was not his finest hour, as a boyfriend or even just a friend. His guilt over the matter was part of why he found some comfort in their recent separation. The coward's way out, he thought.

That he had been a total ass was now being waved in his eyes like a red flag to a bull. He knew that was not what she was intending, but it stung anyway. Now he was the one who needed time to figure out what to say next. "That's horrible, Mary Beth. I am so sorry." He kissed her forehead. "You shouldn't have to go through any of that, and especially not the personal stuff. I should have been there for you, then, and now." Maybe he did know what to say.

Tears welled up in Mary Beth's eyes, and she tried to say more. "Oh Irv." The tears streamed down across her flushed cheeks, and she broke into a full cry—not something she did very often, but there was no holding back the fountain now. She tried to say more, but couldn't. Instead, she buried her head in the curve of Irv's neck, wrapped her left arm around his shoulder, and let loose with a tsunami of hurt. Oddly, it felt good.

Chapter Ninety-Eight

Planning Meeting at the Alderbrook Lodge

Johnny, Irv, and Mary Beth met at the Alderbrook Lodge, on the shores of Hood Canal, a half mile from downtown Union. The lodge was now a five-star resort, after years of use as a somewhat rundown retreat hotel owned by a ministry. It was in a small cove, overlooking its own beach and dock, and the Olympic Mountains, seemingly just a few miles away.

Johnny had proposed on their telephone call last week that they spend the weekend prepping for the hearing upcoming in Belfair; Mary Beth had suggested the Alderbrook Lodge and made the reservations for them. It was Thursday night, giving them several days to prepare for the Monday public hearing on patient dumping. It was only a twenty-minute drive on a two-lane road winding next to the canal to the small town of Belfair. This town was bigger than Union, with a large auditorium and the modern communication hookups needed to broadcast the national news they hoped to create at the hearing.

The three had dinner in the lodge's fancy restaurant and then adjourned to the bar for further conversation. By ten o'clock, they were the only customers left. The bar staff showed them how to work the tap and told them to write down whatever they drank or ate on a notepad, and left for the night. *Button lock the door when you leave.*

The longtime friends were having a great time reconnecting. For all their efforts to stay in contact over the years, through visits, phone calls, emails, text messages, smoke signals, good thoughts and intentions, it was nothing like being together, really together, again. The setting now was a bit more modern and fancy than the living room in the University District home where they once regularly spent long nights chattering and laughing about life, but the context mattered little to them. It was enough that they were together.

The conversation bounced across a multitude of topics, stories, and people. As they ever did. Over the course of several hours, each also got more serious. Life was throwing some curves at all three, and they were thirsty for comfort and advice from their closest friends and advisors. It mattered little that some of the curves had to do with each other. Such was their friendship; no topic was out of bounds.

Mary Beth shared the challenges she was facing keeping the Mason Health Foundation afloat, and how personal some of the attacks had become. She admitted, perhaps for the first time to others, how important this was to her sense of being and the question that had been gnawing at her for most of her adult life—did she have what it takes to be a success in the business world? Would this be her only chance to prove she did? Mixed in, every once in a while, was second-guessing about choosing career over relationships, and the loneliness she felt and was still suppressing.

Irv shared the tenuous nature of his job situation. Things had always worked out for him as far as career and positions, but they were decidedly not right now. He was newly unemployed and had little inclination to get into the fight again. He confessed his screwup of the most important relationship in his life, looking away from Mary Beth as he did so. He didn't know how to put things back together. He used to be a fighter. Now he felt like his mom, slowly dying and unable to resist the downward spiral. This investigation was the only thing keeping him alive at the moment, and that was reaching an end.

Johnny shared his problems too. His days as a member of Congress were numbered, unfortunately just as he found himself in a position to do some bigger good. He shared how the Theory of Irv had infused his political adventuring with a sense of purpose twenty years ago, but only recently had he really started to grasp how much better he could make things for people in an even bigger way. Instead of using this power, he was going to be forced out of his Senate seat. Maybe, he thought, there was still time to make some meaningful change for people—around this investigation. Without this, he was having a tough time being the optimistic adventurer he once was.

Johnny's polemics naturally led their conversation to the upcoming hearing and the reason for them coming together this weekend. He explained the hearing was a key tool in trying to leverage some good out of his situation. But it would take some clever planning, solid execution, and a lot of luck to make it work. Maybe it would also help solve Irv's and Mary Beth's problems too.

He reviewed the basic plan so far. They had talked about this before on the telephone, and there wasn't much new about it. They were going to use the hearing to create a moment of leverage. Exactly how to do that was the point of this meeting, and they all knew it. It was time to brainstorm.

Chapter Ninety-Nine

Prep for the Public Hearing in Belfair

Johnny looked up from his notes resting on the cluttered table and looked at Lance, Nancy, Irv, and Mary Beth. They were in a small diner just outside of Belfair—a local spot out on a county dirt road, perched alongside a small cove of Hood Canal. Doubling as a bait shop, the diner was only open during tourist season, which usually ended in late September. It had decent enough food, but was not the type of place that the reporters or dignitaries staying in the area for tomorrow's public hearing would likely find.

There were only five small tables and a counter with seating for three in the small building. A couple was having dinner at a table near the front, and one elderly man was drinking a beer at the counter.

Johnny was not one to normally focus on small tasks at hand but this moment was an exception to the rule. "Let's take it from the top again. We will convene the hearing at eight o'clock tomorrow, bright and early so we don't miss the East Coast news cycle with the three-hour time difference. I will make some opening remarks using the script that Lance prepared. Profile why we called a hearing on the critical issue of the dumping of emergency room patients and then raising the red flag on the troubling article that will appear in tomorrow's morning paper. Nancy, are you sure the story will run?"

"Yup," Nancy Jones replied. "I just got off the phone with the editor of the *Times,* and they are not only going to run the story in Seattle, but have agreed to provide a hot copy for the *Shelton Herald* so they can run the story in real time down here."

"Did the editor tell you what is in it?" asked Lance.

"He wouldn't let me see it until midnight tonight when it goes to press. He assured me that the story was mostly about the allegations of the patient dump in Mason County that are now coming to light, with a number of quotes from the patient's relatives and friends. It will also link the story to tomorrow's hearing, and after that he will make enough noise to get this inserted into the regular news cycle across the nation early tomorrow. It is in his interest to get as much national air time as possible, so we can count on him doing so."

"Is he biting at all on other charges?" Lance knew it was critical that the broader transgressions at play get life tomorrow, as the patient dump itself would barely last a twenty-four-hour news cycle—if it got mention at all. Bigger conspiracies were what one needed now to shape and tilt public opinion. They had the makings for one here, but it would be hard to go much further publicly without more proof. HealthMost had been working hard to put up a wall around this, and the group hadn't been able to dig up more evidence. Public embarrassment was looking like their best bet to score points—and maybe stop it.

"There will be some references to 'other allegations of wrongdoing.' Probably without any specifics, though, as HealthMost threatened a libel action against them if they make any statements about anything that doesn't have a basis in hard fact. He said that the statements from HealthMost's attorneys were very clear on that point. If we want the paper to say more, we really need to share with them the evidence that we have—without it, the story is little more than rumors, ugly enough in implication to support a prima facie case for slander."

"Well, we will have to take what we've got, Nancy. Remember, we agreed that it wasn't wise to let HealthMost know how much evidence we had on them. The paper would have asked HealthMost about anything solid that we would have provided and let our secrets slip. We are the ones who will have to get the larger ugliness of what is going on out into the public arena, and then the media can help amplify our story. Ideally it will trigger outrage and official investigations, giving it a long shelf life in the public eye. I will have to try to make that case tomorrow though. You got my latest draft on that part of your statement, right?" asked Lance.

Johnny nodded to indicate that he had. "Yes I did. Like it. It throws a lot of mud at them, for sure. I will start by outlining my belief that there is a conspiracy between HealthMost and the federal government to illegally deport Mexicans and South Americans under the guise of a health care program. I will toss out some raw numbers of people involved based on what we learned from the ALI database and speculate that this is why HealthMost is being paid millions by our government. Once that juicy accusation is firmly planted, I will go for the jugular by sharing our belief that this conspiracy also involves dozens of missing foreign nationals who are at least missing, and perhaps dead.

"I will delicately suggest that it is not out of the question that HealthMost even might have had a role in killing them. But without question they have been illegally disposing of their bodies, with one of their graveyards being only twenty miles from here. We've got some photos of the site that we will put up on the media screen—a shot of the massive hole and the public notice with HealthMost's name on it. Our shock and awe introduction will end with me expressing my anger that the issue of patient dumping that led to this hearing has uncovered crimes of an even more sinister nature and that I demand justice, accountability, and punishment on behalf of the American people."

"That should turn some heads at CNN," said Nancy. "I can see the banner on the lower screen now as they show a shot of you speaking at the hearing—HealthMost Kills Migrant Workers for HHS."

"I'll be happier if they show Thrust and the secretary squirming in their seats at the witness table. Right after I make these charges, I am going to change the order of the planned testimony and call on them to testify immediately. I will bury them in accusations and innuendos first," replied Johnny.

"How far are you going to go? Any worries that it is too far, at least without more proof?" asked Irv. It amused him that he was the one suggesting they might want to be a bit more cautious. Just weeks ago, he had chased a corpse around the country to try to get more proof.

"Pretty hard, Irv. Normally, a politician would show some restraint. We are indoctrinated by our consultants to remember that what goes around might come around. Not the bad actions themselves, but the taking off of gloves in the attack. I am a bit of a loose cannon in that regard anyway, as an independent and political outsider. But when we couple this with our press release tomorrow announcing I will not be running for reelection to the Senate and will instead be devoting my remaining time to righting this wrong and assuring there is a vote on new health protections for Americans, there really is nothing holding me back from using my bully pulpit to its fullest.

"They will get their say too," Johnny continued. "Good luck with that though. I will be interrupting them regularly to score some more points for our side. If we are really lucky, one or both of them will say something that we can use to totally blow the lid off this story. All we need is one horrible quote, and that will be the CNN banner headline.

"If not, we've got some other ways to pour gas on the story. The next panel at the hearing will be the son of Helen Neederdam, who will talk about her death and their loss, followed by the head of the local ACLU and local farmworkers' bureau. By noon eastern time I would expect this to be the biggest news story of the day. If it goes according to plan, we will be busy all afternoon and evening doing satellite feed interviews with the major networks."

Nancy liked the plan. "I've got the governor and some other local political leaders on standby too. I didn't tell them anything more than that they should be ready to comment on what will be revealed during tomorrow's public hearing on patient dumping." Nancy knew how to pull the local media strings.

"Wow," exclaimed Mary Beth. "That should blow the top of this thing off! Just imagine the headlines on Wednesday's paper. When do I make my announcement?"

Johnny looked at her. "We've been talking about that. We think it might get lost if we do it today. Instead, maybe we do a follow-up story later this week that adds your news to the mix and keeps the bigger story in the public's eye a bit longer. I know you are anxious to explain away the no confidence vote, but if you can hang on another day or so, I think we can more effectively put that to rest. Okay with that?"

"I am, Johnny," replied MaryBeth. "The hurt and damage are already done, and all I can do now is get things back on track for the longer term. Your approach will allow me to do that."

Johnny smiled. "I do expect that we will be able to blow this up so it stretches beyond the usual nanosecond of public attention. You would think we could get a few days, maybe even a week or more of public outrage."

"That's all?" Mary Beth expected more. "Won't there be an investigation? Consequences? Vindication?"

"We hope there is. But really, it is mostly hope. Our evidence is a combination of hearsay allegations, personal investigation by a disgruntled public employee, and confidential documents that have been stolen from their owners. That is what they will say, anyway, which will pump some oxygen into the fire we start tomorrow. But then will come the justifications for downplaying our story by those with influence who will want to slow down any embarrassing investigations. Remember, our play is not to the proper authorities but to the public. And the outcome is not some official investigation and report, but the other outcomes we have discussed."

"Well, I say we seem ready to go," Irv announced.

"Agreed," declared Johnny. "Let's get some menus and eat our dinner and turn in early. Tomorrow should be quite the day!"

Chapter One Hundred

Temporary Restraining Order

The rapping at the hotel room door awoke Johnny from his deep sleep. He glanced at the clock. It was 5 a.m. His alarm was set for six. He expected to awake well before then, but his excitement over the day to come had left him unable to sleep for much of the night. He had gotten up and reviewed his notes, again, at 2 a.m., and finally dozed off at about three. The knocking at the door put an end to his rest for the night.

"Just a second," he mumbled as he got out of bed and looked for some clothes to put on. There were some boxers on top of the minibar, and he stuck his legs through while stumbling toward the door. "Who the hell is up at this hour, anyway?"

A man in a rumpled sport coat was standing there, waving a piece of paper in his face. Johnny took it from his outstretched arm, more as a reaction than any intentional act, still surprised by the rude awakening. It was then that he heard a click and realized that the man was accompanied by a shorter companion standing off to the left against the wall. He had taken a photo of him being handed the piece of paper, on his cell phone.

Johnny glanced down at the piece of paper, trying to make it out. While the hallway was brightly lit, his room was still dark, and he was still standing halfway in. Without some more light, and his reading glasses, he was having trouble seeing the letters on the document, let alone the words. He took a half step out into the hallway to get a better look.

The man who made the delivery stepped abruptly back, apparently thinking that Johnny presented a physical threat to him. Johnny was a tall fellow, but gentle as a lamb. Then again, maybe not so much once he had a chance to figure out what he was holding.

Johnny looked at the document, still unable to make out the smaller writing. But he could see the larger type. It was from a federal court, and it was labeled "Temporary Restraining Order." Johnny looked up from the document and at the man in front of him. "What the—? Who the hell are you—and what is this about?"

The man backed up some more. He turned and, without saying more, walked quickly back down the hallway, followed by his cameraman and glancing several times over his shoulder to make sure Johnny wasn't following. Johnny was not—he had already backed into his room, turned on the lights, and found his reading glasses. He read through the document.

"Shit," he mumbled. He found his cell phone, which he had plugged in last night when he went to bed so he could make sure there was a full charge for what should be a busy day of telephone calls. It still would be, he thought, just different calls than what they had discussed at the diner only a few hours ago.

He pressed a button on his cell phone, and a groggy hello came through the speaker. "Lance. Sorry to wake you. But I just got served with a temporary restraining order. Looks like we are legally prohibited from making any mention of our allegations against HealthMost, or others, regarding their federal contract with HHS. Can you get the rest of the troops up and to my room? Maybe in about fifteen minutes? Looks like we need Plan B."

Johnny took a fast shower to help him wash off the night's sleep and get ready for the day. Normally, Johnny was the most laid back character in the room. In the dawn hours today, he paced like a caged tiger.

He was anxious for his friends to arrive so they could figure out what to do next. Different scenarios were running through his head, more than he could process so early in the morning. *Maybe coffee will help*, he thought. He found the coffeemaker and brewed up a pot. It reminded him of the days when Irv worked at the roasting plant. Simpler days, for sure.

Lance, Nancy, Irv, and Mary Beth had assembled in Johnny's hotel room by 5:30 a.m. Johnny handed the legal document to Lance, who read the relevant parts of it to the group. "Senator John Gibson and any associates are prohibited from making any public declaration regarding the contract between HealthMost and the federal government." " . . .

this applies to any general mention to the media or others, and specifically prohibits any mention of this at the Public Hearing to be held in Belfair on . . . " " . . . under full penalty of law including potential criminal prosecution under the USC 110-43, relating to national security and defense secrets."

"That's an early mouthful," opined Nancy. "Does it mean what I think it does?"

Lance looked up from the TRO. "If you think it means we can't say a word about the allegations against HealthMost later this morning, you would be right. It is not only a regular TRO, but it's linked by reference to the country's top classified information protections. Meaning that anyone who violates the order of secrecy can be put in jail for an indefinite period of time."

"Wow," said Mary Beth. "They are not taking any chances, are they?"

"No, they are not," offered Lance. "I don't see any way we can ignore this order. And if we do, odds are that we will be the story of tomorrow's news, not our charges, which will continue to be shielded. I don't even want to contemplate what the CNN banner headline will be as they show a clip of Johnny being whisked out of the room in handcuffs. What do you think, Johnny?"

"I am with you, Lance. The best we can do on the legal front is challenge the basis of the TRO. Let's put our lawyers to work on it. But we know, even if we win, that is at best a day or two out. And there's no guarantee we will win. The administration has packed the courts with their people. I have to assume they've lined up the right justices to make sure they will acquiesce to HealthMost's requests—or they wouldn't have been able to get this type of TRO in the first place. There obviously isn't any national security implications to this contract."

"Unfortunately, that means we will have to cut out the allegations regarding deportation and the killing or disposal of bodies, today. We can try to find a different way to get this stuff public, but I can't imagine that will be today. The hearing will have to go back to its original purpose of exploring patient dumping—not that we have told anyone it would be more than that. We can hear from the Neederdam son and our other witnesses and then I can call Thrust and Olsen to testify. See if I can trip them up. Maybe we will get a headline or two that we can use to stimulate some national interest on the *Times* article. I suspect that is about all we can do with today's hearing. After that, well, I think we all know what has to be done."

The group sat quietly, processing Johnny's words and their new predicament. No one offered up more for what seemed like minutes. When Irv spoke, it was really only about fifteen seconds of quiet, but it seemed like so much more.

"Plan B it is, Johnny." They all looked up from their coffee cups and smiled.

Chapter One Hundred One

Thrust Gets Ready for His Win

Richard Thrust looked into the mirror of his bathroom in the suite of the Belfair Inn. He was used to more glamorous accommodations. A suite at the Belfair Inn included little more than an extra-large bathroom and an anteroom with a lumpy couch, a table, and a minibar. Not exactly the Ritz Carlton, but then again, without a guarantee that he could fly in by the time of the start of today's hearing, he didn't really have a choice. Just another reason to hate Gibson, he thought.

It was more the principle of the accommodations than their reality. Thrust got far more enjoyment out of winning than the personal luxuries that came from his conquests. He would display the trappings of opulence, but mostly to make the point that he was the one on top of the world, not those who coveted such things but didn't have his brilliance to attain them.

He adjusted his red tie so it was perfectly aligned in reference to the stiff collar of his newly starched white dress shirt. The cameras would be rolling today, and he must look his best as he consumed his prey.

He smiled. By now, Gibson should be holding the temporary restraining order. Whatever he had learned about the HHS contract was now off limits at today's hearing. What's more, so was any mention or even evidence around their system of disposing of bodies. He still wasn't sure that Gibson had anything to do with the odd breaches in security over the past few months, but he wasn't taking any chances.

The dumpsite was now completely gone, or at least what had been dumped there—not a grain of sand to be had from its past—and now one would only see workers prepping the site for a foundation pour to build a new HealthMost data facility. Whatever remains were in the soil were now spread across vast stretches of the American West. Even if someone knew exactly what had happened, it would be almost impossible now to trace the many trucks and vans used to disperse the dirt piles from the site.

It was simply more proof of his brilliance as a tactician. His underlings thought it enough to move the dirt out of the county; he was the one who insisted on a series of transfers of the piles to faraway locations to ensure that nothing would ever be found. Sometimes he got tired of always being right, but it was his cross to bear, since he was.

He moved away from the mirror and sat down on the lumpy couch. *Not too comfortable*, he thought, *but I won't be the one shifting around in my seat today*. He picked up his notepad on the table in front of him and reviewed his draft testimony for today's hearing.

The basis of his testimony was a report he had commissioned regarding HealthMost's experience with their hospital emergency rooms—a 450-page report that found no problems in diagnosing or treating patients when they presented at HealthMost's 250 emergency rooms across the nation. Indeed, it concluded that patients were receiving top-notch care. Though not by HealthMost's competitors.

The report alleged that there were instances of patient dumping, even egregious examples. But these were transgressions of its competitors. Government should do something about this, but not as a matter of policy that would affect good actors like HealthMost. No, the federal government should enforce its existing laws rather than grandstanding and passing laws that would harm patients.

Thrust had already seen a copy of the *Times* newspaper article. He hadn't been able to stop it from running, and there would be consequences for that failure. But he had made sure that there were independent statements in it questioning whether there actually was a patient dump. After all, it looked on its face to be a tragic accident involving a patient who had left their emergency room without consent. His lawyers had forced the *Times* to include in the article the fact that Helen Neederdam's son was addicted to methamphetamine and had been in trouble with the law. One observer, who mysteriously became available over the last week, alleged that Helen's son had made up the incident so he could pressure HealthMost for a cash settlement. Cash that he would then use to buy drugs.

There wasn't much real proof of any of this in the article. That would have been hard to come by, since it didn't really happen that way. But there was enough to bury the story as one of national import. The references in it would soon be buttressed by Helen's son failing to appear at the public hearing. Thrust had made sure of that with a payout that he could actually use for drugs. What Helen's son couldn't do was say anything about their arrangement, under the terms of their buyout agreement, and especially not since he flew to Guadalajara last night for an extended vacation.

Thrust took pleasure in thinking how much Senator Gibson's hearing was blowing up in his face. It would be a big nothing burger nationally, probably even locally, and the senator would soon be fending off multiple attacks in the national media through a series of video stories profiling his degenerate lifestyle and socialist beliefs. Bridgewater had done a good job in organizing unified political opposition to him from both parties, and while HealthMost had provided most of the dirty money to produce the ads developed by the SwiftBoat operatives, there was ample cover for the corporation in the alliance. Gibson would have to step aside, or get ready to lose. At best, he had about six weeks left as a United States senator.

Bridgewater had encouraged Thrust to leave it at that. But Thrust was not having any of it. Bridgewater was a good enough political hack, but he just didn't have the bigger vision and understanding of what it took to be a true ruler. Prince Machiavelli knew that it was not enough to beat your opponents; they must be left as dead so they may never arise again. Thrust was a little disappointed that he couldn't apply this solution literally. Still, he could metaphorically destroy Gibson by leaving him so utterly debased that he could never arise again.

So, today they would not just walk away from the public hearing victorious. There was little evidence of patient dumping and, if anything, reason to applaud HealthMost's behavior. No mention of any potential wrongdoing or conspiracies, pretty much nothing, other than maybe some wild and unproved ramblings of liberal politicians and groups who wanted to steal taxpayer money to achieve their own socialist and unpatriotic ends.

Instead of walking away with this victory, they would insist on a meeting with Gibson and his staff that afternoon, where they would share a copy of the first video attack ad to get his attention: charges of homosexual behavior, not just with another man, but several underage boys. The message would be delivered through Gibson's campaign consultant, Nancy Jones. She would likely immediately agree to the meeting, hoping there would be some way to deep six the ad. If that didn't work, they had some material on her too.

When they met, Thrust would give Gibson the chance to pull out of the race and resign. They had prepared a public statement for him in which he would apologize for his improper behavior and especially for any suggestions he had made that HealthMost was not the leading health system in the nation. It was drafted over the top, with the hope that Gibson would turn them down.

Thrust was looking forward to the next act in their play—that they had even worse dirt to sling around on Gibson. His family and friends would be taken down with him if he didn't do the right thing, including close friends of Johnny of whom Thrust's investigators had found evidence of bad behavior. Thrust didn't actually know what this evidence was; he was just assuming they had something to hide. He looked forward to their squirming, and for Gibson to realize that his friends would betray him in a pinch.

This was how one dealt with an enemy. Total and utter destruction. Thrust sat back in his chair. *Maybe I will buy and tear this shithole hotel down and put in a clinic. It will teach them a lesson and we can make some more money in the process.*

The stage was now set for today's conquest. He was already beginning to move on to his next conquest, confident in what was to come that day.

Chapter One Hundred Two

The Hearing in Belfair

A hearing that only a few hours ago promised to be a game changer landed with barely a thud. *The Seattle Times* had run its news story that morning, giving Senator Gibson something to point to in his introduction, in addition to his original arguments for opening a series of national hearings on patient dumping. The article was all right; it outlined the tragic case of Helen Neederdam, as expected, without the inclusion of any more pervasive allegations of sinister wrongdoing. It gave a bit too much air time to unproven stories that the claim was actually fortune-seeking by Helen's wayward son, but it was good enough to push forward a charge of bad behavior at the hearing through just a little more personal insult.

There was barely a breath of that to come, though. More like the fizzle of a damp fuse, on a bomb that was now little more than a handful of sparklers duct taped together.

Senator Gibson called Helen Neederdam's son to testify. He was a no-show. No one seemed to know where he was. Sam Bridgewater moved through the room whispering to anyone who could hear that this was proof of the allegations in the *Times* article that morning. Johnny gaveled the room for silence, but the point had already been made.

The ACLU and Farmworker's Bureau reps did their jobs well enough—providing legal and system context to the cost and illegality of turning people away from diagnosis and treatment at emergency rooms. Without direct evidence to the actual allegations of this case, though, they were only shading what was now more a hypothetical than a real situation. There was no news to be had in what they said. Certainly nothing that would take nationally. Johnny tried to provide some color commentary, but his most provocative material was in legal embargo.

Next up was Richard Thrust, CEO of HealthMost, and Secretary of HHS Ben Olsen. It was telling that Secretary Olsen deferred to Thrust and let him go first. While Johnny tried to steer Thrust toward the incident at hand, the lack of direct testimony about this made it hard to pin him down. When he tried to use the national data showing extensive patient dumping, including many cases involving HealthMost, Thrust's retort was a study that HealthMost was releasing that morning showing no illegal or even improper behavior by the company, anywhere in the United States, let alone in this locale.

At the end of his testimony, Thrust seemed to be preening for applause for what a great job his company was doing in treating patients, not defending it from vulgar action. It didn't take long for him to get that applause. The first five minutes of Secretary Olsen's time was made up of mostly praise for both HealthMost and Thrust.

The secretary then spoke to the issue of patient dumping, citing the report released that morning by HealthMost. He outlined it as another excellent example of the public-private partnerships that was America at its best, and supported its analysis and conclusions. He shared that the department had done its own review of patient dumping allegations since his interrogation by Senator Gibson last spring. They had found a few incidents, not at HealthMost but other entities, and were enforcing existing law to resolve these problems. He rejected the need for any policy change.

Senator Gibson tried to score a few points during the hearing. He pressed the secretary on his belief that patient dumps were rare and not that consequential, using numbers developed by committee staff that showed a 50 percent increase over the last year, and ten cases that involved unnecessary deaths. He asserted that he would be proposing legislation to stop this crisis in short order. The secretary denied the picture was a bleak one, citing the HealthMost study. He said that the administration would oppose any legislation on this topic, and that the president would veto it if a bill was sent to him by Congress.

At the end, Johnny made one more play at the secretary. Senator Gibson tried to pin him down with regard to how severe the penalties should be on corporate or public or private leaders who did violate America's laws—patient dumping or other laws. It seemed a strange line of questioning to many. Instead of fact finding about patient dumping nationally or in this area, he had pulled back to raising hypothetical breaches of conduct, and looking for affirmations that such should be prosecuted fully under federal law.

Secretary Olsen tried hard to duck this line of questioning at first, but Senator Gibson continued his attack. Among his arguments was that the president and vice president had run on a strong criminal prosecution platform. Were they now saying they wouldn't be hard on criminals? Secretary Olsen finally bit and stated that such wrongdoers should be prosecuted to the full extent of the law, and more. He was well aware of the ads about to be run against the senator, ads that would allege criminal wrongdoing, and his powerful statement toward prosecution of wrongdoers might be a great sound bite to play when the senator was the target in the public crossfire.

The hearing adjourned at 9:45, well before its expected noon close. There just wasn't that much to say or argue. The rug had been successfully pulled out from what Johnny and his team hoped would be a public moment of reckoning for personal and policy wrongs. Most of the media had left before the end of the hearing; there was little to say about this failed event.

As he stood up at the end of the hearing, Johnny could see Nancy Jones beating a fast track toward him. "Tough time, Johnny. You did as good as you could under the circumstances. I don't think we have to worry much about media follow-up today. I would say we probably want to duck out of them if we do get some requests. They probably would only be bad news for us now—until we can say more about the other thing."

Johnny nodded in agreement. He could see the rest of the team forming about ten yards away and he began to run through what he might say to them. He was wondering if they needed some encouragement—this was a more embarrassing non-event than he had ever imagined. It could have been a great moment; now it was anything but.

"One more thing," Nancy interjected. "HealthMost asked for a meeting with us at 2 p.m. Less a request than an order. They have some things they want to share with us, and I don't think it is a bound copy of their antidumping report. More like the campaign stuff we've been talking about getting ready to hit the fan."

"Who is asking," inquired Johnny.

"Bridgewater. But he doesn't change his underwear without checking in with Thrust. I would expect him to be there, reveling in his victory and being dicktatiously ungracious."

"Well, by all means, let's meet with them, Nancy. I assume your dad will be able to join us?"

"Oh yes. He wouldn't miss it for the world."

"Great. This day still has some wonderful possibilities, doesn't it? Come on, let's go grab a bite with the team. We also have to get ready to announce my departure from Congress. I was ready to throw it out during the hearing, but that would only have made things worse. Maybe after our meeting, things will be looking better for that too."

Chapter One Hundred Three

Post Hearing Meeting with Thrust

Senator Gibson's team gathered at 2 p.m. for the meeting insisted on by Richard Thrust. The early arrivals for Thrust's group had already staked out their spots around the circular table in the Belfair Inn's small meeting room. Richard Thrust would be in the seat toward the front of the room, away from the window that looked out into the pasture to the hotel's rear. Sam Bridgewater had chosen a seat next to that, and on the other side sat HealthMost's Chief Operating Officer Lane Stevens. Thrust was not yet in the room—his emissaries were there, early, to reserve his seat.

Senator Gibson arrived for the meeting a couple of minutes before two. Already gathered were Chief of Staff Lance Givens, campaign consultant Nancy Jones, and friends Irv Tinsley and Mary Beth Collins. And one more person—an older gentleman seated next to Nancy. Bridgewater recognized the face but could not place it. Nor were there any conversations or even introductions. They silently waited for Thrust's arrival.

Richard Thrust strode confidently into the room at five minutes after two. He went directly to his seat and sat down, placing a black notebook on the table in front of him. Both sides were ready to get down to business without any social gestures. Since Sam Bridgewater was the one who had called the meeting, he opened it, introducing Thrust and the HealthMost team.

"We asked that you come before us today," began Bridgewater, "so that we can put to rest this unfounded attack on our company before things get really ugly." There would be no playing around, not with Thrust present. It was how he played the game.

Bridgewater continued. "Senator Gibson, you have tried to do damage to HealthMost Corporation, including at today's farce of a hearing. We've had enough of this and it will stop today. Understood?"

Johnny took command of the opposing team in the room. "I am not sure I do. It was only through some shady legal court order that we were not able to get the real facts on the table. That and whatever you did to get rid of our witness. We will find him, and our attorneys are already challenging the temporary restraining order. If you want to stop this, the only way that is going to happen is that you admit to what you have done so we can fix the damage to those you have hurt."

"Enough, Gibson." Richard Thrust's voice boomed across the room. "I've had enough of your insolence. Here's how this is going to play out. You will resign your Senate seat and apologize for your unfounded attack on me and HealthMost. We have drafted a statement for you—it is what you will say. Or else. Bridgewater, give them a copy." Sam got up and handed over two copies of a draft statement—one to Johnny and one to Lance.

"If you don't agree to do this by the time we leave this room, we will release—tonight—the first of a series of advertisements opposing your reelection to the Senate." That was a lie; Thrust intended for this first video to be released whether Gibson took the deal or not. "I promise you won't like what is in it, or what is to follow. Here's just a sampling."

Lane Stevens flipped open a portable computer and set it on the table so that Johnny and his companions could see the screen. He pressed a button, and thirty seconds of an attack ad on Johnny ensued.

It began with a screen-wide shot of the American flag, fluttering in the wind. "We Americans love our country," the deep, manly voice boomed, "and we will do anything to protect her. But there are those who don't, and it will shock you to know that some of these haters are even United States senators." The screen switched to a picture of Johnny; an unflattering one at that. "While we have been protecting our nation, he has been working with our enemies. He has chosen China as his country of choice." The ad included a clip of Johnny saying some flattering things about China—all part of a trade mission he had taken with the Washington State governor, but the words were clipped to make it suggest he wished he was Chinese. "What's worse, he does this not for money, or even political power, but because the Chinese government provides him with young boys who he can use as he wishes." The visual was a group of Chinese boys running to Johnny and hugging him—part of a reception organized by the State Department in support of the trade mission.

"John Gibson wishes to do to them what he does to the United States every time he darkens the hall of our nation's capital. It doesn't take much imagination to understand what that is. Join us in voting this traitor and child abuser out of office. He belongs in prison, not the United States Senate. Brought to you by the Alliance for America."

Johnny began to object as soon as the ad ended. "That is a bunch of lies and . . . "

"Shut up, Gibson!" yelled Thrust, standing up, his face crimson red. His anger boomed across the room. "I am not here to listen to your whimpering. This is only the first of many such ads—and by far the nicest. As I said, your only choice is to resign from the Senate—today and now—and issue your formal apology to me and my company."

Johnny stayed cool, though staring intently into Thrust's eyes. It was still shocking to see how far his enemies would go in trying to get rid of him. His years as a politician had hardened him to this reality, even as it worsened over the years he was in Congress. He dealt with such attacks by considering them a badge of honor, testifying to his willingness to serve the public interest and not the groups and people responsible for such ads. "And you want me to do this by issuing this statement?" Johnny picked up his copy and began to read through it. "Really, you expect me to say this nonsense?"

"Yes, I do."

"And why should I?"

"Because if you don't, we will release the additional material. And you will see that our research has gone much further. There is plenty to say about just you, believe me. And we will. Maybe you can even take that abuse. But I wonder what you think about the rumors and allegations that will soon start swirling around your little friends here." He nodded toward the other side of the table where Irv, Mary Beth, and Nancy were sitting.

"I believe some of these matters have begun to go public already, such as the reasons for Ms. Collins' vote of no confidence by her board. Terrible thing, that abortion. And stealing from taxpayers—who would forgive someone like that. And Mr. Tinsley—fired from his government job. He was supposed to be protecting the public's health, but instead he was working with cartels to push opioids onto the unsuspecting public. Nor can we forget the deviancy behind Ms. Jones leaving her consulting practice in Washington, DC.

"Believe me when I tell you that we are about to tell a vile and disgusting story about each of your pen pals here. It will make clear why they are your friends and associates. Low character and morals attract the same." Thrust let the imagery float in the room for a time. He wanted to see them all squirm and come to realize that they had been bested.

"So, Gibson. You can ignore our warnings. Or you can stop any further embarrassment by agreeing to our statement and issuing it within the hour. My associates are hoping that you will agree—they want to be done with this problem. Myself? Well, I kind of hope you say no. Nothing would give me more pleasure than destroying you and what you stand for. Your choice."

Thrust sat back down, satisfied that he had framed the option beautifully, a splendid beat down of an opponent and his sleazy friends. Senator Gibson continued to sit calmly, throughout and after Thrust's attack. His team members were more animated. Nancy Jones was glaring at Sam Bridgewater, so much so that Bridgewater stared down at the table rather than having to interpret her hateful gaze. Irv was more restrained; he was admiring Johnny's demeanor, remembering why he always lost to him in card games. Mary Beth's face revealed her astonishment with what had just happened. She was still hanging on to her innocence about American politics, but growing up fast. The old man sat placidly at the table, matter-of-factly listening to the dialogue, his hands folded.

Finally, Johnny cleared his throat and stood up. "I almost appreciate your candor, Mr. Thrust. I thought you were a son of a bitch from the moment I met you, and this only confirms it. But that is almost neither here nor there. What matters to me are the horrible things you have done, and the need for justice to prevail. So allow me to share a couple of things before directly providing my answer to you."

Thrust leaned back in his chair and folded his arms across his chest. He was not used to anyone talking back to him. He would give Gibson a little space to do that, before completely destroying him. They had another video to show, one that made the first sound like an endorsement for Johnny. He wanted to show it, but letting Gibson squirm first would only make it more fun.

Johnny continued. "I will be brief and to the point. First, I don't think it is any longer even possible to make this statement." He pointed at the clock in the wall. "My office released a statement to the press at 5 p.m. eastern time announcing that I will not be running for reelection. That was twelve minutes ago. I imagine it will hit the newswire any second now, if it hasn't already. Your henchman there can check on that for you." He looked at Sam Bridgewater, who had already pulled out his cell phone and was hitting some buttons. "So you see, it would be confusing to issue this statement."

Lance stood up and gathered his belongings on the table. "This is also an appropriate time for me to excuse myself. I have some interviews lined up with the national media over the next hour, that is, until Johnny is available to speak for himself. And a couple of other things to do too." With that, he began to walk out of the room.

"Thanks, Lance. I expect that we will conclude our business here soon." Johnny turned his attention back to Thrust and his associates. "I am sorry to say that we did not have the benefit of your advice, so we unfortunately haven't used any of the colorful language you have suggested in this fine document." Johnny waved the press statement handed out by Bridgewater, and threw it on the table. Bridgewater stared into his phone and caught Thrust's attention, nodding in the affirmative to him.

"So you see, Thrust, I am not bluffing. Now, why did I decide to do this? We could chat about that now, but my guess is that it's a topic for another time. For now, all that matters is that the cat is out of the bag with respect to my future. I suppose you are free to run any attack ads you want, but it certainly would raise the question of why you would be doing so. And I do mean *you*. I understand you have a number of allies—what was it, the 'Alliance for America'—in this campaign smear opposition. Nancy has given me a full report. All the others in this want me to get out of the way so they can run their own candidates, and I suspect they all moved on about ten minutes ago. So if you want to continue with these lies, it will become clear, very quickly, that it is you, and just you, doing it."

The truth in Johnny's words hung in the air for a minute. Thrust was looking at Bridgewater to refute it, but he couldn't. Sam shrugged.

"But now, when you asked for this meeting, I thought it would be to discuss the other matter for today. We didn't understand how you might have heard about it already, but as this meeting has already proven, no one should underestimate your ability to break the rules."

"What the hell are you talking about," asked Thrust.

Johnny smiled back at him. "Why, I mean the lawsuit that got filed an hour ago in federal court. Technically it is called a qui tam suit charging illegal inducements made by HealthMost and its corporate officers in violation of federal fraud and abuse laws.

"You know the ones, Bridgewater," Johnny noted, looking at the former congressman. "I believe you supported these laws as part of the Republican health care reform proposals back in your days as a public servant. As I recall, you even made a floor speech asserting that America's health care problems could be solved merely by eliminating fraudulent behavior. Though I think you were really arguing that thousands of unworthies were cheating the government out of health coverage and needed to be rooted out.

"Back then, you and your colleagues didn't think that federal lawyers would assertively press these cases against these cheats. So, you gave authority to private parties to sue over these claims independently of the government. And you sweetened the pot, so to speak, providing potential treble damages for the lawsuits, and for each claim."

Bridgewater had a hazy recollection of the proposals. He had barely paid attention to the details of the amendments that had been added to a budget reconciliation bill at Republican insistence; they were supposed to be talking points for the campaign trail.

Thrust, on the other hand, was remembering them, in vivid detail. He knew that these laws presented a threat to his company, but never imagined that it would have anything to do with this matter. Alarm bells were ringing as Senator Gibson went on.

"Now, I didn't file the suit, nor did my office. Not that it matters. That was done by a group led by this gentleman." He pointed at the older man sitting at the table. "Allow me to introduce you to Christopher Jones, the class action representative." Chris nodded at the three men across the table.

"You may have heard of Mr. Jones. He is the former director of policy at the Harvard Medical School, one of the leading experts in health care policy in the nation, and someone who has advised Congress on proper health policy for a few decades. As his father did before him. Not that he always got listened to, which is what got him thinking that there must be some other way to get sound American health policy into law in this country.

"He is also . . . " Johnny turned to Nancy and opened his palms to her:

"My dad," she spit across the table. Johnny stopped to let those words resonate.

Chris Jones unfolded his hands and spoke up. "And may I add that I am none too pleased with the personal attack you were suggesting against my daughter, Mr. Thrust."

Johnny began to stick the landing of this meeting. "In short, what we wanted to tell you, and I believe Chris has some documents to share with you, is that a federal qui tam proceeding has been filed alleging multiple breaches of the federal fraud and abuse statutes. It involves the millions of dollars received by HealthMost under a federal contract—and inducements made by HealthMost and its representatives with regard to the medical treatment of clients served under that contract. Thousands of cases, really. Mr. Jones seems to have acquired access to a database that tracked these claims. Some, shockingly enough, seem to have even ended in death. Not that this directly affects the amount of the claims under the fraud and abuse statutes, but it sure will make the case juicier if it ever goes public.

"I was never strong on math, but I do believe the potential damages are quite substantial. Even more than your salary, Mr. Thrust. Of course, when we multiply by three, the number could get really large. What was that number again, Chris?"

"Three billion dollars. That would be with a 'B,' if you didn't catch it," stated Chris. He stood up and retrieved a stack of documents from his briefcase, handing them to Nancy. She smiled as she walked around the table and handed them to Bridgewater.

Johnny continued. "Of course, this is just a courtesy conversation. I am sure your lawyers will want to review these documents and have an extensive chat with you. Oh, and probably your board too. As you know,

Sam, you were also around when we tried to do something about Enron. Remember how we shifted the blame to the board rather than the executives and passed some strange laws insisting on more accountability for them? Interestingly enough, when one reads that together with the unique nature of hospital governance laws, the financial accountability gets wrapped into the accountability of hospital boards for quality of care. Section 8 of the lawsuit speaks to this, and here is where the failure of HealthMost to make patient care decisions on the basis of financial and not clinical reasons may turn out to, how would I say it, bite your ass. Or at least your board's asses. We have taken the liberty, or I should say Chris has, of naming each of the HealthMost board members as individual plaintiffs in this suit. You might find that they are less interested in saving your ass when they are busy saving their own.

"You may think I am making all of this up, but I would suggest you check with your attorneys before saying anything more. I totally agree with what you are thinking too—there is no way that Senator John Gibson could have figured all of this out. That's true—I didn't. But then again, I had the help of my degenerate friends." Irv, Mary Beth, and Nancy waved across the table. "Oh and I should mention Mr. Jones. In addition to the rest of his academic and professional achievements, Chris is also an honors graduate of Georgetown Law School. Never chose to practice, but apparently understands this stuff pretty damn well."

"It was also kind of a hobby for me, John," Chris added. "I even remember when these laws passed and I got to thinking that maybe they have some better use than just for some irresponsible members of Congress to pass the buck." Chris was enjoying the moment. He had a lot of payback to unload, for him, his father, and almost a hundred years of unrequited American health policy ambitions.

"Oh, I should also add that you may be wondering whether this lawsuit might be defended by you through the federal contract that is the financial underpinning of the alleged fraud. Chris told me that a clever lawyer might argue, and maybe even succeed, in asserting that the federal government contract is outside of the scope of the qui tam statutes in that it was not really a matter of health coverage but something else. It would be a creative defense—really, it could even work."

***

Thrust was thinking hard. He was aware of the federal laws that were being discussed. His fast analysis was that this would be a novel application of them, but possible. It had never occurred to him, or apparently anyone on his legal team, that these laws could be applied to their federal contract. His mind was racing to the nature of that contract and how that might stop this legal claim. All they would need was for HHS to play ball and they should be willing—through Secretary Olsen.

Right on cue, Chris nailed the end of this defense to the wall. "But not if the person responsible for the agency who entered into the agreement says otherwise. And right about now, I suspect that Secretary Olsen is considering issuing a statement that makes it clear he did not."

"What do you mean," interjected Bridgewater. Subserviency to Thrust be damned. This whole endeavor was blowing up in their face. Bridgewater's partnership, and probably career, would undoubtedly be one of the casualties.

"It isn't really for me to say, Mr. Bridgewater. But I do believe one reason Lance had to leave us was for a meeting with the secretary. That should already be underway, and my understanding is that Secretary Olsen is being reminded of why it might be best to make such a statement."

"Wait a damn second," Bridgewater barked. "Isn't all of this in violation of the TRO they got this morning? Didn't that prohibit any of this under criminal penalty?" He was looking at Thrust as much as Johnny and his colleagues.

Thrust was thinking hard. It was a shock to learn that Secretary Olsen might not be in his corner any longer. Whatever Gibson had on him must be something good, or he wouldn't have bragged about it.

He began to remember something else about the anti-fraud laws. Yes, there was another way out, he thought. Worth a test run now. "One problem, Gibson, and it is a big one. In order to assert the fraud statutes, there needs to be a patient encounter that can be documented to support it. Olsen can say whatever you want him to say, but without an actual and real patient who was involved and harmed, my corporation will assert that none of these claims are enforceable through this mechanism."

Thrust stared at the senator while he spoke, finding his confidence again. *Yes, this is how we win this. Game on. I will move in for the kill shot now,* he thought. "And without going into any details here, you and

I both know that there is no record of an actual patient encounter under this contract, at least one supported by someone you could locate. You would need a patient who was not deported or is otherwise missing, or some record of it. I don't believe you have any such patient, not one who could appear before a court."

Thrust was expecting Gibson to wilt before him. Instead, he smiled back. Then he extended his arms toward Irv. "Permit me to introduce you to Irv Tinsley. You might know him better as Roberto Hernandez. Turns out he spent a night at a HealthMost emergency room in New Mexico, and some other facility near the southern border. I think he will more than satisfy our need for an actual patient nexus to our cause of action."

Thrust ran that name through his memory bank. No, it couldn't be. But that was the name that had been shared with him when the missing patient in New Mexico had been brought to his attention.

"*Que pasa,*" said Irv. "It was a hell of a couple of nights."

They had been outplayed again. Perhaps Bridgewater could scare them out of going further. "His being there was fraudulent in its own right. Impersonating a patient. That is obscene. I can't imagine a court will allow him to satisfy this legal need for a patient."

This time Irv replied. "Maybe not. Of course, I was acting in my capacity as a public health investigator at the time. I think we could successfully argue that this gave me legal permission to use extraordinary means to uncover wrongdoing. Besides, my understanding is that this would be a matter of fact finding for any court, and that the details of all the patients involved would become public knowledge if they engaged in such an inquiry. Somehow I don't think that HealthMost would want to see that happen—without going into any details here, of course."

Johnny retook the floor and let the words roll off his tongue like a duck floating over slow rapids. "You see that look on Mr. Thrust's face, Sam? That is him realizing that none of what we are doing has anything to do with speaking publicly about those dastardly deeds, unless you force us to establish client jurisdiction. Indeed, this entire court case can be pursued without any of this ever going public. One might even want to make sure that was the case, if you were a member of the board and were personally responsible for this horror and financial misjudgment.

But no, we are not revealing any information protected by the court. No, we are providing confidential information to the court and asking them to protect it. And the country from you! Do I have that right, Chris?"

"Yes, you do, Senator. I've had some of the best legal minds in the nation take a look at what I was filing, and they believe this is an airtight case. A smart person might want to cut their losses and settle it before things get even worse. I mean, really, do you think the TRO is going to hold back on us sharing the public charges about murdering immigrants when it gets attached to this lawsuit?"

Johnny put his finger to the corner of his chin. "Hmmm. Really hadn't thought much about that, Chris. But you make a good point. Anyway, gentlemen, I think we've shared enough with you for one day. I don't need any response from you about this—it is already happening. And as far as your question to me, allow me to quote from my friend Irv from a recent encounter he had with a government official—bite me. It was a pleasure meeting with you and have a nice day, Mr. Thrust. You son of a bitch." Johnny bowed. His colleagues rose and applauded.

Thrust arose, grabbed his notebook, and stormed out of the room. His associates followed, a couple of steps behind him.

By the time they cleared the door, Johnny and his friends were busy hugging each other.

"Now that was fun," offered up Mary Beth.

"Here, here," added Nancy. "Best damn political meeting I've ever had!"

"I thought Thrust was going to split in two when you started talking about the lawsuit," bellowed Irv, laughing. "It was like the wicked witch in *The Wizard of Oz*, liquifying before us."

"Hell of a meeting, Johnny. Hell of a meeting." Irv patted his friend on his back. "By the way, what are you going to do now that you are no longer a politician?"

Johnny looked back at Irv. They both laughed.

Chapter One Hundred Four

Lance Meets with the Secretary of HHS

"What the hell are you doing here," barked Secretary Ben Olsen as Lance pulled out a chair at Olsen's table at the restaurant and began to sit down.

"I am sorry, Mr. Secretary, I believe we have a meeting."

Lance continued to make himself a member of the Secretary's lunch table, as if he belonged. "No," Olsen began to opine. "That is with . . . " His voice trailed off, as he realized he had been set up. His campaign chair had set up a meeting with a wealthy donor who wanted to meet that afternoon. This was mostly why the secretary had agreed to testify before Senator Gibson and the committee far away from DC. Once he had been tricked into agreeing to do it, he justified it with the opportunity to meet with high-end donors in the Pacific Northwest.

Most thought it was to fund the president's reelection campaign committee, but what he was really doing was planting the seeds for his own presidential campaign in 2024. He would need millions, and there was money to be had in this region, and political and business favors to be traded for these funds while he was the secretary of HHS. His understanding was that the donor for this lunch had pharmaceutical business interests and would be impressed by the dismantling of Senator Gibson's criticisms at the hearing.

"You mean Nelson Duncan?" Lance replied. "I am sorry. Nelson is an associate of mine. He got hung up by a celebration in the Bahamas and won't be able to make our meeting today. But he wanted me to step in for him. You should have gotten a text from your scheduler about this change."

The secretary's portable device shimmied, and he picked it up and looked at the text message that had just arrived. Lance could tell from the look on his face that Nelson Duncan's message had arrived just in time.

"Are you hungry? I can get us a couple of menus." Lance waved at a waitress walking by. It was now almost 2:15, and there were few lunch customers left in the hotel dining room.

"Thanks, but I seem to have lost my appetite," said Secretary Olsen. "I think that I will be on my way. It doesn't seem like there is any reason for me to stay."

"Oh, but that is where you are wrong, Mr. Secretary. If you have any desires to remain in politics, you will definitely stay. Or by tomorrow you will have the political half-life of a dinosaur."

"What the hell do you mean," Olsen yelled, pulling his face up close to Lance's and spitting the angry words into his face. "What the hell are you and your boss up to? I will have your damn head on a platter."

Instead of confronting Secretary Olsen, Lance sat back in his chair, picked up a fork from the table and examined it. "Now, now, language, Mr. Secretary. You need to watch that. My understanding was that you are a God-fearing Christian, anxious to spread the word of the Lord among the infidels. I don't think Jesus would have used such language, do you?"

"I don't care what you think, you miserable asshole. I've got a lot of friends who will make sure you never work again if you don't get out of my face and my business."

Lance leaned back some more and scanned the menu the waitress had dropped off. "I hear the crab sandwich is good here. Will you join me?" He put the menu back down. He was enjoying this meeting. "Mr. Secretary, I think we may have gotten off on the wrong foot here. Let me try to set things straight.

"Mr. Duncan is, for real, an associate of mine. We don't have a long history, but did meet earlier this year in Hartford, Connecticut, and found we had some interesting things in common. You may know him better as the son of Nelson Duncan II, and his sister as Judith Duncan. She now goes by her married name of Lester."

The secretary took a deep breath. He knew who this was. Everyone looking for conservative political donors did.

"Yes, that Lester. She and her husband have been the largest single funders of Republican candidates over the last thirty years. I don't think that any Republican candidate who has tried to run for president has ever come close to the nomination without their support. Nelson the Third's dad would have been proud of what she has accomplished; she didn't fall far from his tree. He had these types of ambitions for Nelson the Third, but it didn't quite work out. He kind of got off track with some personal issues. Because of that, he and his dad were never all that close. When he passed away, it was left to Grandma to try to sort all of this out. Turns out that she did know that part of the struggle was that young Nelson had a thing for boys, and then men. She didn't want this to get too much public air, and she worked to find him a place where he might do something positive for the family name and not embarrass it.

"So, she and Nelson cut a deal, decades ago. Nelson got a cushy job running a life insurance company in Hartford, and he would have access to his family trust funds, so long as he kept his sexual proclivities a secret. He did a pretty good job of that. Even got married and somehow sired a couple of kids. Well, we think they are his anyway.

Lance continued to examine the cutlery as he spun his tale. "Not that he changed his ways. As you know, boys will be boys. It all stayed quiet enough. Until things got a little confused by other developments. Do you have any idea who confused things?" asked Lance.

"Not a frigging clue," replied Olsen.

"You just shared a hearing table with him. Yes, none other than Richard Thrust. Seems Thrust needed an insurance plan to implement one of his financial schemes. Thrust put my friend over a barrel and forced him to enter into a joint venture with him. Something to do with a major federal contract with the Department of Health and Human Services. Ring a bell?"

"Still not sure what you are talking about." The secretary could feel the story closing in around him, but was not ready to accept it yet.

"Well, I am sure it will come back to you eventually. Now, it all might have worked out. But it turns out that Thrust was doing some pretty nefarious things through that contract. Not that Nelson knew this or would care much if he did. Really, he had little interest in even being an insurance executive or any of the deals that came along with it, if anyone ever bothered to dig.

"But Thrust was playing him for a fool. Nelson kind of knew that, but wouldn't admit it. So, he swallowed his pride and decided to ride out his last years into retirement, before moving on to spending his dad's fortune. But Thrust had to treat him like him shit, because that is what Thrust does. Now you have to at least realize this!"

Secretary Olsen didn't say anything. But, yes, he understood it very well.

"The normal indignities from all of this might have been something Nelson could swallow. Yet it turned out that the bad things that Thrust were doing were hidden in the files of ALI. And when a certain independent senator from Washington State, and his intrepid chief of staff, figured this out, they got Nelson to turn over the information."

Lance waved off a waitress who was approaching to take their order. He was on a roll. Speaking of which, he was hungry. He grabbed a dinner roll from the basket in front of him and smeared a lump of butter on it, then took a couple of bites and swallowed them down. No reason not to enjoy the moment.

"When they got this information from Nelson, they analyzed it and figured out that some very, very bad things were afoot within the federal government. But they were going to have a hard time proving any of it since this evidence was technically stolen from HealthMost. But then Thrust did us a huge favor."

"What was that?" Olsen needed to find a way into this story that would give him some leverage. Senator Gibson wanted something from him, though he was not sure what.

"Thrust got Nelson dismissed from his position as CEO of ALI for turning the data over to us. It was a huge embarrassment to the family. Even his sister Judith was pissed, and they hadn't talked for years. Seems they thought it was beyond Thrust's class to do something like this. As I said, Nelson didn't really like being the head of a life insurance company, but he thought he was due such things by virtue of birth. And the money served his larger purposes. And he really, really didn't like how Thrust screwed him over.

"So he decided to help us some more."

"I thought he already gave you what you wanted. But it was HealthMost's data," Olsen said.

"Oh no. You are right. We already had that. And it had a different use for us than what we initially thought. But what Nelson provided us had almost nothing to do with his position at ALI. No, it was his underground network in gay America. You see, Nelson still had a thing for the fellas, and the terms of his deal with his mom meant that he had to be extra careful in expressing his sexual preferences. Part of how he ended up in Hartford. But he had plenty of money and he bought his way into networks that would provide him some companionship, with great discretion."

Secretary Olsen began to squirm in his seat, and the color drained from his face.

"Yes, turns out that this is a network used secretly by a number of high-profile individuals. Nelson did a little digging into some rumors he had heard from one of his lovers, and sure enough, one of those happened to be the secretary of Health!"

Secretary Olsen looked like he was going to be sick. "You can't prove any of that. And if you say anything about it, I will—"

"Relax, Secretary. We don't want to say anything about it. Senator Gibson really does think that is nobody's business but your own. I thought your wife should know, and maybe your church, and maybe those Bible thumpers who are behind your campaign. But, hey, Johnny's the boss. But you are wrong—and we can prove it." Lance pulled out his cell phone and tapped a few buttons. "It seems Nelson was able to obtain a video record of a recent tryst of yours—I believe it was in Pittsburgh." He put the phone in the secretary's face. "Sure looks like you, doesn't it? Though the heels don't really do you justice." Lance pulled the phone back and looked at the screen himself, turning it on a tilt. "Looks like you had a good time!"

"What do you want?" Secretary Olsen understood it was not a time for negotiation, but surrender.

"Just one thing." Lance took out a piece of paper. "You see, the senator and some of our colleagues are meeting with Thrust right down the hall, where he is learning that a multibillion-dollar lawsuit is being filed against HealthMost related to the government contract you agreed to with them. Seems the only possible defense to that suit is HealthMost being able to cast this as somehow not being a contract as it appears. All you have to do is issue this statement, and otherwise tell the truth about what that contract really was—a contract to provide health coverage for immigrants."

"That's all?" asked the secretary.

"Why, yes, we just want you to tell the truth. What, do you think we are animals or something? Isn't that what the contract was?"

Secretary Olsen thought back to the first conversations about the immigrant proposal from Sam Bridgewater, and then with Thrust. That was exactly how they had labeled it when the blasted scheme was first introduced. A way to provide health coverage to immigrants and get illegals out of the country at the same time.

"Yes. That is what it was. And is. Is the rest of what it is going to come out?"

"Not so sure about that. Depends on whether HealthMost is willing to settle with us, and a little bit about whether your administration is willing to support some legislative fixes that will make sure something like this doesn't happen again. Who knows—you might even still have a political future."

"What happens to the video?"

"We will hang on to our copy, of course. We can make you a copy if you want one for your records, though. Nothing else will happen to it, ever. Unless you don't continue to tell the truth about the nature of the contract with HealthMost, or don't work with us to fix the damage you have done. We also want the administration's public support for a legislative proposal that we are drafting. In the event you don't do either of these things, you can expect to see the video running on *Meet the Press* and your church's electronic bulletin board."

"Deal," said the secretary. He knew that the consequences of the bigger tale was even bigger than what he could comprehend. But it seemed mostly to do with Thrust, and maybe Bridgewater. And some legislation that he didn't really give a crap about right now. He didn't give a crap about anything other than what was on the video and getting it out of circulation.

Lance extended his hand, sealing the deal with a handshake. "Now, where is that waitress? I really am hungry."

Secretary Olsen wasn't. He got up from the restaurant table and raced through the lobby to a side door into the parking lot. There was a large potted plant next to a fence, bordering a gate into the hotel's small pool. The secretary ran to it, stuck his head over it, and vomited.

Chapter One Hundred Five

The Rest of the Friends' Discussion in Denver

A couple of months before the hearing in Belfair, Johnny, Irv, and Lance had met in the penthouse suite of the Denver Hilton to consider the best way to move ahead with the investigation of HealthMost. Parts of this conversation have already been duly recorded here, but there was one last planning session of note that took place before they headed to their respective coasts.

The three were hoping that the dumpsite Mary Beth was looking at would give them some embarrassing real evidence of the hideous plot they had uncovered. But, before they left the room, they decided that they weren't going to put all of their eggs in that one basket.

Lance was the one who suggested they assume the worst—that HealthMost would cover up whatever evidence they had found, and that they would need far more evidence than what they had now to effectively press any case of criminal wrongdoing or stop what was going on.

Irv pressed him on his assertion. "We've got their database with ALI, we've got my account of what happens to immigrants who go to their emergency rooms, and we even have a site where the bodies are dumped. Maybe even a body."

"All hearsay, and largely unsubstantiated, at least until we see if we have a corpus delicti at the dumpsite. Without that, the rest is your personal account, and we can guess that there would be a major effort to discredit you. I would suggest that this seems to have already started given what you have shared about your conversations with your boss. You, my friend, are likely to be labeled a rogue operative with an axe to grind against HealthMost. I am also not sure we could use the insurance data as the basis for any proof of the crime—it will likely be seen as stolen, and we had to make some suppositions to uncover its true purpose. Not sure a court would go to the trouble of doing that if we are talking legalities here."

"Lance is right, Irv," said Johnny. "Not just from a legal sense, but a political sense. Whatever you have uncovered is big and dastardly, but whoever is behind it—and we can surmise it is at least the higher-ups at HealthMost—will go to extreme measures to hide it. It is no easy feat to wipe flight records off the national air travel database. Makes one wonder if there aren't some folks in high places in government involved."

Irv was starting to get their drift. It wasn't that there wasn't something nefarious and evil at play; it would just be very difficult for them to prove it and do anything about it. Without a body. Which they didn't actually have yet. "So, we are looking for a Plan B in case the dumpsite doesn't give us what we need?"

"Exactly," said Lance.

"What are our options," asked Irv.

Johnny put down an apple he was eating and stroked his chin. "We came up with two. One was to continue to dig and find out how we can make a case against HealthMost in the court of public opinion. It wouldn't have to be an airtight legal case, but would have to be strong enough not to be discredited out of hand. We both think that will be hard, in part because of the powerful forces we seem to be up against, but also because we are about to hit major campaign season. It will be very easy—without clear and apparent evidence—to dismiss whatever noise we make as dirty politics. Many will dismiss it as 'fake news' and we will have another story of misbehavior that is more part of a deep state rumor mill than actionable offense."

"That doesn't sound very promising" offered Irv.

"No, it is not," said Lance. "Again, what we find at the dumpsite may open this door a bit wider. And there may be other things we don't know about yet. So we could take a chance that we can connect some dots down the road and make hay. You should give it some thought. You are the one who put your ass on the line, and you have a lot to say about deciding what we do next."

"Much appreciated, Lance. Let's just think of us as a team. I couldn't have gotten near as far as I have without you and Johnny. What's the other option?"

Johnny continued. "Option two is to run a diversion tactic and hit them where they don't suspect it. And when we do, hit them really hard."

"Uh, sounds good, Johnny. Are we just going to kind of bluff our way through this? I don't see much so far that suggests we are dealing with the type of people who will just fold their cards at the first signs of a bad hand."

"Hear me out, Irv. It gets a little complicated. But it could work. The first part of this is some legal research that we did while you were busy exploring HealthMost's care systems. Remember you okayed us sharing what we had found with a short list of people?"

Irv nodded in assent.

"One of those was Chris Jones, Nancy's dad and also a longtime health policy expert. We swore him to secrecy and were hoping to get some policy angle on care for immigrants that might help us out. On that front, he told us we didn't have much to go on. No one has wanted to take any responsibility for their care, so there is little in the way of laws, policies, or even customs. He said it was quite possible that the administration could construct a reasonable justification for their contract with HealthMost even if we had more evidence that there was criminal behavior associated with it. He is also a lawyer and confirmed that we didn't have enough evidence to prove any crimes yet, at least without a body."

Lance took over the storytelling. "We were discouraged, to say the least. But the next day Chris called us back. He got to thinking about the HHS agreement in a different way. He said if we look at it as a health coverage transaction using federal funds, he thought it possible, even likely, that HealthMost was making illegal inducements to health care providers for purposes of making money. That is fraud, my friend, and covered by special federal statutes that allow for such behavior to be ferreted out and stopped."

"Wouldn't that mean that the attorney general would just figure out how to sweep this under another the carpet? He's already been doing a lot of that, and this would hardly be a stretch."

"Yes," said Lance. "Except for one thing. It is not up to him to decide. One of the major tools provided to help root out such health care fraud is the ability of private parties to bring lawsuits independent of the government. Chris's idea was that we—he—could bring a case as a class action, representing all of the clients covered by the terms of the agreement. He thought we had the documentation that would help create the class too—the ALI file. It might not be admissible in a court for other purposes as a trade secret, but it should be plenty to certify the class and the underlying harm."

"So you are saying we could sue HealthMost ourselves to stop this behavior."

"Yes," said Johnny. "And we can recoup damages to make them pay for it. A lot of damages, as it turns out."

"How much," asked Irv.

"The potential damages is in the millions. Chris thought a reasonable figure just to start was over $500 million." Irv's jaw dropped on the table when Lance laid out the big stakes at play. "And that's not all. There is a treble damages provision intended to really pound down the hammer on fraud. So, maybe $1.5 billion in all. And Chris thinks that if we put the right people on this, it might be even more."

"Wow. That is quite the hammer you two have found. Does he think we can win?"

"We talked to him for a while yesterday by phone. He's been doing more research on this and really believes it is a winner. Almost a slam dunk off of the statute. The one defense that he's concerned with is a public cause justification. That would get applied if the government asserts that this is not a standard health coverage contract but something else. He said that most of these fraud and abuse cases get settled. Most defense lawyers see they are losing cases and convince their clients to buy their way out of even bigger trouble. With the bad acts at play here, that might also be to our advantage."

Irv was wide awake now. He was still hungry and could use a shower. Probably even could use a good dump. The news was too good to stop for any bodily needs, though. "You called this option a diversion tactic. I get it that this lawsuit is what we would hit them with. But what else would they be looking at that would catch them off guard?"

Johnny took the floor. "We were thinking that they don't really know who is lapping at their door. But I'd be surprised if they didn't think I had something to do with it. I have been yanking them around over patient dumping and making a big stink about holding them accountable. All to say that maybe we can use the Belfair meeting to catch them off guard."

Lance continued. "So, what if we make them think that this hearing is our big play on whatever we may have uncovered? They have to wonder if we have much to begin with and might easily assume that our plan is to do a surprise media attack using whatever we've got. It wouldn't be hard to make sure that some of our plan was 'leaked' to them.

"Senator, I was thinking some more about that, and it sure seems like we could use that Bridgewater guy to bite." Lance had been thinking overnight about what they could do to make this option work.

Johnny added his agreement. "Great idea, Lance. Bridgewater would sink that hook through his jaw if we did it right. I think so would HealthMost. Thrust is a power nut and thinks he is the smartest person ever to land on the planet. We just have to give him enough slack to think he has uncovered our true plot and then he will figure out how to make sure we are smacked down at the hearing."

"It won't matter though," interjected Irv, "since the real objective is to do them in with the lawsuit."

Lance pounded his fist on the table as Irv confirmed the true strategy. "Exactly, Irv. We would file the lawsuit while we are in the hearing. We would try to have the hearing work just as they feared. It would be great if we were able to use that event to embarrass them or better yet disclose their illegal behavior. Since we would be trying hard to actually do that, it would be great cover to our lawsuit!"

Irv was almost laughing out loud. "This keeps getting better and better." He got up and looked out the picture window of the suite, over the now busy streets of downtown Denver. Thankfully he had enough clothes on to not fully expose himself to those walking below. "You know, Johnny, this could get even better."

"What're you thinking?"

Irv turned from the window and looked into Johnny's eyes. "A couple of things. For one, you've talked about this antidumping thing and have shared that you wanted to get some legislation out of it. Maybe even your swan song to being in Congress. Maybe it's time to get you your bill and think even bigger."

"I love that idea, Irv. Lance, what do you think?"

Lance nodded his agreement. "I think there is an opening about the size of a pickup truck for us to do something with this. If we think it through and can get the politics aligned right."

"And the one other thing," Irv added. "I think you are going to like this. I am generally familiar with those lawsuits Chris is talking about under the fraud and abuse statutes. Forgot all about them until you reminded me, and I've been remembering what I know about them. I got a heavy dose of them in one of my education conferences for work. If I remember correctly, there is essentially a finder's fee for whoever provides the basis for the lawsuit. I want to say it is as much as 25 percent of the value of the claims. Now, even just 10 percent of $1.5 billion would be some serious cash. If it is ours to figure out what to do with, I would suggest that we are just scratching the surface on what we could do."

Johnny and Lance looked at each other, their mouths agape. Chris Jones had forgotten to mention this part of the law, or maybe wasn't as familiar with it.

"Sounds like it's unanimous—Option Two it is." Johnny put his arm down straight toward the floor like a swan flying over the carpet.

Irv and Lance extended their arms the same way, their hands meeting in the middle. "Go!" they shouted.

There was a lot more to figure out, and a lot to do. But they had a plan. A good plan. No, a hell of a plan.

Chapter One Hundred Six

Mary Beth's Vindication

"Are you ready to roll, Mary Beth? Looks like we have a pretty big crowd out there." Ken Sonnberg, chair of the Mason Health Foundation and its related public hospital district, was peering through the curtains on the stage. They were in the Shelton High School Auditorium, getting ready to begin a press conference.

"Let's do it, Ken." Mary Beth still got nervous whenever she had to speak before big crowds. She could only tamp down so much of her introversion. She had become a very effective speaker, learning how to use her emotions to connect with audiences, rather than hide them. But it still sucked the energy out of her, especially when the crowds were big.

It was also part of the job, and she knew that leading meant having to do public talks every once in a while. She remembered her last public performance—the night of the board's vote of no confidence. There was nothing about that she would want to relive. At least this evening's event would be to share good news. No, great news. No, *fantastic* news. And to put the vote of no confidence where it belonged.

Ken and Mary Beth walked out on the stage and sat down at the table to the left of the podium. Already seated were their guests for the press event—Washington Insurance Commissioner Bill Brewer, the hospital's attorney, Jim Reynolds, and Chris Jones. All three had speaking parts in what was to come. Seated at a table to the right of the podium were the other members of the board: Commissioners Sam Olinsky, Patrick Johnson, and Ginger Bettis.

The auditorium could hold about 200 students in its theater-style seating. There were about seventy-five people in these seats, and about twenty members of the press, who were standing with their cameras, tape recorders, and notepads in the well in front of the stage where an orchestra would provide musical accompaniment to school plays. Seated in the first row of the seats behind the media were Irv, Johnny, and Nancy; next to them were the staff of the Mason Health Foundation.

Ken waited another minute and then stood up and walked to the podium to the right of the table. He pulled the microphone attached to a wood lectern a bit closer and began to speak, looking around at the crowd as he did. He was looking to see if the loudmouth critics in town had dared to come to this event, or if they were still in hiding.

"Good evening, everyone. I am Ken Sonnberg, chair of the Mason Health Foundation. I am also an elected commissioner of Public Hospital District 1 of Mason County, and serve as the chair of that public entity as well. I—and we," he pointed to Mary Beth to his left, and then turning, he pointed out his fellow board members and commissioners on the right, "are excited to make a major announcement about the future of health and health care in our community tonight.

"Before doing so, I did want to make a direct reference to the last public event our board held in this community, a little more than six weeks ago. It was then and there that we took a vote of no confidence, publicly shaming our executive director, Mary Beth Collins. It was inexcusable what happened that night. Rumors and innuendos about her personal life were mixed in with what have turned out to be lies about her professional life. Too many of our community members were quick to believe these, and that led to this board voting three to two to adopt the no confidence vote.

"I was not among the yes votes. But I also want to make it clear tonight that I won't denigrate my fellow board members for their approval of this measure. All felt in good faith that they were doing what was right with the information before them. They now know that much of this information were lies created by an active campaign of a political operative to smear Mary Beth and stop the good work of the Mason Health Foundation. We will provide a bit more information on that later in this conference.

"I should also announce that Commissioner Anne Kastner has resigned from our board. She was the one who made the motion of no confidence. I can tell you that Mary Beth and I tried to talk her out of doing this. She believed that she was doing the right thing at the time. When she saw the real facts and looked back at how this political operative had persuaded her to think the worst of Mary Beth, she said she was ashamed. Mary Beth, I wanted to let you know that I talked with Anne last night about our public event, and she asked that I publicly apologize to you. She hopes you can find it in your heart to forgive her."

Applause rippled through the audience. Mary Beth smiled at Ken and nodded.

Ken continued. "The last thing I want to share about the no confidence vote with you was to let you know that the reason it happened was Mary Beth. She was the one who encouraged me to let it happen, and she even suggested that I make sure it passed. She told me to never tell anyone about this, but, well, I just can't hold on to this secret any longer.

"Why did she do this? In part because of what we are about to announce here. Mary Beth thought it was important to protect the planning that was underway to find a big solution for health for the people of our area and didn't want the controversy of her role to get in the way. Back then, I didn't really understand exactly what she was working on, but trusted that it would be something good and important. Just as she has done for us in the past.

"But the bigger reason she told me then was that she was worried that the attacks on her would get redirected to the Mason Health Foundation—and that it would do damage to the organization, staff, and the people we serve. Six weeks ago we weren't entirely sure what was afoot—including whether it was an attack on Mary Beth or our organization. Or both. Mary Beth selflessly recommended that the board put the public fire squarely on her shoulders, in order to protect everyone else. She hoped that it would ultimately work out, but had no assurance of that. It was one of the bravest acts of leadership I have seen in my public life, and I wanted today to make sure you all knew of it—and what a marvelous leader we have in Mary Beth. I would now ask her to come to the podium to make today's announcement, and I ask that we all show our appreciation for her."

As Mary Beth stood and moved toward the podium, the board members seated at the table to the left immediately stood and applauded, looking at Mary Beth, and doing so in unison with her friends and the staff seated in the audience. Seconds later, the entire audience grasped the moment and stood as well, clapping their appreciation and affection.

Mary Beth moved to the podium and shifted the microphone down to her height, about a foot shorter than Ken. "Thank you so much, Ken. And all of you." The applause trailed off and people began to take their seats again.

"It has been a challenging couple of months. I think you all know that. And I can tell you there were times when it seemed all was lost, and we should just give up. There was a time in my past when I probably would have, thinking that things are what they are, and there is only so much that us regular people can do about them. But then I met some wonderful people, who taught me so much about what life means and how we should live ours." She was looking at Irv, Johnny, and Nancy, and she held out her hand toward them so there was no doubt who she was referring to.

"They are all very different people, but they shared something important to me, as my friends, that helped guide me. Especially in these tough times. One was to know who I was, and to let that blaze my trail through adversity. Another was to keep squarely in target that whatever we do should be for the benefit of others, not ourselves. Running through all their lessons was a theme that it is our values as people and community members that define us, and to let this be the North Star to our behavior.

"My value of hope was what brought me to this community. I was hoping to find myself again, struggling at the time to find myself in some personal and career setbacks. But also the hope that we could do something meaningful for the health of the people who live in this community. It was my good fortune I was chosen to do this job, and to be supported along the way by so many wise and giving friends here. Over the last couple of months, some of them even became convinced they had made a mistake. But they couldn't know that they were reacting to a campaign of lies and deceit—they were just acting on what they thought best for the people who live here. I don't hold any of this against them, and neither should you." Another wave of applause spread through the auditorium.

"Today, we are announcing a major award of funding that will allow us to carry forward the dream of better health for the people who live here into perpetuity. Mason Health Foundation is the beneficiary of the damages awarded in a federal lawsuit filed last month against the HealthMost Corporation. You know this corporation as the company that purchased the hospital here in Shelton last year. Mister Chris Jones, who is seated here to my left, organized the lawsuit, which was a class action brought on behalf of the thousands of people harmed by that corporation. I am not allowed to say too much about HealthMost and this lawsuit—and Chris will share what he can in a few minutes. What I can tell you is that this lawsuit was settled just a few days ago. And one of the terms of the settlement was that $250 million in damages will be awarded to the Mason Health Foundation so that we can continue to grow our work in this region."

A murmur went through the crowd, even among the dignitaries seated on the stage. Most knew that the press conference was to announce an award of funds to Mason Health Foundation. No one was entirely sure of the source, and they imagined it would be an amount in the thousands. Whatever the number of zeroes, it would be a significant addition to the Mason Health Foundation asset base—$250 million was an astonishingly large amount of money.

Mary Beth continued. "I know—that is more money than any of us would ever have imagined. Over the last couple of months, I thought there was a small chance that the recent attacks on us might possibly translate to some payment for our troubles, but never did I think it would be anything like this.

"It will be up to the board of the Mason Health Foundation to figure out exactly what to do with these funds. I've got a few general thoughts that I will share with all of you now in the interest of transparency—but remember, it is the board's decision.

"First, we should think about the future—we have enough funding to make sure that the foundation is available to pursue better health in our community for maybe forever. We should do that.

"Second, our surveys have shown us that almost all who live here in this rural community believe we need and want a hospital. A special provision in this settlement allows us to purchase the Shelton Hospital back from HealthMost for a fixed price of one million dollars. We just need to make that decision within three months of the settlement date. I suggest we do this and will present a motion to the board at its meeting next week to do this." Loud applause came from the audience, and the board members were among those clapping.

"Third was a request from the representatives of the class action. Mr. Jones was the leader, and he is asking that we consider nationalizing our scope of involvement in health and health care. To be clear, he is not asking us to change who we are in terms of our perspective that health care is a local matter. Rather, he is asking us to keep doing that, and in even bigger ways with this award, while also thinking how we might catalyze or organize other organizations like ours across the country. He called it a virtual and community-based health reform movement of, by, and for the people. I will be suggesting we take 10 percent of our award, or twenty-five million dollars, and do that.

"Fourth, even as we act locally to improve health, we must recognize that it happens in a political context that is greatly influenced by Congress and the actions of federal agencies. We do not want to become a political organization, but we do want to make sure that sound and effective health policy will drive what happens with federal decision-making. Mr. Jones and my friend Senator Johnny Gibson both have a lot of experience and have made some recommendations on how we might do that. I will ask our board to consider their ideas and for us to take action in support of health policy change consistent with our values, and that we be prepared to do so even before this year is out, in case there is an effort to effect change nationally.

"Fifth, and last, goes back to that matter of values. Ours has been that not only is health care a local matter, but it is a personal matter. The system should relate directly to people, and our programs and policies have tried to make this so. One of those programs is our personal navigation support service. Johnny, Senator Gibson, helped model how to do this for us. It has been providing benefits to now thousands of people in our community over the past eighteen months. Another was our Mason County Community Health Challenge.

"You might also remember that complaints about what we were doing were in the middle of some of the intrigues of the past few months. That included some allegations of wrongdoing on the part of our foundation; you likely saw the newspaper article that summarized these allegations. The insurance commissioner for Washington State is seated to my left and will be speaking momentarily about this—and will be apologizing for what was an illegal operation in his office.

"I mention that now because the allegation made in those charges was that our service was 'fraud,' because we claimed it was 'free.' We used insurance broker payments from health plans to fund our navigation service, and served all who sought us out without regard to whether we received any commission payments. So it was free to our clients. As was the Mason County Community Health Challenge. And I think the insurance commissioner now completely agrees with that." Mary Beth looked at Bill Brewer, who shook his head in the affirmative.

"My final recommendation to the foundation board is that we settle this for all time by using our new source of funds to pay for our personal navigation services. And that we grow this service to include new languages and new tools and services that will allow our clients to not only choose health coverage plans, but improve the health of themselves and their families. Future Mason County Community Health Challenges might be a part of this. And maybe those commissions can instead be used to reduce the cost of health coverage in those plans.

"Let me stop there. There is obviously a lot more to be figured out, and done. And we will. It is a great day for health and health care in Mason County, our region, the state, and even the nation. I thank you for letting me be a part of this great story. I will turn it back to Ken to introduce our other guests and then we will open this up to questions from the press."

Mary Beth received another standing ovation from the crowd as she stepped away from the podium and moved toward her seat. She stood next to her chair for a minute or so, smiling and then waving at the audience. She directed her gaze to her friends in the first row. And especially Irv.

Ken Sonnberg moderated the balance of the press conference. Chris Jones shared what he could about the class action lawsuit and the settlement. There weren't too many details of the basis of the suit—this was sealed under a confidentiality agreement linked to the settlement. Most of his comments were about the $250 million and the timing and limited requirements associated with it. The insurance commissioner then took the stage and apologized for the improper actions of his office. He said an assistant insurance commissioner had been fired as a result—there was evidence that he had taken his actions against the Mason Health Foundation because of inducements made by an out-of-state political operative.

Jim Reynolds closed out the presentations with an outline of legal actions that would need to be taken to secure the funding and position the board for its next set of decisions.

Ken opened to questions from the media, and those on stage answered these for another half hour. Mary Beth barely remembered any of the questions. She was too happy to finally have the bitter taste of the last few weeks gone from her being. And too anxious to see where things would go next. Sure, in part with the Mason Health Foundation. What a fabulous opportunity that would be.

But also with Irv. It had been nice, no wonderful, having him around every day for the last month. She remembered why they had once become so close and began to forget the reasons why they drifted apart. He seemed to feel the same. Now, all she really wanted to do was leap off the stage and give him a big hug.

Chapter One Hundred Seven

Johnny Gets His Bill

Johnny was amused that he was sitting in the same seat in Senate Majority Leader Thomas Bell's Office he had a few months ago. My how time flies and things change. Then he was about to get his comeuppance; now he was about to demonstrate that the world spins round. He even got a bit nostalgic—this was likely the last time he would ever be here, most certainly as a member of Congress. *Let's make it a memorable meeting*, he thought.

His purpose was to close the deal that was offered at that last meeting, but he might as well have some fun too. He was ready for the vote on his bill. The Senate majority leader had promised him this if he stood aside and didn't run for reelection. Johnny had done his part, and it was time for the majority leader to realize that his part of the bargain was now due and payable.

Johnny expected there would be resistance. At first he couldn't even get the appointment scheduled. His history with Senator Bell's appointment secretary had helped crack through; that and some messages delivered to the majority leader's political action director. The majority leader got and kept his job by keeping his caucus members happy—and this meant supporting their reelection campaigns.

Senator Bell had thought it a useful tactic to send his political hacks at Johnny via his campaign consultant, Nancy Jones. Turnaround was fair play, and Johnny had asked Nancy to deliver her own message back through the campaign consultants for other Democratic senators seeking reelection—Senator Bell was bungling prospects for the future control of the Senate.

Johnny was going to let him know in no uncertain terms that the grumbling Nancy's messages had stirred up could be followed by cruel reality. If the majority leader reneged on the deal for a vote, Johnny would ask his devoted followers to support the Republican candidate in the race for his soon to be vacant seat. Bell would know that this would easily tilt the election to the Republican, as there were thousands of Washingtonians who believed in Johnny and were upset that he was not running for reelection. Fifty thousand would be plenty enough to turn the election, and Johnny had at least twice that many devoted followers without breaking a sweat.

Johnny knew that he had Bell where he wanted him. This meeting was to close the deal and get his vote scheduled. The timing mattered, and he did not want the majority leader or his confidants modifying the legislative package Johnny was putting together. Most of all, it was time to remind Senator Bell that his promise was to put up a bill for Johnny that included "whatever he wants to put in it."

Johnny was sure he had the upper hand when Senator Bell came out to the waiting area personally to usher him into his office; right on time. "John, great to see you," offered Senator Bell while extending his hand in friendship.

"Senator Bell, thanks so much for finding the time to meet with me." Johnny closed his large hands around Senator Bell's and squeezed hard. It was a trick he had learned from his grandfather, and it generally worked, at least with old white men. "I am sure you are busy with the election campaigns."

"Always time for friends like you, John. Come on in the office and let's talk about what you need." They walked into the spacious office, and Johnny settled into the same seat he sat in months before. Senator Bell would remember that was the case, and observe that Johnny had full recollection of their time together and their deal.

"I understand you are looking for a vote on that bill about patient dumping, John." Senator Bell sat down in a lush red leather chair, putting his feet on the top of the desk. "I've talked to my folks, and they said we would be okay with some improvements to those laws. I can even get our votes to pass it, both in committee and on the floor. The politics on this seem to have shifted a bit, and rumor has it that the White House would go along with it. The secretary of HHS has taken the lead on the administration response and is singing a different tune now. Let's work out the details and get it done—it will be a big victory for you. Leaves a real legacy to your time as a United States senator. I might even suggest we name the act after you."

Johnny was impressed that Senator Bell had done his homework and was adding his own sweeteners. The not so subtle message from Nancy had gotten through, and Johnny figured next would be a request for him to support the Democratic candidate in the Washington State Senate race. Johnny was willing to go there, but the deal would need to be sweeter, much sweeter, than this. He would reshape the conversation immediately.

"Senator Bell, much of that sounds good. But it is not enough. You will recall that the deal was that you would make sure I had a vote on my bill, and that we talked about it as 'patient dumping' and whatever else I wanted to add to it. My team has been working on the legislative proposal, and there will be some other things. We don't have the bill language yet, but I can provide you with a summary." Johnny took a set of papers out of the organizer he was carrying and handed it to the Senate majority leader.

Bell flipped through the several pages. Johnny knew it wouldn't take long for him to figure out that the scope of the legislation would be far more than patient dumping reform. "Whoa, cowboy," exhorted the leader. "This is way bigger than what we talked about."

"But it is whatever else I had in mind, Senator. And I don't need to remind you that I have done my part. Since my announcement that I won't be running for reelection, I can see time is short for me to accomplish my bigger ambitions of being a senator. I am less interested in naming a bill after me than passing some real reforms that will help the American people and our health care system. This is what we have come up with."

The majority leader took his feet down from the desk. He folded his hands and placed them on the front of the desk, leaning his chin upon them. Johnny thought the room got a little darker. *Does the majority leader have a light switch somewhere on the floor to help set his desired mood in political negotiations? Not out of the question*, he thought.

"Let's say I give your bill a vote, John. Assuming you can get it out of Committee."

"It will. All I need to make that a sure thing is that you promise your Democrats on the Committee that there will be a floor vote."

"Okay, let's assume that then. I can't be sure that I can muster enough votes to get it through the floor vote if it looks like this."

"I bet you can. With my vote, it would pass 51-49 if all the Democrats supported it. I would think that the vast majority of them would want to do so on its face. Our research polling shows that a plurality of Americans support the reforms contained in this package. I think most of your members would be on their side when they go to the ballot box in another month."

"You might be right about that, John. But what about the five or so who are from more conservative states? And McCormack from West Virginia and Schmidt from Montana are running for reelection. What am I to tell them?"

"To start with, that we've done issue polling in both of their states. Over 75 percent of likely voters in their states like what we are talking about in concept—and half of all Republicans. They can position themselves as thought and action leaders on the number one issue Americans are thinking about as they head into the voting booth."

"And what if that isn't enough—you and I both know that was the case with the Affordable Care Act, which ended up being a very tough vote for Democrats in swing states."

Johnny remembered well—the House switched power to the Republicans because of that vote during the Obama presidency.

"Then you might ask them what they think about winning reelection but being in the minority party. I haven't made any endorsements in the campaigns to replace me—yet. You and I know that I can deliver a hundred thousand votes without even trying. These are people who would have voted for me even if they believed those attack ads you came up with . . . " Johnny wanted Bell to understand he knew of the ads and his active role in them.

"I could probably generate another hundred thousand votes for either candidate if I actually campaigned for them. You haven't given me any reason to get involved in this one way or the other so far, though I am tilting toward the Republican since my Democratic friends who I have been so helpful to over the past year seem to be very involved in the dirty politics around getting rid of me." Johnny wasn't screwing around anymore.

Senator Bell eyed Johnny, his face tightening and his diction losing its folksy drawl.

"So I give you a floor vote on your bill, and get all the Democrats to support it. You give me an endorsement of the Democratic candidate for the Washington State Senate seat. Do I get any say in what is in the legislation?"

"No. But I will be open to floor amendments provided that I approve of them. And I want a favorable Rules Committee action managing the vote." Johnny's team had planned a comprehensive path to getting this bill out of the Senate.

"I won't be able to defeat a filibuster. You can't hold me and my caucus accountable for that." Bell was certain there would be one, the ace in the hole for defeating many previous attempts to get major legislation through the Senate, especially health care reform.

"Let me worry about that; I am confident that I can get enough Republican votes to get the bill on to the floor for an up or down vote. I may not be able to get them to vote for it, but am pretty sure that we have enough to at least get the sixty votes needed to stop a filibuster."

The majority leader wondered what Johnny had in his pocket. Off of this meeting, he had no reason not to believe that Senator Gibson was good to his legislative gamesmanship word. "Okay. Let's say you get it out of the Senate. You are on your own when it goes to the House. Though that shouldn't be a big hurdle over there since everyone is up for reelection. That is if your research on public views about the bill is sound."

"I am counting on more than my research over there, Senator Bell. For now, I will just say we have some ideas. But I do understand that you are off the hook once the bill gets out of the Senate, and I will then announce my heartfelt support to Ms. Flaherty."

Senator Bell shifted back in his chair. This deal was essentially done. "I will need this vote done before mail balloting begins in Washington state," he added.

"Perfect. My ask is that we schedule a vote for the first week in October." Johnny had worked out his timeline before the meeting.

"All right. And good luck with getting the president to sign this." Senator Bell waved around the multi-page document Johnny had shared with him.

"I'll take my chances," said Johnny.

"Fine." Senator Bell stretched his hand out toward Johnny. "We have a deal."

Johnny grabbed the senator's hand and squeezed it even tighter than their first handshake. It made the majority leader break out in a smile. "You know, Senator, I wish you had decided to be a Democrat. We could use some people with balls like yours in this party."

Johnny laughed and strode proudly out of the senator's office. As he was crossing through the anteroom toward the door to the Capitol hallway, Penny approached him. "Well, how did it go?"

"Perfect," said Johnny. "Got time for dinner sometime this week, Penny?"

"Sure do, Johnny. But you should know that I have changed my policy and don't date members of Congress anymore."

"Well, that won't be a problem soon enough." He laughed and looked at his watch. "Right now I have to run. Got an appointment with the minority leader. I am going to be a bipartisan pain in the ass today!" He hugged Penny and strode out of the leader's office, a man on a mission.

Chapter One Hundred Eight

The Process Used to Draft the Bill

It was Irv who first encouraged Johnny to use the opportunity created by the investigation to seek major health legislation. Irv knew little about how one actually makes something go in Congress. Johnny did, largely because of the advice he had received many years ago from the House Parliamentarian to learn the rules of the game, and then use them when he had a chance to do something meaningful. With a little help from Nancy Jones, that is what he had done—and a bill was now on its way for consideration by the full Senate, and, he hoped, toward law.

Johnny also knew that, despite all he had learned about health policy from his friends, that this was not his area of expertise. More importantly, he was thinking big, and figured that they would need a group effort if they were to take full advantage of this opportunity. This task was the bigger reason for Irv, Johnny, and Mary Beth gathering at the Alderbrook Lodge over the weekend before the Belfair hearing.

Their opening discussion was captured earlier and then moved on toward a dialogue to identify the contents of their health care reform proposal. The three friends had gathered for dinner while they waited for the rest of their conspirators to arrive at the lodge. All were an essential part of what was afoot—the task of identifying "anything else he wanted included" in Johnny's ask of the Senate majority leader.

This was only the first step in their legislative play. It would take a lot more than the majority leader's promise to get any legislation into law, and while the odds of success got smaller the more ambitious the legislation, they were ready to try to do a lot.

It was now near 11 p.m. in the bar of the Alderbrook Lodge Restaurant. Johnny, Irv, and Mary Beth were still by themselves. The conversation shifted toward the legislation, led by Johnny. "I think we have a chance to push through some real policy change in health care, but I don't know what it is! I really need you to help me figure that out."

Irv looked at Mary Beth. Mary Beth looked at Irv. They both looked at Johnny. "Of course!" they blurted out, restraining laughs. "When have we not given you cheap advice?"

Johnny couldn't help but chuckle himself. It was a lot more drama than their usual playful banter. "It looks to me like we have a full bar, several hours of privacy, and rooms that we can walk to whenever we get tired. And two more days before we have to head to Belfair."

"When will they be here?" asked Mary Beth.

"Not long at all. They checked in about twenty minutes ago and should be almost ready to come." Johnny picked up his cell phone and texted someone. Seconds later, he looked at it again and added, "They will be here in about two minutes."

Sure enough, they were. Into the bar strode Nancy Jones. She was excited to see Johnny, Irv, and Mary Beth. With her was an elderly man, carrying a briefcase.

"So great to see you. I understand we might have a bit of plotting to do. Just my cup of tea. Though a gin and tonic might be a better way to start. Can I get you something, Dad?"

Nancy turned toward her companion, putting her arm around him and turning toward her friends. "Allow me to reintroduce my father, Christopher Jones. You all met him years ago after the Clinton reform fiasco. Maybe the greatest expert on American health policy around. Johnny thought he might be helpful to our planning."

"You have been bragging about him since the day I met you, Nancy." Johnny walked over and grabbed Chris's hand. "Good to see you again, Professor. I so enjoyed our recent phone conversations about fraud laws that are a huge part of what got us to this night. Even more excited that you can join us in the flesh to do some even bigger plotting for the public good. But first, let me get something for you in the bar."

Chris was smiling. "I can't begin to tell you how much Nancy has talked about the three of you over the years. Your reputations precede you, most famously. And if the plan she described to me is anything close to what she shared, it is my great honor to be with you tonight. Make that an Irish whiskey and ice, Jameson's if they've got it, Senator. I also wanted to let you know that the court documents are ready to go. We should discuss exactly when we should file. But we are ready, and think we have an open and shut case. It is very promising, to say the least."

Johnny nodded. "Fantastic!"

The group got their refreshments and settled in around a large, circular table just outside of the bar. Mary Beth had rolled in a large portable grease board from a nearby conference room. Johnny, Irv, and Mary Beth had spent some time planning how to use this time on their telephone conference last week. This meeting would be a lot more structured than how they plotted things in their youth. But Mary Beth now had skills that she didn't have then. It would be a good time to use them.

Mary Beth had developed a real expertise in facilitating planning sessions for groups, especially political groups and not-for-profit organizations. Under Nancy's tutelage, she had created a repertoire of unconventional approaches to facilitation. Almost all who participated in her sessions found her techniques fun, and unusually productive.

She began by framing their goal: to outline the elements of a legislative package that Johnny might introduce before the United States Senate—and try to get passed into law. She drew a big green circle in the middle of the grease board. "This is what we hope to fill in by the time we leave here on Sunday."

She had Johnny explain where things stood with the notion of a legislative proposal. He told them he would announce that he was not seeking reelection on the afternoon of the Belfair hearing. The price for this deal was that he would be allowed to bring a health care bill up for a vote. He explained that it was originally going to be legislation about patient dumping, but that the Senate majority leader had cracked the door for it to be "anything" that Johnny wanted.

Mary Beth wrote down on the lower middle of the grease board some key questions relating to this. They would come back to these questions later, she said. Chief among them was the legislative strategy to get any bill passed. First, they were to focus on what might be in it. Others added some issues to her parking lot list on the bottom of the grease board.

Now, it was time for each of them to report on their homework. She had asked them to bring a list of their best ideas related to what such a bill might look like: legislative ideas, principles, values, wild-ass suppositions, literally anything. They would go around the table, and each of them would offer up one item from their list at a time, and then would have one minute to explain it. Only clarifying questions would be allowed for this round. Then, the next person would bring up their item. They would keep going around the table until all of their lists were exhausted.

Mary Beth would write short descriptions of the individual contents of each person's list in the four corners of the grease board as they shared them with the others. Once they exhausted their lists, they would see what they had on the full board—and try to figure out what a bill might look like from these ideas.

Irv went first. His list was the product of his longtime philosophical thinking about health care change. He had been thinking about this question for many decades and had developed a set of philosophical building blocks for creating meaningful change of the health care system:

"One. *It's not the money, stupid.* That is, the system is so influenced by money, and much of its design problems are related to bad and conflicting financial incentives that have to be corrected and aligned to create effective and efficient reform. But the primary aims of the health care system are not financial—they are about health. Doing this well requires us to stop making the pursuit of better health and health care be primarily about money.

"Two. It's about health. A corollary to number one is the clear and unambiguous understanding that the objective of the health care system is and must be to produce health, not just more medical care. Of society and each of us individually. The definition of health should be in sync with the World Health Organization's: a state of complete physical, mental, and social well-being, and not merely the absence of disease or infirmity.

"Three. It takes both personal and collective responsibility to create health. We need to pursue both of these at the same time—and reject attempts to limit our progress to one or the other. That is the partisan and ideologic trap that gets in the way of progress.

"Four. Health care is exceptionally personal and should be centered on each person. Medical care as a system must be rebuilt around the needs of people, not the institutions and people working within the system.

"Five. The answers to our problems must be built from hope and be reinforced with accountability of all. We need to embrace the possibilities and aspirations for a healthier future, rather than obsess over the demons of the past."

There were questions from the group to Irv about what his building blocks represented, and how to use them for the task at hand. Chris asked whether these were intended to be legislative proposals. "No," shared Irv. "These are just windows into the type of thinking that will produce meaningful answers." He explained that it was more than unlikely their bill would be the last and best word on how to reform health care. He thought their legislative ideas would be a first step, hopefully a big one, toward creating a better system and make it easy for future advances to be added on. He had some practical and discrete ideas for the legislation, but to him, it was crucial to advance these ideas while keeping in mind they were just building blocks with longer term design implications.

Johnny went next. Surprisingly to Irv and Mary Beth, he was less philosophical and more practical in his approach to the homework assignment. Perhaps it was all those years of hearing about people's problems and considering failed legislative proposals to do something about them. His list was somewhat the opposite of Irv's—a laundry list of practical policy solutions, but certainly more expansive and creative than those typically debated in halls of government. He brought five ideas to this planning session; there were more if they needed them, he added:

"One. Strengthen the duty to treat by providers, especially those infused with public advantage or necessity. The antidumping statutes that were the topic of the hearing fit with this, and specifically making sure that not-for-profit and public hospitals with ERs and getting public benefit from these designations behaved appropriately.

"Two. A public option, preferably a Medicare buy-in. It would be hard to create or sustain a single source of health coverage in this nation. One government program is probably not the right answer for us anyway. But there needs to be more and better choices than the ones provided through the ACA marketplace exchanges. A public option should be created, and Americans should be able to make their own choice about it. The easiest and best model to do so is by allowing any American to buy into the Medicare program at its actuarial value. Let that 'choice' compete with those offered by private health plans, and we will reset the base of American health care at a greatly more effective level of cost and performance.

"Three. A health care lottery. Health coverage is a mixed system. In part, it is collectively insuring for true insurable events across society—catastrophic and unanticipated events that one can pool to lower individual risk. But it is also about prepaying for services and products that many expect to use. One way to focus the system is to provide alternative and fairer ways to deal with the insurance element. While it will be hard to legislate out the ability of people with high wealth to acquire whatever they need if these things happen to them, every American should be able to have a fair chance to get such full assistance by virtue of a national lottery for expansive health services of a catastrophic nature should they not have the resources to pay for the care.

"Four. Diversity and disparities in health. For too long, the greatest suffering and inequities of the American health care system have related to race and ethnicity. These must be rooted out and changed by shining an exceptionally bright light on them and by linking accountability systems to them, including financial rewards and penalties.

"Five. A national competition. We need to promote a better health system collectively and through our own personal responsibilities. Let's bring both of these out through an annual national health competition. Besides, it could be fun."

Chris said he brought a list with him, and that it was already conveniently written up. He held up a red book and told the group his dad, and Nancy's granddad, was part of the staff who helped to create it. He thought it the most important treatise ever produced on the future of American health care—and his list would be each of the five recommendations of the committee. Irv immediately knew that Dr. Jones was referring to the Committee on the Cost of Medical Care, and its five tenets:

1. Medical service through organized groups
2. Strengthen the public health service
3. Costs should be managed on a group basis
4. There should be strong state and local coordination of health care
5. Professional medical education

Mary Beth didn't consider herself to be much of an expert on health policy, or at least those policies that came from government via laws. Her list was more a set of conventions that she felt the group needed to apply to make this process worthy of their time and effort. She wanted to do what was meaningful and right, rather than what might be convenient. The list included some of the "Not Lists" she had used in other brainstorming sessions over her career:

1. "This is the way we've always done it."
2. "You can't do that."
3. "It won't work."
4. "That's how the system is set up."

Nancy Jones had a list, she said, but it was always the same item—she kept repeating it every time the circle made its way to her. It was "the broken window theory." She explained, each time, that it had more to do with the political implementation of whatever they came up with, and she would say more when they came back to the parking lot issues.

The roundtable of ideas took about a half an hour. Mary Beth then tasked the group to have at it. "What might this list tell us about what should be in Johnny's legislative proposal?"

It was one of the easiest and fun facilitation jobs she ever had. Some of the most astute observers of American health policy, politics, and the human condition were sitting around the table. They were comfortable in their thoughts, which had been formulating for many years.

Just as important, they were comfortable with each other. There was no need to impress or lobby anyone else—it was all about finding the best idea. Breaking through this barrier was usually what Mary Beth had to do in her facilitations. Now, she just had to keep the conversation moving.

Nor was that a great challenge—they had the room until breakfast. By 5 a.m., they had agreed on a ten-point legislative proposal, in concept. They agreed to review it again the next day, with the benefit of sleep and the arrival of Johnny's chief of staff, Lance Givens, to the group.

If they couldn't explain it to him, then they would need to redo it. Presuming that they still could, and Lance didn't reject it, they would deem the ideas as "worthy" and ask him to take the lead in drafting up a bill that would satisfy their ten-point proposal. If things went according to plan, Johnny would need bill language in another month or so.

They were about to call it a night and adjourn when Nancy reminded them that they still had parking lot issues on the board. Or at least hers, she emphasized. She had been an active participant throughout their brainstorming session, but the broken window theory had never come up.

They sat back down so Nancy could explain it to them. It was late, and all were getting tired, so she gave a brief description. The theory was a fundamental model for creating big change in American society that she had learned at Harvard. She had occasionally tried to apply it, but had mostly observed the failure of policy makers to do so as they tried to do big things.

The broken window theory suggests that major policy change is created by three distinct elements, using a window as a metaphor. First, the window must be opened to create a chance for the change to occur—this was the political system. In this case, it was Johnny who was opening the window with his legislative deal with the Senate majority leader.

To solve whatever problem, there must be a policy answer to it, a solution that one can in concept pass through this open window. It wasn't enough to just create a political movement without this answer—and it must be worthy ingredients of an effective solution. In this case, it was the ten-point legislative proposal that they presumably would be trying to move soon.

The third part of the formula was the most overlooked, she shared, and perhaps the most critical: The window must be opened, and stay open, wide enough to allow a suitably large idea for change to be passed through it. This, almost inevitably, required the greater public to become comfortable and involved with the solution, as big change usually spoke to something that people cared greatly about. If people weren't allowed to weigh in, they could be influenced to think the worst of things that they might otherwise support. This public judgment not only allowed larger ideas to be offered as solutions, but would help defend them from subsequent efforts to fight them.

If the window was not sufficiently open through public support when the policy ideas were passed through, it would break—the "broken" part of the theory—leaving metaphorical shards of glass that would sever the lifeblood out of any legislative proposal to solve the social problem, when introduced or further down the road.

Chris picked up where Nancy left off, sharing his experiences with health care policy and its historic resistance to big change. He realized, once he had heard this theory, that many of the past failures of health care reform fit this model to a tee. He offered up some examples—Clinton Care, the repeal of Washington State's comprehensive health reform law, even the Committee on the Cost of Medical Care.

The group got their second wind and talked about the broken window theory. It spoke to them. Yes, they needed public support for what they were proposing. Mary Beth asked why Nancy had made it her one and only idea for the brainstorming.

"Because I don't know enough health policy to be all that helpful in formulating what should be in this legislative proposal. But I do have some ideas for how we might find and amplify that public judgment. And let's be clear—we have to do so quickly to fit with the timeline Johnny is giving us. This is what I've been thinking about. Want to hear them?"

"Yes," they shouted in unison.

"Where's that coffee pot?" asked Johnny. "I have a distinct feeling that this is something we need to really hear."

Chapter One Hundred Nine

Thrust Goes to Prison

The heavy iron door shut behind Richard Thrust as he walked through the main entranceway of Texarkana Prison. As it closed, the reality of his confinement began to hit him. He was realizing that this was not even a security door, just a minimum security entranceway. Soon he would see some real doors that would hold him in place over the three years of confinement awaiting him.

He had pled guilty to fraud charges; a set of separate allegations related to but distinct from the class action lawsuit brought by Chris Jones against HealthMost Corporation. That lawsuit was settled, quickly and quietly, once the HealthMost board of directors realized the jeopardy that the immigrant health contract with HHS had put them in, organizationally and personally.

Thrust had tried to get them to defend the suit aggressively, but to no avail. They surely could have dragged the litigation out for a few years, and who knew what might happen before the end date of the litigation. Witnesses die, or forget; old grievances get replaced by new grievances. Thrust was hoping to stretch it out long enough to find another CEO position. Then, it would be their problem to deal with, not his.

The board didn't bite. In part because of the inference from Chris Jones that the real purpose of the contract would become public knowledge during any trial, and that this scandal might take down the company totally and permanently. Truth be told, while this did concern them, what really scared them was that they would personally be implicated in the scandal. Public ridicule toward them and their families was not what they signed up for, nor were they anxious to find out if they might be personally responsible for a share of the damages and fines.

So, they served up Thrust and other executives with dirty hands around the transaction. Thrust berated the board when they told him of their conclusion, reached in an executive session held without him. He called them fools and cowards, and threatened them in every way known to man. By then, though, they were listening to their new corporate counsel, not Richard or anyone left on the Thrust management team. The new HealthMost attorney assured them that Thrust was now more bark than bite.

The deal Thrust then struck with the board, Chris Jones, and the attorney general was that he would plead no contest to fraud around some of the financial transactions related to the immigrant health program with HHS. The larger purpose of this agreement would be kept confidential, as would the terms of his sentence and the settlement agreement Jones's team had with HealthMost.

HealthMost agreed to pay $1 billion in damages, and a $250 million finder's fee to Chris Jones, which he had in turn assigned to the Mason Health Foundation. It was hard to identify all of the harmed parties of immigrants who were deported, or worse—in fact most of them had disappeared from record once they left HealthMost's control. The few who were identified received a financial award and were offered a track to United States citizenship. The rest of the damages were placed in a trust dedicated to helping pay for the cost of health care for immigrants to the United States. A non-profit trust was formed to manage this money.

HealthMost would be allowed to maintain its business, but with some major constraints—the membership of the board would be subject to review by the court. The board chair would be selected by the court and the terms of the agreement dictated that the first new chair would be a consumer representative.

The new corporate counsel was named the successor president and CEO, and she promptly fired all of the senior executives who once reported to Thrust. The newly named chief operating officer was given specific instructions by the CEO and the board to review all other management positions across the organization and make sure that these employees were of the highest ethical and moral character.

Some board members were surprised that there were not more strings attached to letting them stay in business. They would soon learn that other strings were to be attached, but not just to them—all organizations wishing to make money out of providing health care to Americans would be affected through legislation brought to the Senate by one John Gibson.

Thrust himself would have to serve three years of a seven-year prison sentence in a minimum security institution. It would be as easy a ride as possible in the federal penal system. More important to him was that the limited disclosures would make it possible for him to work again. He had plenty of money salted away and would be financially secure for life, but he knew his rightful place was as a captain of industry. He would rise again, he thought, and have his vengeance upon all concerned.

His first stop within the prison was at a desk, where he left all his personal belongings. The sergeant on duty made a record of all of these things, including jewelry, shoes, clothes, wallet, and even the magazine he read on the Uber ride to the prison. The guard put these belongings into a bag marked with his name, and asked Thrust to read and sign the list.

Thrust was struggling to keep his cool, now standing naked before the desk sergeant and two guards who were waiting at a doorway to the inside of the prison. He did his best to look dignified, signing the document with his flowery signature, the one he used when he signed important agreements. The sergeant stuck it in a file in the desk and tossed the bag of materials into a chute behind the desk.

"This way," said one of the guards. Thrust hesitated as he looked through the bars of the door. "Get a move on," said the guard. Thrust took his time moving through the door, and the guard then grabbed him by his arm and yanked him through. "I meant now, asshole. Stand over there."

Thrust saw he was being asked to move toward a bare concrete wall on the other side of the room. The floor slanted down to a drain in the floor. He strode over to the wall, with his head held high as he attempted to use his iron will to prevail over the guards. It mostly looked foolish to them, as it just exaggerated the distance between the chin on his largish head and the hand he had put over his genitals trying to cover up.

"This is the fun part," another guard said as he picked up a hose in the corner. The other guard tossed him a plastic bottle of what seemed to be soap. "Put some of that on and then hold on, big fella. We're gonna hose you down." In a matter of seconds, a strong flow was surging through the hose, and the guard began to pelt Thrust with its stream. He rubbed a little soap on himself.

"Don't forget your hair, big boy. And get some up your ass crack. We want that to be shiny clean. You didn't put anything up there, did you? Dan here is quite adept at cavity searches." The guard turned up the water pressure, and the stream was forceful enough to push Thrust toward the wall. "Okay, now turn around."

The water was turned off. The other guard threw a towel at him. "Dry off." He gave Thrust about fifteen seconds and then told him to throw the towel on the ground by the drain. Dan walked toward him and gave him a stack of clothes to put on. Thrust put on his prison garb—blue pajama bottoms with an orange T-shirt. There was a pair of white socks and some shoes that were more like slippers.

"Oooey. Doesn't he look fine in those duds."

"Sure does. I hear he was a bigshot executive, ran some health care company. Well, we are going to have to get you a secretary."

"I hear Bruno learned how to type. Maybe they can become bunkmates?"

The guard laughed. "Maybe. Come this way, Dick." He motioned to Thrust to move through a next set of doors out of the room and presumably to his cell.

Thrust stood tall and barked back at the guard. "My name is Richard."

The two guards laughed together. "Hey, Dan, it is going to be fun teaching this douche that they are all just dicks to us."

Chapter One Hundred Ten

Bridgewater's Fate

The collapse of the HealthMost conspiracy, and its fallout, was a devastating failure for Sam Bridgewater. It led to the immediate cancellation of the lucrative lobbying contract with HealthMost Corporation. Soon, rumors were floating about possible criminal and civil prosecutions related to its governmental affairs activities, and Bridgewater was a centerpiece of these rumors.

His lobbying firm discharged him by a vote of the partners. It mattered little that his was one of the names on the door of the firm; they just peeled him off the door and sent him packing. They wanted nothing to do with him anymore, and nor did most of Washington's political community. His name was toxic. It was made worse by the reputation he had justifiably earned for being willing to use any means to win. Playing dirty meant you had to be a winner, or face the consequences of not being on top. He was now, clearly, a loser.

Sam had completely cut his ties to his family decades ago and had not spoken to his parents in over ten years. He was single and did not date much; he used prostitutes to relieve his sexual needs. Nor did he have any friends in the community, or anywhere. Sam had always been a loner, from a very young age and throughout his Washington career.

He was hoping to rebuild a client base. People like a comeback story, he thought, and he would just have to wait out the moment. He had saved millions of dollars from his work endeavors and could live comfortably enough until then. But he was anxious to get back in the game—it was all he really had.

About a month after the Belfair hearing and the beginning of the end for his HealthMost contract, he began to suffer severe headaches. At first he figured it was just the stress of the moment, and he would find relief with painkillers. Pills did little to stop the headaches, and if anything, they were getting worse.

He hadn't been to a physician for over twenty years and went online to find a specialist. He would be paying cash, since his health insurance was linked to his job and had expired with his termination. *No worries,* he thought. *I have plenty of money to pay out of pocket.* He also got a series of brain scans ordered by a neurologist.

The diagnosis was bad news, far worse than his work defeat and the demise of his career. He had a glioblastoma, a brain tumor. It was growing, and quickly. The neurologist gave him a grim prognosis—six months to a year at most to live. Maybe a lot less. He could offer a few experimental treatments, but they were unlikely to make much of a difference.

Sam was stunned. He recalled that this was Arizona Senator John McCain's diagnosis, and that despite optimism and excellent health care, the prognosis proved accurate. If Senator McCain, with all his contacts and resources, couldn't find a solution, how would he? Alone with his diagnosis, Bridgewater went into a deep depression.

Help came from a surprising source. Irv Tinsley had been closely following all matters related to HealthMost and the lawsuit; he was out of work and had plenty of time to do so. He also wanted to make sure there were no surprises that might interfere with the final implementation of their plan.

Through his research, he discovered that Bridgewater had missed some court appearances, and rumors were floating that it was because of medical reasons. He dug around, thinking this might be a ruse. Instead, what came back through one of his traplines was that Bridgewater had been diagnosed with a glioblastoma.

Irv knew what that meant. He found Bridgewater's home phone number and called him up. Sam was surprised to hear from him. No one else had reached out to him. Now, an adversary and someone he had done much harm to, was calling and asking about his health.

He was suspicious and somewhat reluctantly agreed to meet Irv the next week. Irv was in DC to visit with Johnny around a new foundation being formed. Johnny was a candidate for the executive director position and wanted Irv to check it out with him.

THE THEORY OF IRV

Sam and Irv met at a coffee shop in the afternoon. It was an awkward greeting between the two.

Irv saw the discomfort of the moment and cut right to the chase. He told Sam that whatever he had done to him, or his friends, or others was now moot. Irv knew that he was facing a life-ending disease and wanted to offer contacts and advice.

"Why," asked Sam, "after all I've done to you?"

"Because that is what those of us in health care do," said Irv.

He gave Sam the name, telephone number, and email address of a physician with the Mayo Clinic. Mayo was doing some groundbreaking research work on glioblastomas, and if there was anything that could be done for him, they would know of it or be the ones to do it. He reminded Sam not to get his expectations up—that was where Senator McCain had been treated.

"If there is nothing to be done," he told Sam, "let me also give you some information about end-of-life care." He had several pamphlets and a page of website addresses that Sam could use to find out more, and he encouraged him to reach out to those organizations if his diagnosis remained the same.

Sam was curious not only about Irv's motivations, but why he was reaching out with this information. "Isn't this the type of information that the health care system would generally provide to someone with my diagnosis?" he asked.

Irv asked him whether he had received any of this information from the health providers he was seeing. The answer was no.

Irv told him this was not surprising to him. He explained that the medical care system had struggled for decades in helping patients square up to the grim reality of impending death. So much energy and focus on cures made it hard for much of the system to want to even acknowledge that they might fail to save any patient. It was one of the great system failings of health care to consistently help patients and their loved ones navigate the end-of-life phase.

Irv wasn't planning on going too far into the history of all of this; he didn't imagine it would be of interest to Bridgewater given what he was processing. He seemed interested, though, and it wasn't like they had a relationship to take the conversation in any other direction.

Irv described for Sam how one of the quieter revolutions going on within health care, almost exclusively outside of the political fights about health care, was changing cultures and practices to help people prepare for death. He told Sam that almost everyone asked preferred to die in their own home, yet denial and system problems led to most people dying in hospitals, hooked to machines and extraordinary efforts to preserve their life.

Sam still seemed interested, so Irv went on. "It is really a big system issue that needs fixing. Mostly because people are not dying the way they want to—and we must be far more respectful of their choices rather than what medical providers might want to do. Secondarily," he explained, "it is also a huge cost issue for the American medical care system—end-of-life treatments are extraordinarily expensive.

"Don't get me wrong," said Irv, "if that is what you want, to be in a hospital or to undergo experimental treatments, you can probably do that. I am just here to tell you that you have a choice, and there are organizations and providers that will help you make, and honor, your wishes."

None of this had remotely occurred to Sam. He was still wary of Irv's motivations, but he had not found anyone else to help him work through these issues. He sized Irv up. Someone like Thrust might be capable of exploiting this moment, he thought, but not the man before him. He thanked him, clumsily. Sam had not shown much gratitude over the course of his life and didn't really know how to do it.

Sam contacted the physician at Mayo that afternoon, and a couple of days later flew to Minnesota for some additional tests and a consult. It was too late. He returned home and contacted one of the organizations on Irv's list in the DC area—Death with Dignity. He met with a team at Death with Dignity to discuss and plan for what was to come.

They helped Sam find his way through the difficult process: figuring out what he wanted to do with his time left, and how he wanted the end to come. He did a lot of writing, poetry. It helped him find his way through to his end and resolve, as best he could, his life experiences and choices before.

He called up Irv to thank him for the advice and referral. He apologized for all that he had done wrong to him, his friends, and others. He shared more of his personal story than he had ever shared with anybody ever before and asked if Irv would be okay with talking some more, as the end neared.

Irv said yes. They talked by phone once a week over the next month. That was until Irv got a phone call from Death with Dignity. Sam had passed away the night before, in his DC apartment with a hospice nurse beside him. He had died in comfort, and before passing had asked them to call Irv with the news. "He said that you were the only friend he ever had. He also wanted you to know that he was gifting his entire estate to the Mason Health Foundation, in the name of his deceased brother. He hoped he was finally able to do some good. The memorial service will be next week," the nurse said.

Irv flew out to DC for the service. He was the only one in attendance.

Chapter One Hundred Eleven

Irv Gets His Whole Life Together

Irv rolled over in bed and looked at the clock. It was 8 a.m. Mary Beth had left a couple of hours ago. She had a meeting in Olympia with one of the governor's aides, and had kissed him on the forehead as she left.

It had been several months since the announcement of the financial award to the Mason Health Foundation. Since then, the money had been deposited, the board had accepted her recommendations, and she and the foundation were off and running on their move to improve health and health care in the area, and even the nation.

Irv was proud of her. Mary Beth was so talented, in her understated way. Johnny and he had dominated the conversations over their decades together, but both now realized she was the real brains of the operation. While they were talking, she was listening, and processing, and figuring out how to make their high-flying schemes practical and useful. Irv and Johnny had a role in helping her get the money into the foundation, to be sure, but she was the mastermind of its creation and how to invest the new funds.

Irv stretched in bed and sat up. No reason to get up and go. He had no appointments, other than playing guitar and doing some writing in his journal. It was his new life. His pay from public health was about to run out, and he could be soon collecting modest unemployment insurance benefits. He was ostensibly looking for work in his field, but was mostly biding his time. He had time to reflect on his life choices now, and he was going to take advantage of that.

He had already achieved a high level of success, even when judged under the tough grading curve of the Theory of Irv. It amused him that the pinnacle of this was not the result of some plan, but the random assignment of a case to him as investigator on call. Even then, he was about to get fired from that job, and soon was, but before that happened, he was off on a secret investigation into one of the most disgusting episodes of health care mismanagement and fraud in national history.

It was a team effort to make this investigation a raging success—but he knew and was incredibly proud that but for what he did, it never would have been uncovered and stopped. What's more, in doing so they had triggered several major streams of big change that offered hope that health and health care would be much better for millions of Americans. Not that they could talk openly about how all of this came about under the terms of the legal settlement, but the hushing up of any public story about this didn't make what had happened—and his pivotal role in it—any less real.

Stopping HealthMost, and corrupt federal government officials, was a great thing. The huge financial damages, and what Mary Beth and the foundation might do with them, was another. And Irv took even greater satisfaction in how he had helped Johnny leverage the situation into a comprehensive national health care form legislative package that had become law.

Really, what more could one do to fulfill the Theory of Irv?

Just as satisfying to him, maybe even more, was that the events had forced him and Mary Beth together again. No longer were they getting together for occasional phone calls or weekend visits. He had moved into her small cottage home in Shelton days after his firing and before the Belfair hearing. He hadn't left, other than to return to his Seattle home to pick up his guitars and some other belongings.

It wasn't like she was encouraging him to leave either. Quite the opposite. They picked up where they had left off before things went sour in the time of her cancer treatment. Irv had tearfully offered up his mea culpas for how badly he had handled that. Mary Beth had waved even that off. It was not time to look back, she said. We've been through enough together and apart, and let's just enjoy where we are now, she said.

That was exactly what they were doing, and it was going spectacularly well. So much so that they were making plans for their future together. Mary Beth now had a steady job, and a raise in salary, and they would pool their resources and buy a new home in the northern part of the county in Union. Their new home would be only miles from the HealthMost dumpsite. Somehow that seemed fitting.

Mary Beth would be home in the early afternoon, and Irv was going to surprise her by cooking a nice dinner. Stir-fried vegetables and crab Rangoon. He was becoming a decent enough cook now that he had time on his hands, and someone to cook for.

The bigger surprise, though, was that he was going to ask her to marry him.

"Well, what's your answer?" he asked Mary Beth. She had jumped off the couch and flung her arms around him, giving him a big kiss.

She momentarily pushed away from him, but was still hanging onto his shoulders, and looked sternly into his eyes. "Why, that is a big yes, you idiot." They kissed again.

"Just had to make sure," he said. "I wasn't sure that this was something you wanted, or not. All these years together, and we never really talked about it."

She was now sitting in his lap, smiling and running her fingers through his hair. "That's funny, we never did." She thought about it, getting a bit more serious. "Maybe that's because for so many years it seemed unnecessary. We were a couple and there wasn't any reason to make that more definitive or legal. And then we had these last few years, where things were so unclear. Now it seems like we should, if for no other reason than to declare that period of our life over."

"It's strange," added Irv. "Without that, this, or a whole bunch of other things, it probably wouldn't have happened."

"But it did. Not that I want to talk about any of our stuff that has happened. I just want to move ahead. And getting married seems a wonderful way to do that."

"So, what would you like to talk about?" he asked, giving her a big kiss.

"Let's see, how about how you make crab Rangoon? And our ceremony and party—oh, we should do it at our new house on the back deck." They had found a small house with a large backyard looking out over Hood Canal and the Olympic Mountains. It had a deck that would be a wonderful place for a party.

"Great idea," said Irv.

"And I have a surprise for you too—if you want to talk about it."

"What's that?"

"Well, I had some time in the car with our board chair and Jim Reynolds. We were meeting with the governor's staff to work out the final details of our purchase of the Shelton Hospital. We are ready to go and will announce the transfer to our foundation in a couple of weeks."

"Awesome. I assumed that your meeting would go smoothly. You are the hottest thing in health policy in this state since the start of group practice. And they have never seen you in your bedtime scrubs!"

"You idiot. Stay focused here for a couple more minutes, if you can. On the way back, we talked about something that I had been thinking about, but wasn't sure how to bring up the topic with them. And then they were the ones who brought it up."

"Okay." Irv was now giving her a quizzical look, not sure where the conversation was going. "What's that got to do with me?"

"Well, we need someone to become the hospital administrator at our newly purchased hospital. They asked me about you."

Irv just looked at Mary Beth, processing her words. A minute or so passed.

"Well, don't just sit there like a bump on a log. What do you think? I know you've been thinking what to do next career-wise. If anything. I was thinking before they ever brought it up that you knew more about hospitals and health care than anyone I know."

Irv was still thinking. Truth was, now that he had played such a big role in creating change in the health care system, maybe it was time to get back to solving the day-to-day challenge of providing health care to people. He had been reflecting on his time as assistant administrator at the hospital in south King County.

It was really satisfying work. What had torn him away was not his dissatisfaction with it, but the calling to solve the problems he was encountering upstream, in a bigger and more impactful way. He now understood that this was when the deeper implications of the Theory of Irv had started to form. How could he imagine ever doing more than what he had just done to achieve it? He had begun to think that afternoon of going back to just helping to manage health care in a smaller way.

"Isn't it a problem that you and I are together? Getting married will make it legal together, too."

"That's what I was wondering about also. Really, that and whether you wanted to do something like this were the only reasons I could think of why I shouldn't suggest you as the man for the job. Ken and Jim told me we would have the job report to the chair of the Mason Health Foundation, and not to me. We would essentially be two related divisions of the same organization, working together. Jim would have us sign some legal documents disclosing our relationship, and there may be some occasions when we would have to do the same. Other than that, we would be good to go. You will need to apply and interview, but I don't think there is any question that it is your job if you want it."

"Awesome." He gave her a big hug. "That is a yes, by the way. Didn't want to leave any doubt about that."

"I am so happy, Irv. Shall we cover the recipe for the crab Rangoon?"

"In a little bit. I couldn't help but get fascinated about the idea of working under you. We won't get to do that in the worksite, but maybe we can do a little role playing about that now." He began to unbutton her blouse.

"Oooh," said Mary Beth. "This will be a performance review for the ages." She wrapped her arms around him as they kissed.

Chapter One Hundred Twelve

Johnny and the Olympic Institute

Johnny looked out over the desk in his office to the Capitol Building just a few blocks away. He had a great view of it from his large and elegant office. Funny, he thought, far better than any desk, office, or view he had during his decades as a member of Congress. The lot of being an independent in a two-party system.

He tucked his long arms behind his head, pushing his feet against the corner of the desk so that he could lean back and take in the view of the Capitol. He could see the fields in the front of the building facing the Capitol Mall and the Lincoln monument. People were milling about a series of tents on the mall, while others were jogging or biking the trail on its perimeter.

These were his tents—part of the first national health competition being conducted under the Federal Health Care System Revival legislation passed last year. He gushed with pride whenever he recalled the story of how this legislative idea became law.

The national competition was one of ten primary proposals in the health care reform proposal conjured up by him and his friends at the Alderbrook Lodge last August. The national competition was even more of his baby than the others because he had taken a job promoting and running it.

The Olympic Institute was founded in December of last year and was proposed to be the national not-for-profit organization that would organize the first annual national health competition beginning on September 1, 2021. A grant awarded by the Mason Health Foundation enabled a quick organization of the event. Johnny was appointed as the first chief executive officer of the institute, which got its name from both the notion of the Olympic Games and the Olympic Mountain range in Washington State, right down the road from the Mason Health Foundation.

Johnny knew the mountain's peaks well from his time living in the state. Now that Congress was not ruling his schedule, he was able to spend even more time in Washington, looking at the mountains from a small cabin on the shore of Hood Canal. Its main attraction was that it was only a half-mile trek up a thousand-foot-high hill to Irv and Mary Beth's new home. Penny from Senator Bell's office would accompany him on his trips out there; they were now an item, and she was a private citizen again.

He was happy to be able to spend more time with Irv and Mary Beth. It warmed his heart to see them happily living together again. Married now. He never really understood the rift that grew between them. Thankfully, that was in the past. The universe was far more in order when those two were together.

Individually, they were both doing well too. Mary Beth had finally gotten full confidence in herself and was letting her instincts, beliefs, and brains loose. She not only could be an executive director, but she could be one of the best damn executive directors ever.

Irv was quite content with being a hospital administrator, and it was important work. Hospitals were sacred places that held the lives and well-being of so many in their organizational hands. Even with the latest legislative changes in place, health care remained a complex undertaking. There was always something new and different going wrong, and it was Irv's job to solve these problems.

Johnny was also able to let go of his conviction to solve the whole of the system's problems. He had done more than his share of that and could now deal with problems arising from the normal course of humans interacting than the utter failings of the American health care system. Irv had begun to write too, sharing his views about how those working in the system could further advance reform of the American health care system.

Mary Beth had talked Johnny into taking the position as the CEO of the Olympic Institute—and he was glad he had listened to her. Who better than he to make sure that the annual health competition included in the Theory of Irv legislation be done right, consistent with their wacky thinking that August night? Someone had to reach out to states and organizations across the country and help them figure out how to create their own programs that fit with the general framework of the national challenge. He would meet hundreds of people doing this, and his basic message would be the same—they need to find their local way to health and health care in their communities.

He didn't make all that much as CEO, but it was enough to maintain a second home in the nation's capital and a comfortable lifestyle. Like Irv and Mary Beth, he had agreed to cap his annual salary at $150,000 per year. None of them had gotten into this for the money, and that would be more than enough for each to live on. It would make it easier for them to insist that other executives be careful about excessive compensation when they worked with them.

Besides, imagine having such a fun time and getting paid to do what they did. Johnny was reveling in running the national health competition. It was a six-week affair, and they were now in the middle of the first year's games. It would end with a closing ceremony on the national mall in mid-October.

The design of the national competition was structured around a few core concepts. One was to make it easy for individuals and organizations to join in the national competition. They could enroll, at no cost, on a national website run by the Olympic Institute, where they could report their health activity each day, or on a weekly or monthly basis, using friendly software.

Importantly, they could get credit for what they had done in the reporting time period for both healthy living and healthy systems actions, in the form of Health Miles.

Healthy Living was generally an area where participants could get credit for taking greater personal responsibility over their lives and health. One could get credit for physical activity of all types; the miles were adjusted to a standard unit within the software so that all forms of activity were acknowledged. But one could also achieve Health Miles by losing weight, obtaining needed Clinical Preventive Health Services, drinking water, making their decision to enroll in a health plan, or a host of other things that individuals could do to improve their own health, as agreed on by a national panel of health experts convened by the institute.

That was a creative enough notion, but even more so was providing Health Miles for Healthy Systems actions. There were a multitude of ways that participants might join with others to collectively improve health. One important way was to join in the activities of organizations who had become partners in the challenge. Another was to answer Healthy Systems questions presented on a daily basis during the national competition—questions that were educating thousands of Americans about the broader determinants of health, and how they might help improve these determinants.

States, communities, organizations, businesses, social clubs, all could not only participate in the national challenge but construct their own sub-competitions within it. The driving logic was to create a fun way for people to engage in their health where they were most comfortable and likely to do so.

Three weeks into the first national competition, it was looking to be a big hit. Participants had logged over five million Health Miles, enough to travel to the moon and back over ten times. Johnny was upscaling how they would close the first year competition in just a few more weeks, and how they might improve it for the second year. It would get bigger and better over time.

At times, he would also reflect on the other nine legislative elements of the Federal Health Care Revival Act, or what he privately called the Theory of Irv legislation. It was still early, but initial indications were that these other pieces were also showing promise to greatly change American health care for the better.

He knew that these ideas weren't perfect or complete. That was fine, Johnny thought. Their aim was to get the change process moving and to orient this around what it did for people rather than the health care system, politicians, or investors. Much like the prescription laid out by the Committee on the Cost of Medical Care in 1932. That was good.

To think, it was all triggered by the discovery of a body in a run-down shack in eastern King County, Washington. Johnny laughed out loud, thinking about how maybe that shack would be reconstructed and placed in a museum next to Abe Lincoln's log cabin home and George Washington's wooden teeth.

Chapter One Hundred Thirteen

The Theory of Irv Bill

On October 15, 2020, the United States Senate had voted to approve Senate Bill 813, the Federal Health Care System Revival Act, by a vote of 51-49. The voting record vote noted the defeat of an attempted filibuster, with ten Republican senators joining with the Democrats to pass a motion to proceed. Senator John Gibson introduced the bill, along with ten other senators, five from each party.

The bill was sent to the House of Representatives, which conducted an expedited review of the proposal. Within a week, the bill was considered by the House under a rule forbidding any amendments to it. It passed, without amendment of any type, by a vote of 300-125. Immediately thereafter, the House adjourned so that its members could close out their reelection campaigns back in their districts.

On October 28th, days before Election Day, the president signed the bill into law. Observers were surprised. The secretary of Health and Human Services stood by his side at the desk when he did this; on his other side was Senator John Gibson. Immediately to Senator Gibson's right was Chris Jones, a longtime health policy leader, who was holding a photo of his father, Patrick Jones, in one hand, and an old red bound copy of the Final Report of the Committee on the Cost of Medical Care in the other.

Newspaper stories and articles at the time explained how this federal legislation made it through Congress. All noted the leadership of Senator Gibson . . . and got many other parts of the full story wrong. Senator Gibson was not saying much at the time, preferring to let the legislation move through the process without him telling stories about how it came to be. That could happen another day, when the time was right.

Years later, the full story was finally told. Or at least parts of it. The relationship to an investigation of a suspicious death, a tainted immigration program, and the misdeeds of a health care corporation. A federal contract, sleazy government agents, and political games.

One aspect of the story that stayed under the radar for years finally came out. That is how an extensive digital advocacy network had been activated to build public will to support the legislation. This network told the story of the need for health reform among the American people, in a non-partisan way.

A political consultant named Nancy Jones was the lead designer for this effort, and it built from her extensive experimentation of how the Internet, social online networks, and digital spread of messages could help win political campaigns. She had been cutting new ground in this through her campaign work for candidates, including Senator Gibson. Now, she added the notion of "issue advocacy" to its application.

Pivotal to this was a trusted network of influentials and social connectors who would spread an understanding of what was good about this bill across the country, and especially to states that had key elections on the ballot that fall. The Mason Health Foundation in Washington State had such a network and had advised and funded parallel efforts and networks in the key battleground states for the race for the presidency.

MHF was a trusted partner in this and was able to fund this work through a major award it had received to improve health in its own state and the nation. The terms of the settlement proceeds that were the source of the money had dictated that some dollars be used for this purpose.

Nancy had worked with the head of this foundation to retain college students across the country to help build the social network. It found great grassroots favor by avoiding the zero sum game politics of past health reform efforts, and proposing a new and unique set of solutions. Instead of the usual ideologic propositions, the proposal was to find non-partisan and practical ways to make health care work better for people.

Other organizations and leaders jumped on board, such as patient advocate groups and individual health care providers, and shared information with their members and networks.

Polls were undertaken by state, and published through the regular media and through the national digital network. They showed that the great majority of Americans—well over 70 percent—agreed that there should be bipartisan solutions to health care, and that the provisions of this legislation fit that prescription for change. The force and swiftness of this message, so close to the election, was one that neither Democrats nor Republicans could reject outright. When they or their surrogates tried to do so, the digital network of advocates took them on in the court of digital opinion.

The president had to decide whether to sign the bill before the election. To veto it was sure to mean his demise—the battleground states were resoundingly in favor of giving this new set of ideas a chance. Signing it would give him a chance to run with health care reform, rather than against it. Since health care was the single most important issue to American voters, it created a way to reshape the politics of his campaign. So, he signed it. Maybe not enthusiastically, but with a smile as the ceremony was rebroadcast on news programs, and through Nancy Jones' national digital network, across the United States.

What was in it, you might ask? Here is what was shared with Senate Majority Leader Bell, as Senator Gibson met with him to request a committee and floor vote on his legislation in early October:

Summary Bill Description: The Federal Health Care System Revival Act

Be It Enacted by the Congress of the United States of America:

Section 1. National Health Goals. A set of Five Health Goals will be Established by Congress. These will be established with simplicity and clarity, and be measured by clear metrics that will show where the United States stands with respect to the achievement of such goals over time. The president will also provide a plan for achieving these goals, over the short and long term, and submit this to Congress as part of his annual budget proposal. Congress will set specific annual accountabilities within these Health Goals and their Plans, and direct federal health care spending to these aims.

Section 2. One National Health Goal Will Address the Cost of the American Health Care System. It will be framed around the percent of the gross domestic product applied to health care over time, with a standard definition over time of what to count within that calculation. This rate shall not exceed 17.5%, and if it does, Congress will be required to cut government program expenses such that it falls below this level. Congressional and Executive Branch salaries will be reduced by the percentage amount of the excess. The annual rate of increase in total American health costs under this goal shall not exceed 3% per year.

Section 3. Regional Health Budgets. To assure the proper investment of governmental resources into health care, regional health care budgets will be assigned to seven different regions of the nation, and adjusted based on age and other health risk factors within these regions. Each state within a region will be required to work within the overall region to fit their expenses and plans into these regional budgets. Each state will also develop a process of local health planning that will be part of its input into the regional budget spending plan. Regional budgets will be adjusted based on the regional performance for key national health priorities, such as the achievement of national health goals, the rate of elimination of health disparities related to race and ethnicity, and the annual National Health Competition.

Section 4. Public Option. Medicare will be made available as an option to any individual in the nation looking to buy health coverage. The premium will be the actuarial equivalent of what it costs for Medicare for any standard eligible. There will be two potential buy-in options: Part A for hospital costs, and Part B for other costs, consistent with current Part A and Part B features of the Medicare program. There will be no federal subsidies to help people buy into this program; such subsidies will, however, be continued through federal support to the expansion of Medicaid.

Section 5. Strengthening of Federal Antidumping Statutes. A duty to treat will be added to the current Duty to Evaluate and Stabilize Patients in past federal law. This will apply to all not-for-profit or governmental hospitals with emergency rooms. Any not-for-profit organization violating the statute will immediately lose their federal tax exempt status upon breach of this duty, and will be fined. A national pool will be created to assist hospitals who experience catastrophic losses due to treating uninsured or underinsured patients under this new duty, funded by fines and a premium surcharge of 1% on all health plan contracts across the nation.

Section 6. National Health Care Lottery. Any American who experiences a catastrophic or life-threatening diagnosis shall be eligible to enter into a national health care lottery. The lottery will randomly assign applicants into a winner pool, with random chance being the only determinant of being granted public support and access to heroic or expensive medical interventions approved by their health care providers, and desired by the patient.

Section 7. Public Health Funding. The Health Improvement Fund created by the Affordable Care Act is reinstated, and funding restored. These dollars will be used in great part to fund the core public health function of surveillance and monitoring for major public health risks. It will also be used to assure the nation is prepared to respond to any major public health risks, such as pandemics or natural disasters with major health consequences. It will also be used to finance the free availability of those services included in the most recent federal Guide to Clinical Preventive Services, should these not be available to all through health coverage or other arrangements. Local health departments will be required to undertake local prevention planning in their areas, with these plans submitted to the regional budget entities created under Section 3.

Section 8. Professional Education. The federal government shall also create a series of federal grants and loans to students wishing to pursue careers in the health professions. These dollars will be allocated through the Regional Health Budgets created under Section 3. Funding support will be prioritized for those students committing to serve at least five years of their career in medically underserved rural or inner city communities. While making sure that education for these professionals is based on science and best education practice, another express goal of the federal government's support is to create an oversupply of health professionals across the United States.

Section 9: A Patient Centered Design Institute Shall Be Developed within the National Institutes of Health. Congress shall provide annual funding to the Institute, whose charge shall include researching and testing innovations that will fundamentally redesign American health care to be organized around the needs of individual patients and their families or surrogate and support systems, rather than the institutional or professional elements of the health care system.

Section 10. An Annual National Health Challenge Shall Be Conducted Each Fall. Participation and scoring in the challenge will include both collective Healthy Systems objectives and the achievement of

Healthy Living personal responsibilities by participants. Winning scores will result in additional funding for health within the regional budgets created under Section 3. A national not-for-profit organization will be awarded a grant to host the competition, built off the concepts of President Kennedy's national fitness program of the 1960s.

On leaving the bill-signing ceremony, reporters approached Senator Gibson and began to ask him questions about how this bill became law. A *New York Times* reporter asked him what they should call the legislation, telling him that some were beginning to call it the Gibson Health Act.

"No," Johnny said. "That is not what it should be called. And I would greatly appreciate it if you could see fit to give its rightful name."

"What's that?" the reporter asked.

"The Theory of Irv."

Chapter One Hundred Fourteen

Afterword

This book is a novel about health care. It is a work of fiction to educate readers about what is wrong with the American health care system, why it is that way, and what might be done about it.

It is a product of my personal passion to help fix it, expressed first over a four-decade career in various settings of the health care system, with some, maybe even many, successes along the way, but without the major and big reform that was truly my aim. Maybe this is my last chance to spur big change, or perhaps it will just allow me to get a few things off my chest so I can move on to new things.

Let's start with a few words about the American health care system: few social systems in world history have delivered such a stark contrast between good and bad. On the one hand, American health care achieves the near impossible on a daily basis, saving lives and bringing comfort or cure to millions. It has taken medical challenges equivalent to putting a person on the moon and made them commonplace experiences. It has figured out how to transcend what we once thought the biologic limits of our bodies, and perhaps even life itself someday. We live substantially longer than our ancestors and experience our mortal being in a better and more comfortable manner, generally speaking. American health care has been a huge contributor to these advances and should take a bow for these amazing achievements.

On the other hand, American health care confounds our commonsense judgment regarding how such a system should function. Within a service sector that by nature should deliver the most intimate and personal of human interactions and experiences, it depersonalizes these experiences to the point of incredulity. We find ourselves frustrated with our contact with the system, from the care we are provided to the bills we get in the mail. It leaves us shaking our heads, wondering how this could be and questioning the ability of any system so built to really be all that good for us.

This has bred enormous distrust of the system, a disgust that has risen to such heights, many of the incredible advances are now taken for granted or, even worse, are under suspicion. Where once germ theory and the ability to produce vaccinations were seen as a godsend for people and their children, many now perceive them as tools of the devil, part of a conspiracy to poison us or steal our money. This is just one of many ways distrust of the system pokes its head up. When things go wrong, for example, we are all too ready to seek justice outside of its boundaries, from political action to lawsuits.

The system is massive, and very expensive. One may argue that is not necessarily a problem, as spending more on our health and health care is perhaps better than investing in other social alternatives, like wars or frivolous entertainment. Yet, it is extraordinarily expensive, as noted in several chapters in this book. For sure, the growth of the system has been monstrous in its rate of increase, for decades now. The cost of American health care is now so great and still rising that it is gobbling up a tremendous share of our societal resources, rapidly squeezing out our ability to spend them on anything else.

What's worse, for all these resources applied, we have far less to show for it in terms of health than other nations, who spend a lot less than us. We are decidedly first in the amount of money we spend per capita on health care in the United States, and two on the list is a distant competitor. Yet the output is mediocre at best—we rank thirty-seven in international health rankings. Quibble with the methodological details of this ranking if you want, but really, what if we ranked twentieth? Still a humongous effectiveness problem.

There are also wide gaps between who wins and who loses in the American health care system. While regularly battling allegations that it is socialistically inspired, the difference between haves and have-nots is profound. It is generally true that those with incredible wealth are able to acquire the best and brightest to deal with their health care problems. Those of us with less resources are frequently left to get what we can based on the uneven experience with factors such as health coverage policies, personal ability to navigate the system, the nature of the clinical problem, and, sometimes, just blind luck.

Many working in the system attain incredible wealth—a point of friction since most of this money is coming from the rest of us in the form of taxes to government, insurance payments, or direct payments from our own pockets. We might feel better about this if the product was not so uneven.

None of this says that "fairness" is an attribute of our system—and fairness is a deeply held value in America, at least as to its desires for its health care system.

We know who most frequently is on the outside looking in. Health coverage and money matter, but the real dividing line is race and ethnicity. In virtually every way, non-white people in America receive less and do worse in terms of health, including in receipt of medical care.

Overall, the American health care system has become the poster child for non-systems. It is fragmented, disjointed, and unconnected—unable to be pulled together by government regulation or the Invisible Hand of Adam Smith. Users find it to be a maze of confusion. Many—no, make that most—eventually fall through its cracks or encounter its dead ends at some point in their health care journeys. Remarkably, even those who work within the system, such as hospital administrators or physicians, are astonished to discover how obtuse and unfriendly their own systems of care are when they need it for themselves or their family.

American health care has earned its mediocre to bad reputation, and needs a radical overhaul to become efficient and effective. I believe there is little debate about this fundamental conclusion.

The search for answers has been elusive. The good news is that we spend a lot of our civic and political energy trying to find them. But this has done little to actually solve anything. Instead, it has mostly served the political and ideologic divides and those who profit from this. Health care has become a major talking point for campaigns and shock radio or TV. Great for controversy and fundraising and get-out-the-vote drives, but not so much to find and implement real and practical solutions.

Part of the blame for this is not health care but the challenges of our contemporary representative government. Special interests and money rule the day, with the blessing of the United States Supreme Court.

Among these interests are health insurers, health care systems, and professional trade associations. Stopping change is always on someone's agenda, and the odds are stacked in their favor to succeed.

Once in a blue moon a major health policy idea gets passed into law, sometimes at the national level and sometimes the state. More typical, though, are tepid and incremental policy solutions, usually isolated to some symptom of our dysfunctional system than some root defect.

Incrementalism not only makes it harder to get traction toward real change, but it regularly adds new complications and confusion to an already incoherent system. Over the past fifty years, American health policy has seen a bewildering array of government-based, market-based, and intermediary fixes, regularly passed without much attempt to integrate these contradictory forces with what is already in place. The net result is a system of opposing incentives and controls that confound our attempts to make it work as users, regulators, or managers.

There is also an opportunity cost to our efforts to fix health policy, while regularly failing. One might say this is the cost of doing business in a democracy. But in terms of health, it is worth noting that if we really cared about health as the outcome of our health policy, in many cases we would focus our attention on exactly these other issues more than medical care. For example, education, the environment, or housing.

To be sure, much has been written about health care problems and how to solve them. Most of this is serious policy analysis by expert, or alleged expert, authors—some of it very good, others more hyperbolic and air than convincing reason.

But for all the writing, there remains little useful conversation among the regular folk of our nation as to what can be done to solve these problems. To some degree, it is because of the complexity of the system, its problems and solutions. My guess—and part of the premise for this book—is that this topic is not the type of thing many people want to explore or study in depth—it is serious, dry, and appeals only to a small segment of people.

Meanwhile, we need many more people to become knowledgeable about the issues at play so we can have a meaningful dialogue about the solutions needed in this nation, rather than continue to rely on our divided politics and the media to shop simplistic solutions through talking points within their isolated bubbles.

This is why I wrote this book—to educate people about health policy and our national and local policy choices. It is written as a novel with the hope that entertainment in the form of a fictional story might inform and inspire meaningful conversation, debate and eventually action.

The Theory of Irv is the product of my own educational and work experiences with health care, for now over forty years, in a variety of settings, roles, and geographic locations. Much of my work has been in the field of public policy, broadly speaking. Interspersed among the fictional storyline are major snippets of real policy issues, debates, and history. My hope is that it is clear which are real and which are fictional fabrications. These issues are worth talking about, even if made up.

I have been fortunate over my career to have encountered many interesting people and experiences. It has given me, I believe, some unique insights into health policy and the big questions that we face. It has certainly given me a lot of material upon which to base my fictional accounts.

It should be noted that health policy is referenced here in a broad way—a principle of action adopted or proposed by a government, party, business, or individual as to what to do in particular situations. Too many believe health policy is limited to what our governments do through formal processes like passing laws in Congress and state legislatures. Far more of our day-to-day lives are affected by regulations and rules adopted outside of legislative bodies. Add to the mix court decisions, private policies set by business, and programs created by not-for-profit organizations, and you see policy in the broader sense used in this book.

Just like any novel, the characters are mostly fictional, except where historical figures are identified. Characters are based on composites of different people I've met or worked with, and for those of you who see yourself in my writing in a good way, thanks for lending part of you to me, if indeed it is you.

Unfortunately, I did draw from real-world examples when I cast the villains in this story. I may have exaggerated character defects to make my point, but in many cases, not so much. They are all composite characters, however, so if you see yourself or someone you know as one of these characters, rest assured you are at least partly mistaken.

But to be clear, the bad apples within the health care system are a very small number of people in a huge system. Indeed, one of my greatest frustrations with the system defects of health care is that the vast majority of the thousands of people who I've met and worked with over the years are smart, caring, and hardworking. For me, over 90 percent of those in health care are wonderful people who see things regularly go wrong in spite of what they do because of the defects of the system—maybe the most important evidence that health care is a poor system.

My friend Emily Friedman was writing and speaking about hospitals as sacred places before her untimely death. I agree with her, and it is the reality that the people who work within hospitals and really the entire health care system should be doing God's work is my driving passion for the cause.

Many stories within this book are based on real work from across my career. I tried to present a mix of the types of issues that the system covers and the important answers we must find. I am sure there are important ones that I've missed.

Many of the examples are real policy proposals or programs that were advanced by the Washington Health Foundation, a not-for-profit I started up in 1992. I was president and CEO for twenty years. Much of the Mason Health Foundation story is a reworking of the WHF history and work, with great liberties taken in the story telling to keep things moving and interesting.

This matters in part because the Washington Health Foundation is trying now to revive itself. My hope is that we will soon have new ideas and programs to add to our storyline. But it is also important to know that some of what one may view as crazy ideas that could never happen have been tested by the Washington Health Foundation, with great success. The Washington Health Foundation will also be the beneficiary of any proceeds from the sale of this book. An account of WHF and its work is available at the following website: washhealthfoundation.org. T

I debated which solutions to emphasize in this novel, especially the legislative package offered in the closing chapter. I have given years of thought to this question, and have extensive thoughts and notes on exactly what needs to be done—most in far greater depth than presented in the last chapter and elsewhere.

But, since the point of this book is to flatten the nature of the problems and solutions for accessibility to the reader, I chose to be brief and general. Still, the fundamental points are ones I do assert as the solutions and principles we should seek, based on my long experience and contemplation. I have debated writing more about the solutions in a more serious form and may do this someday.

One final note of importance. I began this book over eight years ago. The beginning was based to a large extent on my personal involvement with the SARS issue, including while I was in China. Yes, a pandemic. I found the time to conclude the book during the lockdown in March and April of 2020 as the world dealt with the plague of COVID-19. While I appreciated the focus it brought to my writing, there were far better ways to get me over the hump. I also imagine that the outcome of this time might have profound implications for our thinking about the issues with the American health care system, along with the eruption of national attention to issues of race just a few months later. I am only in the early stages of my thoughts about these new developments and have decided to end this book now so I can turn my thoughts to those important questions.

There are many recognitions necessary for this book. After all, it is the product of my experiences and the hundreds, if not thousands, of wonderful people I have met along the way. Some have been leaders of major health care organizations across the nation; others served in more mundane roles as supply clerks, janitors, vice presidents, security officers, directors, note takers, or whatever. Still more have been clinicians of all professions who do the truly amazing work of taking care of people. Thanks and God bless them all.

There are a special few who I must note explicitly: Bob Sigmond, who introduced me to the Committee on the Cost of Medical Care, Rufus Rorem, and a whole lot more with practical, insightful, and humorous mentoring, beginning with my fellowship with the American Hospital Association and the Blue Cross Blue Shield Association. Leo Greenawalt, who gave me the opportunity to try much of the crazy-ass stuff described in this book, and other things that were just as risky and crazy. Gail Warden, who made me understand that leadership is for introverts too. Again, there are dozens, if not hundreds of others who have been so vital to my learning and I thank them all.

On the personal side, I thank my loving wife, Jan, for her support and love all these years. Relevant to the book is that she was the student coordinator for the University of Washington Masters of Health Administration program in the book. It was during my time there that I wrote a paper titled "The Theory of Irv" that I have retaken for this book. Notwithstanding, I was able to leave with a degree and eventually a wife—not a bad haul for in-state tuition.

My parents also were pivotal in this journey. Both were in health care, my mom as a nurse and my dad as first a hospital dietitian and eventually an assistant administrator. It was at Mount Sinai Hospital in Hartford, Connecticut, that I first was introduced to health care as a thing when I was only a couple of feet tall. That experience began my journey.

My dad was also a helpful critic along the way. As I worked hard to create big change in the health care system, I would visit him after his retirement. He would tell me how awful the system was now that he was seeking care and that somebody should fix it. I kept telling him that I was trying—and increasingly needed to confess that whatever I was doing hadn't taken yet. Still trying after all these years.

About the Author

Greg Vigdor has spent his life working within America's health care system, trying to improve it. He has now chosen to write about the system with the hope that this will stimulate the type of change that will be good for the people and communities of America.

Born in Hartford, Connecticut, Greg has lived in cities across our nation. His times in Washington, DC, Seattle, Washington, and the American Southwest are important settings for this novel.

Greg has worked in a range of positions and sectors in American health care, providing him a broad and deep perspective on the many issues of the full system. He has served as a policy leader, lobbyist, health care manager, CEO, and many other roles.

One of his more prominent positions was as founder and CEO of the Washington Health Foundation. He created WHF in 1992 through a Rural Hospital Assistance Program. Greg raised funds and soon added to the Foundation's rural leadership work with a variety of statewide and urban community programs applied across the state of Washington for the next twenty years.

Major achievements were helping over 10,000 Washingtonians each year to access health care services through client support services, providing millions of dollars of support to local communities to improve health locally, and rolling out an array of innovative leadership programs aimed at big system reform. These included the Transforming Health Care, the Healthiest State in the Nation Campaign and Center for People's Health programs.

In 2013, Greg became the President & CEO of the Arizona Hospital and Health Care Association. His first assignment was to help pass Medicaid Expansion for Arizona-the first Republican controlled state to do so. In 2016, he took on the challenge of preserving the access protections of the Affordable Care Act by insisting that a replacement must be in place before any repeal. In the absence of such a proposal, he led a statewide effort in Arizona to convince Senator John McCain to vote no on the repeal proposals before Congress.

Other important roles over his career included Executive Director of the Association of Washington Public Hospital Districts, Vice President for Policy and Advocacy at the Washington State Hospital Association, Director of Public Policy for the New Mexico Hospital Association, and Director of Nursing at Mount Sinai Hospital in Hartford, Connecticut.

Greg's academic credentials include a Masters of Health Administration from the University of Washington with the Program Nomination for Outstanding Student in 1983, a Juris Doctorate from the George Washington University National Law Center with Honors in 1981, and a Bachelor of Arts from the University of Connecticut with Distinction in Political Science in 1976. He was chosen to be one of two Fellows for the American Hospital Association/Blue Cross Blue Shield Association prestigious national Health Leadership Fellowship in 1984.

Greg has written and spoken extensively on health and health care topics. He has been recognized for his leadership and innovative approach to health problem solving and he continues to explore new ways to improve health in a volunteer capacity. Among the most important roles in this regard is his current service as the now volunteer President of the Washington Health Foundation and author of The Theory of Irv: A Novel of American Health Policy.

About the Washington Health Foundation

The Washington Health Foundation (WHF) is an important organization linked to the ideas within this book.

It is a not for profit leadership organization created in 1992 by author Greg Vigdor. For twenty years, he served as its President & CEO while WHF became the source of a variety of innovative policy and program efforts to improve health and health care.

Many of the solutions described in the novel were tested or used by the Washington Health Foundation. WHF's website holds the deeper story of these efforts, and should be consulted for more information. (washhealthfoundation.org)

Greg has chosen to publish his novel through the Washington Health Foundation. The importance of this is that all proceeds from the sale of the book will go to the benefit of the Washington Health Foundation, and its effort to revive itself to do more good for the people of Washington and the Nation.

Made in the USA
Monee, IL
16 December 2023

49481212R00331